Navigating Solutions for a Healthy, Sustainable Home

THE SMART LIVING HANDBOOK

Creating a healthy home in an increasingly toxic world
Melissa Wittig and Danielle King
Foreword by Professor Peter D. Sly

All correspondence to the publishers
The Smart Living Handbook
PO Box 4224
Briar Hill 3088
Victoria Australia

First published 2014

© Melissa Wittig and Danielle King (content assigned)

With thanks to:
WordLaundry - Editor
Sharon Westin-Shaw Graphic Design – Book design
Canva.com - Illustrations
Nicola May Design - Graphic Design - Adverts (pages 332 and 334)

The right of Melissa Wittig to be identified as the author of this work has been asserted by her in accordance with the Copyright, Patents and Designs Acts (Australia).

The right of Danielle King to be identified as the author of this work has been asserted by her in accordance with the Copyright, Patents and Designs Acts (Australia).

The right of Belinda Thackeray to be identified as a professional contributor of content to the Low Allergy Sustainable Garden section has been asserted by her in accordance with the Copyright, Patents and Designs Acts (Australia).

This publication is copyright. All rights reserved. No part of this publication may be reproduced, distributed, or transmitted in any form or by any means, including photocopying, recording or other electronic or mechanical methods, without the prior written permission of the relevant author/s or contributor, except in the case of brief quotations embodied in critical reviews and certain other non-commercial uses permitted by copyright law. Any person who does any unauthorised act in relation to this publication may be liable to criminal and civil claims for damages.

This publication is designed to provide accurate information in regard to the subject matter covered at the time of research. The nature of some content is subject to changes in the market place, local rules and regulations and individual circumstances. It is sold with the understanding that readers use the content for informational purposes only and not intended for the treatment or diagnosis of individual disease or issues. Please visit a qualified professional in the medical, local building, sustainability, housing or other specialty sector regarding your specific need before acting on information.

This publication does not endorse any of the findings and methodology in the scientific studies referenced. References are made to these studies to illustrate the varied findings associated with products, chemicals, pollutants and sustainability issues in Australian homes and the potential health concerns associated with them.

ISBN: 978-0-646-92300-0

A Catalogue-in-Publication is available from the National Library of Australia.

Bulk orders available –
Email: info@healthyinteriors.com.au
or
Email: info@greenmoves.com.au

Dedicated to

...a future where our children
can live a healthy, affordable, and sustainable life,
in surroundings free from health altering and environmentally damaging
pollution and substances.

For you:

Lane, Paige and Ryan

Thank you to our partners and families
who have missed many days and nights with
us for this book to be brought to life

Melissa and Danielle

Testimonial

Finally a book that recognises the relationship between energy efficiency and health in the home!

Well written, in plain English, this is a great reference book for consumers, homeowners and industry professionals.

As an education tool it will help new home owners to make not only the right decisions, but also potentially save a considerable amount of money.

For those who already have been living in their home for a long time, this book is an eye opener and a trigger for action! - Jan Brandjes

Who is Jan Brandjes?

Jan Brandjes is an environmental building consultant with over 30 years of international experience in energy efficient building and indoor air quality issues. In Australia he developed a number of concept homes under the labels of 'Ecohome', 'The Sunbury Healthy House' and 'The 'Economical Home'. His main focus is now on training and educating industry and consumers of the benefits of sustainable and healthy buildings.

About the authors

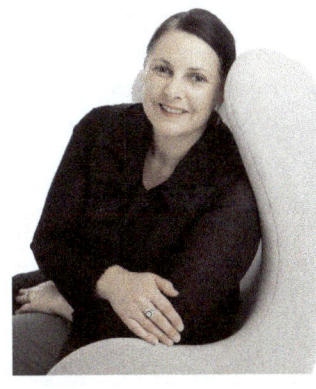

Author - Melissa Wittig

Melissa Wittig is an accomplished 'health focused' interior designer, author of the Healthy Home app, writer and mother. With a passion for healthy indoor environments it was the culmination of her professional property/design experience and role as a mum that ignited the development of her business, Healthy Interiors.

Melissa has a Diploma of Interior Design and is a licensed estate agent with a Grad Cert in Human Resource Management. She has combined her property, design and logistics skills to specialise in educating consumers about designing and creating healthy homes.

Melissa has shared her knowledge on television and radio and has articles published in various mediums internationally. Speaking engagements have included the International Industry Seminar Series for Decoration & Design/International Furniture Fair in Sydney, Australia and state-based exhibitions. The Healthy Home app written by Melissa was a finalist in the 2013 Australian Mobile Awards and has been featured in Australia's leading sustainable magazines.

www.healthyinteriors.com.au

What made you choose to work in the sustainable living sector?

Having worked in the property sector followed by the design sector, I recognised that in many areas of both industries (professional and individual) consumers are making decisions that create a lasting legacy for buildings, occupants and communities. At the same time as recognising a professional need for sustainable principles, I was faced with personal health challenges within my family that were linked with environmental causes or triggers.

As a result of research and identifying a documented link between health and the home environment, as a mother and professional I felt compelled to explore a healthy, sustainable approach to design and interiors.

Melissa's story

When I was studying in the field of property and human resources as a young adult, a career in sustainability and healthy interiors was not on my radar. After working in the property sector and further studies in interior design, it was parenthood 14 years ago that started a deep interest in the way we lived and the connection between the health of our family and our home environment. Research over many years along with personal and professional experiences has culminated into a career that has reinforced my belief that everything happens for a reason.

My health-focused interior design career is what I like to think of as my silver lining to years of health challenges within our family. These challenges have inspired my research over the years – findings of which have helped create a healthy and sustainable design ethos in my work.

An interest in issues associated with healthy homes is something that runs deep and personal. As a young woman I was diagnosed with polycystic ovarian syndrome (PCOS) which at the time was largely unspoken about with very little information available. Some research suggests links to environmental pollutants, such as outlined in the Endocrine Society's statement of 2009. As a consequence of PCOS, I struggled with pregnancies, a miscarriage, and when finally blessed with children we were challenged with their skin issues, allergies and recurring respiratory problems.

My journey of discovery into products, materials and finishes in our home began while I was reading the label of a major brand baby shampoo bottle as my daughter bathed. I was shocked by what I found. The realisation that harmful ingredients were present in products that we had trusted opened a floodgate of questions about all our household products. These led to further questions, and the discovery of a disturbing amount of documentation from authorities that linked chemicals used in the home with health concerns. Material safety data sheets and product labels became essential reading. After investigating the consumables we were using in our home, I moved on to explore materials and finishes we had used to renovate our home with, before we had children.

It became very obvious that our home had been filled with many indoor environmental toxins, and the quality of our indoor air was compromised from our consumables, common daily practices and the way we had renovated our house. Our home had been contributing to our health challenges, and in some instances triggering them.

The more research I found (across many disciplines) highlighting the connection between the home and health, the more motivated I was to learn more. I would have valued knowing what I now know before we bought our first house, before we had our children, before we exposed our family to things that could have been avoided. If I'd known these things, we could have eliminated some of our health challenges. I wish someone had given me the information in this book which is the very reason I wanted to write this for you. Creating a home and a family are two of life's treasured experiences; hopefully with these insights you can make informed decisions to navigate your family through what is becoming a complex world of consumerism.

Helping families design, create and live well in healthy homes is rewarding. It's also extremely satisfying to know that many of the healthy choices for us also benefit the health of our environment and can improve the value of our home.

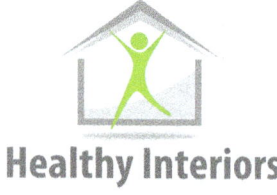

Author - Danielle King

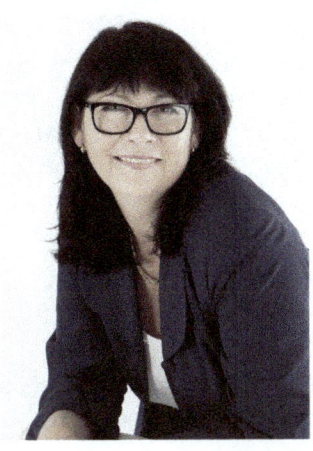

Danielle King is a well-respected and highly qualified sustainability consultant and trainer focused on sustainability and efficiency in the built environment. As founder and director of Green Moves Australia, she holds an MBA and a Diploma of Sustainability. She is also a qualified trainer and accredited sustainability assessor with a Cert IV in Home Sustainability Assessment. She is a member of the Sustainability Advisory Board at the Building Designers Association of Victoria (BDAV), a founding board member of the Green Building Institute (a non-profit organisation for sustainability training for building related trades) and sustainability partner for the Build & Renovating Expo Melbourne.

Danielle has presented many seminars on sustainable building topics and written numerous journal articles that have been published in a variety of media.

Through consulting in the field daily and teaching sustainability topics for reputable organisations including Swinburne University, the Housing Industry Association and local councils, Danielle is able to offer in depth knowledge with practical, creative and efficient solutions.

www.greenmoves.com.au

What made you choose to work in the sustainable living sector?

Returning home to Australia after many years working in the financial IT sector in the UK provided a great opportunity to escape the corporate world. With my business suits donated to the op shop, the world starting to feel the effects of climate change and a new son to look after, I realised I needed another, more meaningful 'job' (besides being a mother). For many years I had been concerned about the state of our planet and the impact from our actions as humans. What was our son going to have to live with later in life due to our actions over the decades? How could we help mitigate the problems and prepare him for what is fast shaping up to be an uncertain future, from food security to liveable habitat? Why do most of us live in homes that neither take advantage of the local climate nor use renewable materials and cost a fortune to run?

Everything I looked at pointed to sustainability in one form or another. It wasn't long before I had enrolled in further education to re-skill into the emerging field of sustainability, focusing on the built environment. We all have homes. Generally speaking they could be more comfortable, run more efficiently and have lower impacts on the environment. This is something we all can do, something that will make a difference, something that really matters.

So for my son's future, for all the children and for their children, I chose to work in the sustainability industry. I love every minute of it!

Danielle's story

Being brought up with a healthy respect for limited resources had a significant impact on how I view things. It was always 'turn off that light, don't waste power', 'turn that tap off properly, don't waste water' or 'no we don't need to buy that'. It instilled a basic need to be efficient with what we had and that waste of any sort was just stupid. So sustainability and efficiency was (by stealth) embedded from a young age.

However I only recognised this some 20 years ago when a work colleague called me a 'greenie', after I had complained about the amount of waste in an office I was working in and offered some solutions. I had never considered myself an eco-warrior, but realised that was what was actually needed. However, a significantly different approach is required to create change in a very financially focused world.

After working for many years as a senior program and project manager in the financial IT industry, the time for significant change came when my partner and I returned to Australia and our son was born. This coincided with more damning scientific evidence on human impact on the planet, and our country's leaders doing little to deal with it. The realisation that we are probably the first generation ever to leave the world in a worse state than we inherited it was shocking. It became very clear that if anything was to be done, we would have to do it ourselves and not rely on leaders, governments or industry.

With this new consciousness combined with my keen interest in property and a passion to leave the world a better place for all of our children, a change was in order. I decided to leave the corporate world and researched and re-educated myself in the sustainability sector. As a key interest has always been the built environment, that became the focus of my studies.

I hadn't really thought much about it in the past, but a home designed for European climates being built in Australia just doesn't make sense. Such homes would use a lot of fuel and be expensive to keep comfortable inside. However this is the reality across much of current Australian housing.

I had built my first new home aged 20 and have embarked on several renovations over the years in a variety of climate zones. It quickly became apparent how the needs of the home change in line with the local climate, stage of life of the occupant and level of financial freedom available. This is something that only recently is seeing proper consideration, yet can make significant impact on the enjoyment, comfort and cost of a home.

In 2005, the minimum housing performance regulatory requirements were implemented throughout Australia. This was designed to improve comfort levels and reduce the amount of fuel required to heat and cool a home. As a result, many of those in the building industry found they needed some additional education to understand the impact of good design, the importance of insulation and the effect on the environment. This is improving today (and I am one of the many educators in the field) but is only recently becoming a priority to the industry, due to regulatory changes and increased consumer demand for efficient homes.

Research has demonstrated more knowledge leads to more informed decisions being made in relation to key items such as design, appliances and materials used. Documented studies have also demonstrated the benefits of thoroughly considered and well-designed homes. When consumers realise that a home could cost them $10,000 per year to run, as opposed to another home that could cost just $2,000 (or less) a year to run, it encourages significant thought.

My devotion to the field is fuelled by passion, enthusiasm and need. There is so much potential and so much still to do, it's overwhelming at times. I continue to learn and take great pleasure in sharing that knowledge. It helps others become better informed, more aware and empowered to take action in whatever way they can. With a little knowledge, some good guidance and by opting for responsible, healthy materials, we can enhance, rather than impede, our presence on the ground.

Creating efficient, sustainable and healthier homes is not only better for ourselves. It's better for our planet, and we don't have other planets to choose from. I want to leave a better environment for my son, and future generations to inherit. And we can all make it happen, with a little effort, together.

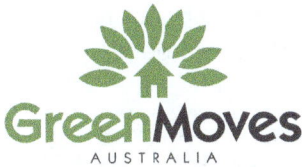

Professional contribution

Low Allergen, Sustainable Gardening Section

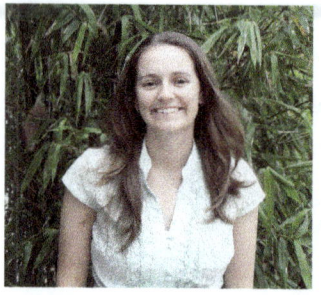

Belinda Thackeray

Belinda is a Sydney-based horticulturist and environmental educator with over 20 years of practical experience in horticulture, bush regeneration, design and education. Belinda has qualifications in horticulture, environmental studies (environmental education), bushland regeneration, workplace training and assessment, permaculture and e-learning.

Belinda is a mum to a young family and is passionate about gardening education and the nurturing of edible plants. Belinda works for Eden Gardens & Garden Centres as education manager, designing and delivering horticultural education enrichment programs with sustainability messages to adults and children. In 2009, she assisted with the design of their asthma and allergy friendly garden.

Disclaimer

This book is designed to provide information on healthy, sustainable and efficient housing attributes. Its primary purpose is to assist people to navigate consumer choices, to make informed household decisions that support efficient use of resources, promote wellbeing and support the environment.

This book is sold with the understanding that the publisher and authors are not engaged in rendering medical advice.

In addition, as every site is unique we recommend that you seek site specific advice for your home.

It is not the purpose of this manual to reprint all the information that is otherwise available to authors and/or publishers, but instead to compile, complement, amplify and supplement other texts. You are urged to read all the available material, learn as much as possible from varying opinions and sources about creating a healthy sustainable home, and tailor the information to your individual needs. For more information you can refer to the many resources listed within and at the back of this book.

Every effort has been made to make this book as complete and as accurate as possible. However, there may be mistakes, both typographical and in content. Therefore, this text should be used only as a general guide and not as the ultimate source of information on this topic. Furthermore, this book contains information on this subject matter current only up to the printing date. The purpose of this book is to educate and inform. The authors and publishers shall have neither liability nor responsibility to any person or entity with respect to any loss or damage caused, or alleged to have been caused, directly or indirectly, by the information contained in this book.

Website currency

Web resource links provided herein are subject to changes by the parties responsible for those websites. Weblinks are current at time of printing.

A note on spelling

UK English is used throughout this publication, except for when quoting directly from, and reproducing names of, sources and organisations from the USA. In those instances the American spelling is retained.

Foreword

Being provided with a safe and secure environment is a fundamental right of childhood. This means more than the provision of four walls and a roof! Before going to school, Australian children spend as much as 80 percent of their time indoors, in their home, so the home environment plays an important role in determining child health. There is increasing evidence that exposure to a variety of environmental toxicants in early life can set the scene for chronic diseases in later life. Chronic non-communicable diseases such as asthma and chronic lung disease; obesity and Type 2 diabetes; cardiovascular disease; and neurocognitive and behavioural problems are reaching epidemic proportions in Western society and environmental exposures in early life are likely to play a major role in increasing the risk of these health problems. Children are more vulnerable to toxic environments than adults are. The way children interact with their environment increases their risk of exposure and their developing physiology means that they receive a higher dose of any toxicant, relative to their body size, than an adult does in the same environment. In early life, children are frequently less able to detoxify environmental chemicals and pollutants, making the provision of a safe home environment for children a major imperative.

The Smart Living Handbook provides a wealth of useful and readable material on how to go about creating a safe home environment for children. This book is not, and should not be, a reference for the health problems associated with toxic exposures in the home. It is, however, a reference for those wanting to understand what a healthy home environment is and how to go about creating one. Clearly, many parts of the book are better suited to those building a new home as many of the construction tips can't be retro-engineered into existing homes. However, there are also many excellent sections and tips that can be applied to existing homes to improve the environment they provide for the occupants. The authors have wisely chosen to provide links to many additional sources of information that will ensure the longevity of the book. One may ask why we still need books in this electronic age. The Smart Living Handbook shows why books that gather a large amount of information and present it in a user-friendly fashion will always have a place. I congratulate the authors on their achievement.

Professor Peter D. Sly
Director, Children's Health and Environment Program,
Queensland Children's Medical Research Institute,
The University of Queensland.

Acknowledgements

The authors would like to thank the many people and organisations that offered their guidance, expertise and encouragement in relation to the content of this book.

- Alternative Technology Association
- Asthma Australia
- Aus Floorworks Pty Ltd
- Australian Building Codes Board
- Australian Consumer Association CHOICE
- Australian Geothermal Energy Association
- Australian Government, Water Rating (WELS), WERS, EER
- Australian Institute of Refrigeration, Air Conditioning and Heating
- Australian Sustainable Hardwoods
- Australian Paint Approval Scheme (APAS)
- Australian Passive House Association
- Australian Water Association
- Australian Window Association (AWA) and WERS
- Australian Institute of Refrigeration, Air-conditioning and Heating (AIRAH)
- Brandjes Environmental Building Consultancy
- Carpet Institute of Victoria
- Clean Energy Council
- Commonwealth of Australia, Bureau of Meteorology
- Commonwealth of Australia, Department of Industry, Your Home
- Commonwealth of Australia, Department of Health
- Commonwealth of Australia, Energy Rating Website
- Commonwealth Scientific and Industrial Research Organisation (CSIRO)
- Earp Bros – Innovative Tile Solutions
- Eco Decisions
- Ecospecifier – Global GreenTag
- Eden Gardens & Garden Centres
- Engineered Wood Products Association of Australasia (EWPAA)
- Environmental Defense Fund
- USA Environmental Protection Authority
- FSC® Australia
- Glass and Glazing Association of Australia
- Good Environmental Choice Australia (GECA)
- Green Painters Australia
- Livable Housing Association
- Nicola May Designs
- Public Health Association of Australia
- Richmond Lighting
- Rural Industries Research & Development Corporation
- Solar Air Heating Association
- State Government of Victoria, Australia, Sustainability Victoria
- TLC Indoor Gardens
- US Department of Energy
- Victorian Building Authority (VBA)
- Water Efficiency Labelling and Standards (WELS)
- Whittle Waxes

The authors would like to thank those who provided permission for their images or illustrations to be used within the content of this book.

Table of contents

Dedicated to iii
Testimonial iv
About the authors v
   Author – Melissa Wittig v
   Author – Danielle King vii
   Professional contribution x
   Disclaimer x
Foreword xi
   Acknowledgements xii
Introduction 3
What is sustainable living? 5
   Missing ingredient in the healthy lifestyle mantra 6
   Toxic soup social experiment 9
   International recognition – your home air matters 13
   Green vs. healthy – do you know the difference? 17
   Living by assumptions 18
5 step approach to creating a healthy, sustainable home 27
Step 1 – Build it/renovate 29
   What makes an energy efficient, sustainable, healthy building? 29
   Site considerations 31
   Know your climate 32
   Design principles 37
   Design considerations – for sustainable lifestyle outcomes 41
   Fire protection consideration 43
   Passive heating and cooling 44
   Insulation and draught-proofing 46
   Condensation – a cautionary word 56
   Windows and glazing 57
   Water 70
   Renewable energy for the home 79
   Livable housing 89
   Adaptable homes 91
   Tips for building or renovating a sustainable, healthy wet zone 92
   Tips for building or renovating a sustainable, healthy kitchen 95
   Site health tips 97
Step 2 – Products & furnishings – interior materials 101
   Our home – a big mixing bowl of ingredients 101
   Sustainable timber 103

- Timber coatings 107
- Plastics and your health 109
- Flooring 110
- Cabinetry – furniture 123
- Benchtops 126
- Paint 131
- Window coverings 136
- Furniture 138
- Water ware and plumbing 140
- Water filtration 143
- Lighting 146
- Appliances 160
- Heating and cooling systems 188
- Indoor plants 215

Step 3 – Our behaviour – consumer choice 217
- Shop wise - resources 220
- Beware of 'green wash' 223
- Shop wise tools 224

Step 4 – Lifestyle practices 231
- A healthier sustainable home 231
- Creating a healthy child's space 238

Step 5 – Maintaining a home for efficiency & health 241
- Maintenance summary checklist 241

Low allergen and sustainable gardening 245
Investment sense 262
The healthy home quiz 265
Checklists 287
- Healthy home checklist 287
- Asthma & allergy home checklist 288
- Healthy home renovating checklist 294
- Extreme heat healthy home checklist 295
- Healthy home maintenance checklist 297
- Draught-proofing checklist 298
- Build and renovate checklist 300
- What to look for in a home checklist 302
- Energy smart checklist 306
- Water smart checklist 309

Conclusion 312
Glossary of terms 314
References 317

Introduction

> Warning: these insights may just change your life!

One of the most important things we can do for ourselves and our families is to create a healthy home environment that is safe, nurturing and supportive for our physical and emotional needs.

With the popularity of television home makeover and renovation shows we find ourselves living in a culture that is promoting the concept of interior design and decoration as a form of consumption. On the flip side, we are being encouraged to consider the environment, minimise waste, recycle and live a more resource efficient lifestyle. Modern home messages are fraught with inconsistencies that are impacting on industry, public health and environmental reform success.

The way we build our homes is evolving. The building industry is striving to encourage homes that are energy efficient, airtight and well insulated to minimise energy consumption and reduce occupant utility costs. The creation of airtight homes introduces the complexities of indoor air quality and health, along with increased pollutant exposure from the products we are building with and placing in our home.

Criteria for the ideal home are constantly changing in the 21st century. We are bombarded by consumerism and technology and in a fast paced global environment we have little time to contemplate the impact our homes and our actions may be having on our health.

A home is a space that we retreat to, to rest, recover and rejuvenate and socialise. Many aspects of our homes are within our personal control, with some occupants having more control than others. Structural design, building materials, finishes and colour, furniture and daily practices all contribute to our emotional and physical health. Too often the development of a home is based upon an aesthetic approach without conscious thought to materials, efficiency, environmental impacts, social impacts of purchases and the short and long term health impacts on our families.

We cannot avoid chemicals or pollutants as we move about the world but we can make a choice to reduce them in and around our homes.

Over the past few years the connection between the home environment and human health has gained attention, with the blogosphere blooming with believers. This book is not intended to take a detailed scientific approach to issues. It is written to provide easy-to-digest considerations to the aspects of the interior environment that have been linked to health and living efficiently and sustainably, when decorating, renovating or building.

A home is more than its beauty or visual appeal. This book aims to be a valued resource highlighting general issues for consumers, such as the health of buildings, interior related purchases and household decisions, especially those that impact on human health and sustainability within the indoor environment. First home owners, existing home owners, renters, mothers-to-be, new parents, existing parents, the elderly, the ill seeking cleaner living solutions, asthma and allergy sufferers, industry students, and any discerning consumer will find it useful.

We explore why there are concerns about the way we live today, who says there is cause for concern, and provide industry insights to navigate the plethora of home related interior products in the market place.

You may find that some concepts or suggestions are repeated throughout the book. This is because healthy, sustainable lifestyle principles are intrinsically linked to many facets of the home environment.

Indoor health is impacted upon by the lifestyle and buying decisions made by those building the home and the occupants. The link between indoor environmental health and energy efficiency is evident when we examine our reliance on energy-consuming lifestyle products. There are many things to consider when choosing products for the home such as health impacts, operating costs and environmental impacts. At a time when the costs of living are increasing, finite resources are being depleted and pollutants being used to manufacture products are increasing, there is much to learn to become a savvy shopper.

As we explore many different products you will find that in most cases, specific brands are not mentioned as this can be problematic with product changes, product model updates and company changes. However, the information provided in this book is aimed at giving you the resources and tools to be your own best advocate as you navigate products for yourself into the future. You can visit the **www.healthyinteriors.com.au** or **www.greenmoves.com.au** websites for supplementary information.

Whether you are building, renovating or renting, in a home or business environment, this book of strategies embraces a holistic approach to healthy sustainable living and offers the many ways you can reduce your bills and minimise your exposure to pollutants linked to disease. It's a smart way to live.

What is sustainable living?

There are many definitions of sustainability. Some commonly referenced are:

'Development that meets the needs of the present without compromising the ability of future generations to meet their own needs.' Brundtland Report, 1987

'Sustainability is improving the quality of human life while living within the carrying capacity of supporting eco-systems'

Caring for the Earth: A Strategy for Sustainable Living Switzerland, 1991

'Enough ...for all ...forever' World Summit on Sustainable Development, 2002

A common understanding is that sustainable living includes the grand goal of managing our environmental, social, and economic impacts on the world so that we meet present needs, while ensuring the ability of future generations to meet theirs.

It's worth noting that human health hasn't been referenced above. We explore this issue further in the book.

Our past

There have always been minority groups in society that have taken an active interest in so-called 'green' housing and lifestyle options. However the majority of Australians' lifestyles have morphed into what they are today as a result of industry influence, and the building industry has been effectively dictating how we live.

In many definitions of sustainable living, the focus is on the planet and global resources, the goal being to save the planet from destruction as a result of human activities and behaviours.

It is significant to note that in the past the definitions of sustainable living rarely includes reference to human health.

Today

The dictionary defines sustainable as 'able to be maintained at a certain rate or level'.

Today, Australians are faced with increasing rates of asthma, allergies and cancers among many other health concerns, many of which have been linked to environmental, biological and chemical pollutant triggers or causes. Authorities and industry continue to encourage Australian families to make sustainable lifestyle choices to protect global resources with a view to protecting the planet for future generations. Meanwhile families are faced with personal challenges and their ability to sustain their own health.

Missing ingredient in the healthy lifestyle mantra

Generally, in childhood and during the teenage years, one has little prescience of one's mortality. As adulthood kicks in and all that comes with it, we gradually become more aware of our lifestyle choices and consequences. A greater consciousness of our actions and choices generally evolves as we age and for many a connection between lifestyle and longevity emerges. We start to wonder how to live a healthy life for as long as possible.

For many, first-time parenthood is a sudden arrival at adulthood. It can be like someone has handed you a pair of finely-adjusted eye glasses bringing a new perspective on the world. Our basic instinct is to shield our children from the world and all its hazards, including increased pollution.

Current obesity statistics and health issues in our society are a constant reminder that a healthy diet and exercise are essential to minimising health risks and living longer. This is where we have stopped short in our quest for overall good health.

Combined personal parenthood and professional experiences to date have revealed many life lessons. One of these lessons, or truths, that impacts on everyone's lives in many ways (including one's health) is that old adage that **'money makes the world go around'**.

We need to see past convenience and clever marketing by challenging information and be our own best advocate.

There are people who have thought about their place in the world and have come to the conclusion that they want to leave the environment a better place. However, there are other people who have not found the time, motivation or inclination to explore the impact they are having on the environment right now.

While it would be ideal if everyone understood where their landfill goes and what happens to the chemicals flushed down the drain, our daily lives are too different to expect that everyone will reach the same page in life at the same time.

What we can be assured of is that everyone's health is challenged at some stage, and many of the features of our lifestyles, and in our homes, contribute to our health.

There are a few things at a basic level that we all have in common.

Living essentials list:

1. We all sleep and wake – usually in our home
2. We all consume food and drink
3. We all move around.
4. We do all of these things in a place where we store our belongings and sleep for many hours in a day – our home.

Although these things are fundamentally basic, it is these very basic elements of our lifestyle that we all have in common. They have a significant impact on our health and the health of our home.

Authorities have been focused on motivating consumers to make changes to their lifestyles that support the 'health of environment', such as recycling household rubbish, using reusable bags when shopping and buying energy efficient appliances. While these initiatives are needed for the health of our environment, the message stops short of immediate personal gain which is a huge motivating factor.

While we all share our environment and understand that changing our behaviour will help the common good for a healthy environment, the immediate gain from actions is largely not appreciated or valued.

What if there was a way to give families information that would inspire them to make choices that resulted in healthier families (immediate personal gain) and a healthier environment?

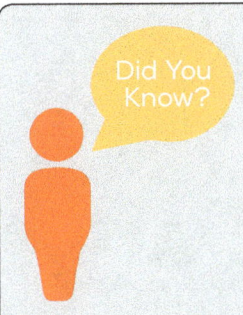

The Development of World Health Organisation (WHO) Guidelines for Indoor Air Quality Report 2006 stated:

There are many potentially hazardous compounds released indoors due to combustion, emissions from building materials, household equipment and consumer products. Microbial pollution comes from hundreds of species of bacteria, fungi, and moulds growing indoors. Indoor air quality management is made difficult not only by the large number and variation of indoor spaces but also the complex relations of indoor air quality and the building design, materials, operation and maintenance, ventilation and behaviour of the building users.

The missing ingredient in the healthy lifestyle mantra is a healthy home. An essential ingredient to good health is to consider the environments we are placing our bodies in for many hours a day.

Our lifestyle

The word lifestyle refers to 'the way a person lives'. In order to achieve a healthy, sustainable lifestyle we need to look at the parts of our lifestyle that are intimately connected. Our home environment is a large part of our daily life. When we look at the total influence a home has on our life, we reveal several layers.

The home is a building shell lined with materials, containing spaces and products that are used in a variety of differing ways, on a daily basis over time. To create a home that supports good health, we need to consider the health aspects of the products used and occupant practices at each stage of the home cycle.

Points 1 and 4 of the living essentials list involve our home, yet our home environment is not often promoted as being linked to the attainment of good health. While we may care for our body by eating well and exercising, it's unlikely that we take the time to consider the potential impacts from environments we spend time in each day.

Our home is an environment that we consistently return to for extending periods of time daily. Again, how often do we question products that we take into our homes to identify unhealthy pollutants that we may be inadvertently inhaling, ingesting or absorbing?

The desire for good health is universal - a shared common goal. A healthy home contributes to this goal and indirectly has a positive impact on environmental health.

To reduce environmental pollution we don't need everyone to study environmental science or become sustainability gurus. Highlighting how unhealthy choices around the home impact on personal health allows people to see that in helping themselves by removing toxins in their life, they are also helping the environment.

Healthy homes enhance liveability, embrace good design and lifestyle principles, foster environmentally responsible choices, and promote quality of life outcomes directly reducing costs associated with sickness.

On this basis, our health is intrinsically linked with sustainable lifestyle success.

A healthy home is the missing ingredient to improved family health and positive environmental outcomes.

A personal experience

'Manufacturers don't have to disclose all the ingredients used in their products.

'After experiencing a family member's allergic reaction – and subsequent hospitalisation – to a drink product, we contacted the consumer help line on the back of the label and advised them of the reaction. When we requested a full list of ingredients to try and establish the irritant, we were deferred to the legal department and advised that they would not supply full details as some ingredients were protected under 'trade secret' laws.'

Melissa Wittig

Toxic soup social experiment

We are surrounded by manmade items every day. We assume that what we have available to purchase is okay for human health, yet this is not necessarily the case.

Our product choice when renovating, building or decorating is wide and varied. However, a concerning aspect of this pleasure is that labelling laws in many instances do not adequately enable consumers to make informed decisions about whether something is going to harm them or not. If everything was labelled like cigarette packets are now, what would packaging on products we buy look like?

Starting with food products, there are labelling loopholes that allow manufacturers to create and sell foods without having to disclose all the ingredients used in their product.

When our children are young we teach them not to put things in their mouth if they don't know what it is or where it has come from, yet on a daily basis we are buying food from people who don't have to disclose what has been used to make it. In times where only whole food ingredients were used to create foods, the excuse of 'secret blend' may have been more acceptable. But when our food can contain chemicals in the form of additives, colourings and flavourings it seems wrong and harmful that we don't have adequate rights to know what we are eating.

According to Dr Sarah Lantz in her book *Raising Chemical Free Kids* (2009):

'Of the 296 additives with a current international numbering system (INS) approved for use in Australia, at least a minimum of 25 are banned in some other countries. Approximately 50 have been linked to cancer, 55 or so can trigger asthma, more than 30 are thought to cause hyperactivity and/or learning difficulties in children and 80 may contribute to kidney or liver problems.'

This is food we are choosing to eat. If we are eating foods with undisclosed ingredients it seems optimistic to expect that we have detailed labels concerning the materials and finishes we buy to build and furnish our home with.

As you stroll through the local hardware store or homewares shop, look at how many products do not contain labels outlining the materials or ingredients used to make them.

It is important to remember when choosing products for the home, that many products have the potential to break down or release particles over time that may end up in our household dust. The dust within our homes affects the health of our home because dust is inadvertently circulated through lifestyle practices and can be ingested or inhaled.

Everyone has at least one mattress in their home, so this is a good example of a product to look at when demonstrating how health attributes are often forgotten. When buying a mattress it is common to focus on the size and comfort of the bed. This is a place where we spend around eight hours a night, where our body needs to rest and rejuvenate. In researching this book we did not find one mattress label that details the full list of materials and treatments applied. The potential health impacts of this product are considerable. There is a big difference between how individual mattresses are made and inadequate labelling makes this a difficult purchase. How does a consumer know what they need to compare to make an informed decision if attributes are not labelled?

When making a decision on a mattress you are deciding which of these attributes/combinations you want to lie on, and breathe up close and personal with for around eight hours a night.

Mattress materials

- **Core materials** are very different in their characteristics and emissions, e.g. polyurethane foam, natural latex, styrene-butadiene rubber (synthetic latex)
- Different **adhesives** are used between suppliers, with varying emission levels
- **Covering material** varies – natural fibres, synthetic fibres such as polyester, nylon, plasticised fabrics
- Some **coverings** are subjected to chemical applications such as toxic dyes, stain repellent treatments, wrinkle resistant treatments, pesticides, fire retardant chemicals and anti-microbial treatments
- **Padding layers** may be a polyurethane foam or synthetic fibre pads – whether bonded or unbonded, bonding batting is usually treated with resin to hold fibres together

As you can see from this list, your purchase will result in potential exposures to pollutants that you may not have thought about and are potentially not on the label. It is unlikely that you will find a product completely free from chemicals, however you can make informed choices that will lower your exposure significantly.

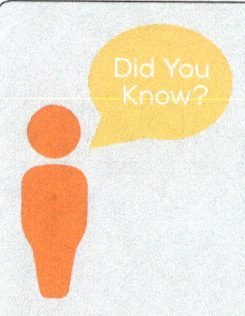

Did You Know?

'Flexible polyurethane foam is made in a slab process combining chemicals known as isocyanates and polyols with other chemicals that act as stabilisers, catalysts, surfactants, fire retardants, colourants and blowing agents, each of these chemicals is associated with a host of environmental and health hazards'. (Bader, 2007)

Isocyanates are irritants to human tissue such as the eyes and the respiratory tract, and have been associated with inducing asthma among other serious health concerns. Solvents used in many of the adhesives have also been linked to health concerns ranging from respiratory tract irritants to carcinogens.

If we start to explore the stories behind all the products we buy, we find similar surprises throughout the home. Currently there is no effective way for Australians to compare the chemical and pollutant levels of products we buy on a daily basis. The onus of buyer beware currently falls firmly with consumers as we unknowingly fill our homes with a range of chemicals and pollutants. Shouldn't the responsibility of declaring a product's history be on the manufacturers and suppliers?

In Australia we value our freedoms, and detailed, accurate labelling is a form of freedom of information. Many families unknowingly fill their homes with pollutants and live among a plethora of chemicals. At the same time our health system continues to be challenged with the increase in allergies, asthma, illness and cancers. Many homes can be likened to a toxic soup that inevitably spills into the environment in the form of household waste.

Asking questions and demanding information about products before buying will encourage suppliers to seek this information from manufacturers, inevitably inducing changes to labelling (retailers will tire of having to chase details for buyers) and allow us all to make informed decisions.

In the following pages we provide you with tools to be able to navigate products in an informed manner.

International concerns

What others are saying:

World Health Organisation (WHO)

'The occurrence of indoor sources of various chemicals and the chemical's toxicity leads to identification of certain compounds for which indoor sources and exposures are driving the health risks of specific population groups in Western countries.' 2006

'Air pollution is now the world's largest single environmental health risk...

The new data reveals a stronger link between both indoor and outdoor air pollution exposure and cardiovascular diseases, such as strokes and ischaemic heart disease, as well as between air pollution and cancer. This is in addition to air pollution's role in the development of respiratory diseases, including acute respiratory infections and chronic obstructive pulmonary diseases.' 2014

Environment Australia – Indoor Air Quality Report

'Indoor air quality is recognised as a significant environmental and health problem in most countries. Modern populations typically spend 80–90 percent of their time indoors, whether at home, work or elsewhere. Coupled with the common research finding that pollutants in indoor air occur more frequently and at higher concentrations than in outdoor air, it is clear that indoor air is the major source for environmental exposure to air pollutants. The result of such exposure is a spectrum of illnesses ranging from mild to severe effects (e.g. mild irritation/lethargy, impaired respiratory development, asthma, cancer) that cost communities heavily in suffering and economic loss.' (Brown, 1997)

'The health impacts of many chemical components in building materials are not well understood. Many chemicals present in indoor air environments have not been thoroughly tested and little is known about their long-term health effects.' (Meek, 1991)

Environment Australia - State of Knowledge Report, Air toxics and indoor air quality in Australia, 2001

'Health effects that may be experienced by the occupants of buildings with poor indoor air quality range from severe effects (asthma, allergic response, cancer risk) to mild and generally non-specific symptoms.'

International Society of Indoor Air Quality and Climate 'Indoor residential chemical emissions as risk factors for respiratory and allergic effects in children: a review.'

'Most research into effects of residential exposures on respiratory health has focused on allergens, moisture/mold, endotoxin, or combustion products. A growing body of research from outside the US; however, has associated chemical emissions from common indoor materials with risk of asthma, allergies, and pulmonary infections...Associations, some strong, were reported between many risk factors and respiratory or allergic effects. Risk factors identified most frequently included formaldehyde or particleboard, phthalates or plastic materials, and recent painting. Findings for other risk factors, such as aromatic and aliphatic chemical compounds [e.g. chemicals found in adhesives, PVC flooring and carpeting], were limited but suggestive. Elevated risks were also reported for renovation and cleaning activities, new furniture, and carpets or textile wallpaper.' (Mendell MJ, 2007)

Mount Sinai Hospital, USA

'Scientific evidence is strong and continuing to build that hazardous exposures in the modern environment are important causes of diseases in children...Indoor and outdoor air pollution are now established as causes of asthma. Childhood cancer is linked to solvents, pesticides and radiation. The National Academy of Sciences has determined that environmental factors contribute to 28 percent of developmental disorders in children.'
(Icahn School of Medicine at Mount Sinai Hospital, New York, 2013)

'...Toxic chemicals in the environment – lead, pesticides, toxic air pollutants, phthalates, and bisphenol A – are important causes of disease in children, and they are found in our homes, at our schools, in the air we breathe, and in the products we use every day.' (Mt Sinai Hospital, New York, 2014)

Oregon Environmental Council Report – Children at Risk

More and more studies demonstrate that exposure to toxic chemicals during infancy or childhood can affect the development of the respiratory, nervous, hormone and immune systems, as well as increasing the risk of cancer later in life. One study has shown that children who are exposed to pesticides before age one are four times more likely to develop early persistent asthma, for example.

'Phthalates are among the most frequently found contaminants in human bodies. Babies exposed to a certain phthalates in utero are born a week earlier on average than babies without exposure. Men with high levels of phthalates in their urine tend to have low levels of sperm production. DEHP is a probable human carcinogen, but the carcinogenicity of other phthalates is unknown at this time. A very recent study suggests a link between phthalates and asthma.' (Doll, S. 2004)

The American College of Obstetricians and Gynaecologists

The ACOG released a media statement in 2013 about the effects on reproductive health of toxic environmental agents. It stated in part:

'The scientific evidence over the last 15 years shows that exposure to toxic environmental agents before conception and during pregnancy can have significant and long-lasting effects on reproductive health.

Linda C Giudice, MD, PhD, president of the American Society for Reproductive Medicine, said: 'For example, pesticide exposure in men is associated with poor semen quality, sterility, and prostate cancer...We also know that exposure to pesticides may interfere with puberty, menstruation and ovulation, fertility, and menopause in women.'

Other reproductive and health problems associated with exposure to toxic environmental agents:

- *Miscarriage and stillbirth*
- *Impaired foetal growth and low birth weight*
- *Preterm birth*
- *Childhood cancers*
- *Birth defects*
- *Cognitive/intellectual impairment*
- *Thyroid problems'*

(American College of Obstetricians and Gynaecologists media release 2013)

International recognition – your home air matters

The World Health Organisation estimates that one in eight of total global deaths is as a result of air pollution (7 million people in 2012) and that indoor air pollution contributes to the development of respiratory disease, acute respiratory infections and chronic obstructive pulmonary diseases. They have also attributed indoor air pollution as contributing to deaths associated with stroke, ischaemic heart disease, COPD, lung cancer and acute lower respiratory infections. (WHO, 2014)

Once we look at the cocktail of chemicals used to create our home environment from the building materials, décor materials, furnishings and consumables we can start to appreciate how many chemicals surround us.

In relation to toxicity of materials in the home you may have heard the thrown away line, "well I am not going to eat it", yet the reality is that you don't have to eat something for it to make its way into the body.

All of the materials, furnishings and products that we surround ourselves with have three routes of potentially affecting our health – through ingesting (eating them), inhalation (breathing it in) or absorption (through the skin).

What is unknown to many people is that materials, furnishings and products that we bring into our homes can release gases or fumes that can pollute our indoor air. Many of these gases/fumes have an obvious odour yet many do not. These gases/fumes are referred to within the industry as Volatile Organic Compounds, otherwise known as VOCs.

Defined by others as –

"Volatile organic compounds (VOCs) are chemicals containing carbon that evaporate into the atmosphere at room temperature." (Department of the Environment, 2008)

"Volatile organic compounds (VOCs) are emitted as gases from certain solids or liquids. VOCs include a variety of chemicals, some of which may have short- and long-term adverse health effects. Concentrations of many VOCs are consistently higher indoors (up to ten times higher) than outdoors." (USA EPA, 2009)

There are two different categories of VOCs:

1. Natural VOCs – eg scents from trees, flowers, organic matter, natural oils
2. Human made otherwise referred to as Anthropogenic VOCs –these are caused by human activity. *"Every process which involves the manipulation and the production of hydrocarbons emits VOC's. For example oil refining, solvent release, painting and industrial combustion are some of the many anthropogenic processes that produce VOC's."* (Whittle Waxes, 2013)

We surround ourselves with anthropogenic VOCs throughout our home, e.g. flooring, painted surfaces, carpet, furniture, toys, clothing and other household items.

Not all natural VOCs are safe, and not all anthropogenic VOCs are unsafe. This is why it is easy to get confused.

'Eye and respiratory tract irritation, headaches, dizziness, visual disorders, and memory impairment are among the immediate symptoms that some people have experienced soon after exposure to some organics.' (Environmental Protection Authority (USA EPA, 2009)

'The ability of organic chemicals to cause health effects varies greatly from those that are highly toxic, to those with no known health effects. Exposure impacts for all pollutants vary

depending on the extent and nature of exposure combined with a person's age, size and state of health at the time.' (USA EPA, 2009)

To avoid being overwhelmed let us focus on a few common VOCs that have been highlighted as particularly dangerous from products within the home environment. These are: formaldehyde, benzene, phenol, toluene, acetone, xylene, ethylene glycol and polybrominated diphenyl ethers (PBDEs, or flame retardants). These can be found in everyday items from furniture, carpet, nail polish, hobby supplies, paints, cleaners, textile treatments, through to office products.

According to the Environment Australia Indoor Air Quality Report (Brown, 1997), there are two major causes of pressures on indoor air pollution:

1. (low) building ventilation rates
2. (high) emission from pollutant sources

The quality of indoor air in a house is impacted upon by everything within the home. Most materials have the potential to release gases at some stage in their product lifecycle. The complexity of measuring the levels within homes arises from the fact that each person's home is unique with its own complex cocktail of emissions based on the products inside, combined with emissions from occupant daily practices. What we do know is that many individual VOCs are health hazards at certain levels and when many VOCs combine within an enclosed space there is increased risk of harmful consequences.

There is no quick, easy answer as to which products off-gas the most and how long the off-gassing of individual products occurs for. Within industry some suppliers choose to have their materials or products chamber tested to measure the VOCs a product emits, particularly for building related materials. The results of chamber testing are presented in the form of an emission certificate. This is not a mandatory requirement for many materials and products that we purchase. The testing is often performed voluntarily and is usually something that you need to ask for if it is not mentioned on product labelling.

Knowing and recognising that when you smell an odour from a product means that it is potentially a harmful gas, is a huge step forward in understanding the connection between things in our environment and their impact on our health.

The 'new car odour', 'new carpet smell' or the overwhelming scent that emits from the local department store shoe section are all great examples of VOCs – a warning from your nose to your body.

As a developed country we are exposed to the plethora of existing and emerging untested chemicals that reach into our homes.

According to 'The Development of WHO Guidelines for Indoor Air Quality Report' (2006):

'Review of the occurrence of indoor sources of various chemicals and the chemicals' toxicity leads to identification of certain compounds for which indoor sources and exposures are driving the health risks of specific population groups in Western countries.'

'Poor indoor air quality is an international issue, although recognised by the World Health Organisation as difficult to manage due to 'the number and variation of indoor spaces but also the complex relations of indoor air quality and the building design, materials, operation and maintenance, ventilation and behaviour of the building users.'

Indoor chemical exposure is not a new topic; hazards have been identified and much research published for many years. With increasing rates of cancers, asthma and allergies and the public health system under enormous strain it is essential that we look at the way we live and take notice of the WHO's research that our homes and the way we live are potentially making us ill.

'CSIRO estimates that indoor air pollution costs the Australian community in excess of $10 billion a year in illness and lost productivity' (CSIRO, 2000)

The commercial building sector is moving forward with the roll-out of green and health focused attributes for office buildings as there have been significant benefits recorded for both the environment and the health of those working in these environments. This is great for industry and beneficial for workers' moral, motivation, productivity and health.

The quality of indoor air is an essential component of greening commercial buildings. It has been widely documented and recognised commercially that clean air benefits health and productivity.

Over the past 10 years and particularly the last five as the commercial green building movement has progressed, it has been exciting to watch important building and health issues surface in the commercial sector; yet frustrating at the same time, as there remains an inadequate focus on the residential sector to communicate these issues to families. Particularly when those in our society who spend many hours indoors at home, such as babies, small children, pregnant women, the elderly and the ill, are those most vulnerable to pollutants.

Infants and young children are at most risk of adverse health effects from household chemicals and pollutants due to their size. Children are more vulnerable than adults due to their respiration rate to size ratio, size of their organs and their organs' capacity to eliminate toxins effectively. Small children also spend more time indoors, more time on the floor and they have greater hand to mouth behaviours than adults. These are fundamental reasons why as adults we need to give deeper consideration as to what we expose our children to and the type of homes we create for our family.

Many homes are being designed or remodeled without fundamental long term health considerations that can assist with preventing family illness. Materials, finishes and products can contribute to serious illnesses. The most common sources of pollution within the home originate from building tasks and the materials used, household products, occupant activities and outdoor pollutants. These sources all contribute pollutants into the indoor air we breathe.

Some aspects relative to maintaining occupant health (such as providing adequate ventilation to prevent mould) have been included into the National Construction Code (NCC) of Australia (Volume 2 Part 3.8 Health and Amenity), previously called the Building Code of Australia (BCA). However the NCC does not currently include any mention of VOCs within the home.

The relative humidity of indoor air as well as surface condensation provides favourable conditions for the survival and growth of biological pollutants such as bacteria, viruses, mites and fungi. The relative humidity of indoor air also impacts on off-gassing.

The rate of growth of organisms and the speed of chemical reactions are very much determined by combinations of temperature and humidity.

Ideally ventilation of dwellings should strive for levels of humidity (and temperature) that are comfortable but also minimise the growth of organisms and off-gassing.

According to a report by Sterling, Arundel and Sterling titled 'Criteria for Human Exposure to Humidity in Occupied Buildings', the optimal conditions to minimise risks to human health occur in the narrow range between 40 percent and 60 percent relative humidity at normal room temperatures, as shown in the graph below.

It can be seen below that off-gassing increases dramatically after 55 percent relative humidity. It can also be seen below that with greater humidity there is an increase in biological pollutants such as dust mites and moulds.

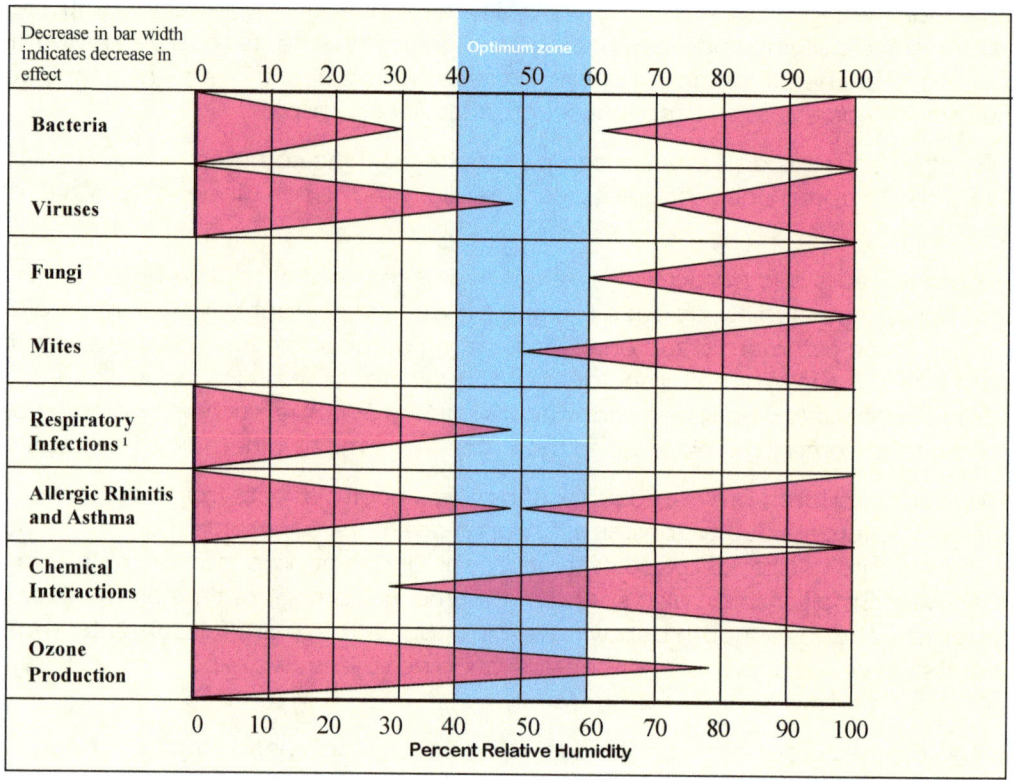

Optimum relative humidity ranges for health. Supplied by Theodor Sterling Associates, Vancouver

As we all move into an era of changing our homes to be more sensitive to environmental impacts, we also need to focus on assessing how our homes are affecting our health.

Creating homes that are affordable, efficient, healthy and environmentally friendly is the modern day housing challenge.

Green vs. healthy – do you know the difference?

The label 'green home' is a broad one. Considering 'green' or 'eco' initiatives within the design process of new homes has become second nature for many in the industry. Energy efficiency, sustainable product selection, material end-of-life considerations and environmentally sensitive practices are often the main focus.

There is a fundamental consideration that is often forgotten in the design, construct and occupy process, and that is the health attributes of products and project decisions.

In many instances a 'healthy' product will also be a good eco alternative, however not in all instances. Therefore we would like to highlight that a 'sustainable' home and a 'healthy' home are two different attributes of a home environment. The ultimate objective is to achieve both – a healthy and sustainable home.

The ideal outcome when selecting building materials is to choose materials that have both environmental and health attributes. From an environmental perspective it's beneficial to choose a material (or finish or furnishing) with the following questions in mind:

- Are materials used sustainably sourced or from a renewable source?
- What is the embodied energy? (The energy used to collect raw materials and processing required to create the product)
- What finite resources are required for processing e.g. water?
- What is the pollution contribution from the manufacturing process?
- Is the product beneficial for energy or water efficiency of the home?
- Can materials be easily and efficiently recycled at their end of use/life?

There are entire organisations dedicated to exploring material life cycle assessments and environmental attributes of materials in the building industry. Companies also use their product labelling to highlight environmental attributes, making it increasingly easier for consumers to compare brands and corporate eco ethics.

In reality, we are time poor and don't have time to research every product before we buy, so many decisions are made after reading the information on a product label. But beware; marketing gurus are good at their job, so ask questions about products beyond the label content.

Independent certification of products is a great way to assist you to make product choices as this means someone has independently assessed the product against criteria. Look for independent certification logos on labels. Once you have identified the certification company name it's a great idea to look them up online to view their award criteria as each certification body looks for different things in a product. Often there is an assumption that if a product is certified as being eco-friendly then it is also a healthier option – this is not always the case. We look at certification labels later in this book.

When building or renovating a home it's essential to keep in mind that human health is potentially impacted by things in the environment that can make their way into the body by inhalation, absorption and ingestion. When choosing products to build or renovate a home opting for products with minimal toxicity (and low/no VOC) makes common sense.

Living by assumptions

Each day we are bombarded by images of Australian politicians in the media. These images of public representatives and government department staff at work debating issues, making decisions and coordinating public affairs has lulled many people into a false sense of security about the safety and protection network the government provides consumers.

Do you make any of the following assumptions?

- I can trust all products that I purchase will do no harm
- People are not allowed to sell products that are dangerous to my health
- I can trust the companies making products because 'they' wouldn't sell products that are harmful to people
- The government accurately and strictly regulates all products sold in Australia
- All imported products are tested and known to be safe before they can be sold in Australia
- If homes could make people sick the government would definitely be advertising health campaign messages warning people of hazards

Unfortunately all of the assumptions above are false.

The cigarette industry is a great example of this – you can easily walk into a store and buy a cancer-causing product. For many years cigarettes were sold without health warnings despite an understanding they were detrimental to health. They continue to be manufactured and sold even though they are now widely accepted as a known carcinogen (thankfully they at least now have a warning that can't be missed).

Cigarettes alone are an example of a consumer product with a known link to disease estimated as having a $318.4m total net health care cost to Australians in 2004-05 (Cancer Council, 2013) with additional impacts on non-smoker health from second and third-hand smoke/pollutants, particularly in the home environment.

A look at consumables such as cleaning products will reveal that many of these products lining the supermarket shelves have very little information about what they are made from. They contain warning and poison labels and choose to hide behind 'trade secret' laws that prevent consumers from knowing what they are using in their home and exposing themselves to.

Cleaning products and other household items such as building products (paints, stains, adhesives etcetera) textile treatments, air fresheners, and many other consumables, contain a plethora of chemicals.

The word chemical is generic and lots of people turn off when talking science, so let's keep this basic and relevant.

There are currently around 38,000 chemicals approved for use on the Australian Inventory of Chemical Substances (AICS) list.

The Australian National Industrial Chemicals Notification and Assessment Scheme (NICNAS) assesses existing chemicals on a priority basis in response to concerns about their health or environmental effects, or both.

Thousands of chemicals in use have not been tested as being safe to human health and are currently being used for products we use in our homes.

Aside from chemicals produced here in Australia, we should consider the additional range of chemicals that make their way into our homes that have been imported. For example, in the United States alone, more than 80,000 chemicals are approved for use with approximately 2000 new chemicals approved each year.

According to America's Environmental Working Group:

'...an analysis of the United States EPA's approval process has found that the agency has been making critical decisions even though it has not received health and safety data for 85 percent of the new chemicals concocted by the chemical industry. The federal government's regulatory framework places the burden on the EPA to show that chemicals are unsafe instead of forcing chemical companies to show that their creations are safe.' (EWG, 2013).

Essentially what this all means is that things we buy can be made from ingredients that are not tested as being safe for human health.

Anecdotal feedback received from clients include concerns about a selection of consumables. For example:

Leather couch - skin irritation, headache and nausea

Imported timber sideboard - strong odour from the stain and caused nausea, headache

Candles - asthma symptoms, headache, nausea

Bed – headache, nausea

Toy plastic play mat – headache, nausea

Blinds – headache, nausea, eye symptoms

Bamboo flooring – headache, nausea, coughing

Consumers are unknowingly taking chemicals into their homes, unable to accurately assess their risk at the time of purchase. Compared with the indoor environment of homes many years ago, the modern home has an increasing range of pollutants finding their way into our lives, and our bodies.

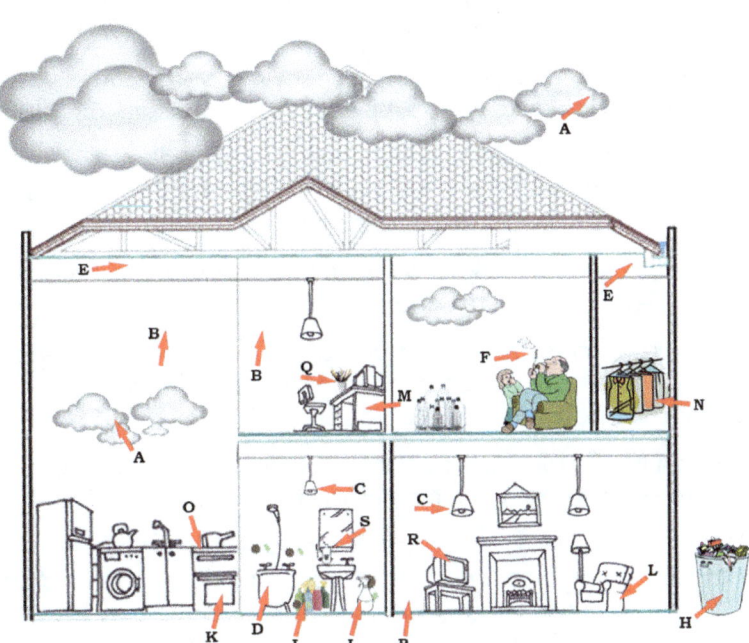

Pollutants in the home

Traditional Home
1. Dust — A
2. Lead — B
3. Mercury — C
4. Molds and Bacteria — D
5. Pollen — B
6. Asbestos — E
7. Tobacco smoke — F
8. Combustion pollutants — K
9. Pests — H

Modern Home
1. Particulate Matter — A
2. Lead — B
3. Mercury — C
4. Molds and Bacteria — D
5. Pollen — B
6. Asbestos — E
7. Tobacco smoke — F
8. Combustion pollutants — K
9. Pests — H
10. Acetone — I
11. Ammonia — J
12. Benzene — I
13. Bisphenol A — I
14. Carbon Monoxide — K
15. Chlorine — D
16. Endocrine Disruptors — L
17. Formaldehyde — M
18. Perchloroethylene (PERC) — N
19. Perfluorooctanoic Acid (PFOA) — O
20. Pesticides — P
21. Phthalates — Q
22. Polychlorinated Biphenyls (PCBs) — R
23. Solvents — I
24. Toluene — S
25. Volatile Organic Compounds (VOCs) — A
26. Triclosan — I

At right, is a summary of where the pollutants listed can be found in the home. On the following page are some quotations from various industry authorities about associated health concerns.

Modern home

Note - Effects of exposures noted are dependent on the amount and length of toxic exposure, person's size, age and condition.

Acetone – paint remover, nail polish remover, detergents and cleaning products, by-product of cigarette smoke.

'Mount Sinai Medical Library of Medicine states that breathing high levels of acetone can lead to intoxication, headaches, fatigue, stupor, light headedness, dizziness, confusion, increased pulse rate, nausea, vomiting, and shortening of the menstrual cycle in women. Furthermore, it might cause nose, throat, lung, and eye irritation.' (Mount Sinai – Acetone Fact Sheet)

Ammonia – synthetic fibres, pesticides, some foods and drinks, cleaning products – glass and oven cleaners, fertilisers.

'Children with asthma are especially sensitive to ammonia. According to the Asthma and Allergy Foundation of America, irritants – like ammonia fumes – can aggravate inflamed and sensitive airways. When ammonia fumes are inhaled, the airway is constricted, and the lungs have difficulty moving air in and out.' (Mount Sinai – Ammonia Fact Sheet)

Benzene – plastics, resins, styrene, nylon, dyes, adhesives, coatings, paints, detergents, pesticides, cigarette smoke, vehicle emissions.

'Brief exposure (5-10 minutes) to very high levels of benzene in air (10,000-20,000 ppm) ... can cause: Affects to the central nervous system, rapid breathing and heart rate, dizziness, tremors, sleepiness to more serious symptoms.' (Mount Sinai – Benzene Fact Sheet)

Bisphenol A – plastics used for bottles, containers, tin linings, toys, personal care products, wallpapers, decals, stationery.

'In children, scientists have found an association between phthalates and changes in reproductive hormones and increased allergies, runny nose, and eczema.'
(Pediatric Environmental Health Specialty Units, 2008)

Carbon Monoxide – product of incomplete burning of gas – exposures from space heaters, gas cooktop, fireplaces and cigarette smoke.

'When a child breathes carbon monoxide it can harm the blood's ability to transport oxygen. Exposure to high concentrations can cause, headache, dizziness, vomiting, confusion and trigger asthma. This can damage major organs and lead to death if exposure is severe.' (Mount Sinai – Carbon Monoxide Fact Sheet)

Chlorine - drinking water, swimming pools, disinfectants, cleaning products.

'Some people may develop an inflammatory reaction to chlorine called reactive airways dysfunction syndrome, a type of asthma.' (Tox Town, PERC, 2014)

'Chlorine reactions may include itchy, red skin or hives (itchy bumps). This is not an allergy but is actually 'irritant dermatitis' (like a chemical burn), caused by hypersensitivity to this natural irritant. Chlorine is also drying to the skin and can irritate existing dermatitis.

'Chlorine may indirectly contribute to allergies by irritating and sensitising the respiratory tract. Studies have suggested that frequent swimming in chlorinated pools and exposure to cleaning products containing chlorine may increase the risk of developing asthma and other respiratory allergies, both in adolescents and in adults.' (American College of Allergy, Asthma & Immunology, 2014)

Endocrine disruptors – plastics (flooring, window coverings, wallpapers), resins, detergents, insecticides, herbicides, fumigants, adhesives.

'Many chemicals are known to act as endocrine disruptors.

'Endocrine disruptors have been suspected of contributing to a range of adverse health effects in humans, including reproductive and developmental disorders, learning problems, and immune system dysfunction. Several recent trends in human health may be related to endocrine disruptors in the environment: widespread occurrence of neurobehavioral dysfunction at birth and in childhood; an increasing incidence of testicular cancer in young men; an increasing incidence of congenital malformations of the male reproductive tract; the increasing incidence of breast cancer; and declining sperm counts.' (Mount Sinai – Endocrine Disruptors Fact Sheet)

Formaldehyde – composite board products – mdf, ply, particle board, flooring, adhesives, carpet cleaner, paper, plastics, fabric softener, dish-washing liquid.

'…Exposure to children can occur, especially in rooms with manufactured wood furnishings and plastics…

'The fabric finish that provides a permanent press quality to new fabrics can be source of formaldehyde poisoning. They [children] can absorb it through their skin from touching treated clothing or bedding for extended periods of time, but formaldehyde levels on the fabrics significantly decrease with each wash.

Exposure to low levels of formaldehyde can irritate and burn the eyes, nose, throat, and skin. In women, exposure can cause menstrual disorders. Some people are more sensitive to the effects of formaldehyde than others. The most common symptoms include irritation of the eyes, nose, and throat, along with increased tearing…' (Mount Sinai – Formaldehyde Fact Sheet)

Lead – old paintwork, old ceramic items, imported painted items, window blinds, cosmetics, crystal.

'Children with blood lead levels above 20 μg/dL may exhibit gastrointestinal related symptoms. This includes poor appetite, nausea, vomiting, abdominal pain and constipation. These children may have difficulty with learning and school performance, in addition to behavioral problems such as hyperactivity. Children may develop anaemia and may also have problems with growth. Severe lead poisoning, with blood lead levels above 60 μg/dL, may be associated with neurological symptoms such as changes in mental status, difficulty walking, seizures and coma.' (Mount Sinai – Lead Fact Sheet)

Mould – derived from moisture

'Exposure to mold can cause allergies, trigger asthma attacks, detrimentally affect the function of vital human organs and increase susceptibility to colds and flu. Common symptoms include congestion, runny nose, coughing, and irritated eyes; new or worsening asthma; flu symptoms; headaches and, fatigue.

'All molds, dead or alive, can provoke allergic reactions in sensitive individuals'

'Children may be at particularly at risk in mold exposure. A study in 2004 found that mold exposure in infants and young children can lead to the development of asthma.' (Mount Sinai – Mold Fact Sheet)

Particulate Matter (Dust) – microscopic airborne particles found indoors and outdoors, dust, smoke and fumes.

'Acute exposure to particulate matter may irritate the eyes, ears, nose, throat and lungs. Respiratory symptoms such as coughing, wheezing and shortness of breath may be seen as well. The symptoms vary from person to person and depend on the particular components of the pollutants.' (Mount Sinai – Particulate Matter Fact Sheet)

Perchloroethylene (PERC) – dry cleaning, scouring agent in textiles, aerosol products, printing inks, adhesives, sealants, paint removers, leather treatments, polishes and silicones, spot removers, shoe polish.

'Perchloroethylene is listed as 'reasonably anticipated to be a human carcinogen' in the Twelfth Report on Carcinogens published by the National Toxicology Program because long-term exposure to perchloroethylene can cause leukemia and cancer of the skin, colon, lung, larynx, bladder, and urogenital tract. ...Short-term exposure to low levels of perchloroethylene can cause dizziness, inebriation, sleepiness, and irritated eyes, nose, mouth, throat, and respiratory tract.' (Tox Town – PERC)

Perfluorooctanoic Acid (PFOA) – non-stick products, products designed to repel soil, grease and water, carpet, furniture, food wraps, sprays for leather, paints, clothing, cookware and cleaning products.

'A draught EPA Science Advisory Board report issued in 2005 found that PFOA was a likely human carcinogen.' (Natural Resources Defense Council, USA, 2011)

Pesticides – insecticides, fungicides, herbicides.

'Although specifically designed to kill insects, unwanted plants, and fungi, many pesticides are also highly toxic to the environment, to humans, and particularly to children. Because the chemistry of pesticides is highly diverse, they are capable of causing a wide range of adverse health effects. The effect of these chemicals, depending on the specific pesticide or combination of pesticides an individual or population is exposed to, can involve virtually every organ system in the body. Pesticides have been shown to cause a wide range of adverse effects on human health including acute and chronic injury to the nervous system, lung damage, injury to the reproductive organs, dysfunction of the immune and endocrine systems, birth defects, and cancer; these effects can manifest as acutely toxic effects, delayed effects, or chronic effects.' (Mount Sinai – Pesticides Fact Sheet)

Phthalates – polyvinyl products (PVC) such as flooring, wallpapers, decals, flexible plastics – furniture, toys, clothing, food storage containers, flexible plastic pipe, plasticised films, personal care products, stationery, fragrances.

'Many doctors and scientists are concerned about phthalates because they can act in ways similar to hormones naturally found in our body. Hormones help control how our body works. Most of the health information we know about these chemicals comes from animal studies.' (Mount Sinai – Phthalates Fact Sheet)

'People are exposed to phthalates by eating and drinking foods that have been in contact with containers and products containing phthalates. To a lesser extent exposure can occur from breathing in air that contains phthalate vapours or dust contaminated with phthalate particles. Young children may have a greater risk of being exposed to phthalate particles in dust than adults because of their hand-to-mouth behaviors.' (CDC, 2013)

'Human and animal studies have found links to birth defects, decreased sperm counts and

damaged sperm, increased risk of developing behavioural problems, premature birth, and respiratory difficulties in children with bronchial obstruction (such as asthma).' (Healthy Child, 2013)

Polychlorinated Biphenyls (PCBs) – plasticisers, paints, fluorescent lighting, electrical appliances, lubricants in electrical equipment (Australia banned PCBs in 1975 – a persistent organic pollutant), though it is still found in items made prior to the ban.

'PCBs are considered a toxic persistent organic pollutant (POP) that can be found in the environment and animals, 'bio accumulative through the food chain and pose a risk of causing adverse effects to human health and the environment. They are listed under the Stockholm Convention on Persistent Organic Pollutants (POP) for phasing out and eventual elimination.' (NIP, 2013)

'When building materials get old, they break apart and produce contaminated dust. These materials can also slowly emit low levels of PCBs into the air. In most cases, the health risk from intact building materials is very small; therefore there is no need to remove PCB containing materials if they are intact. However, these materials must be removed if they begin to deteriorate. ... The EPA has determined that PCBs are probably cancer causing.' (Mount Sinai – PCBs Fact Sheet)

'PCBs have been demonstrated to cause cancer, as well as a variety of other adverse health effects on the immune system, reproductive system, nervous system, and endocrine system.' (USA EPA, 2013)

PCB may still be found in products produced prior to the ban such as fibreglass thermal insulation material, felt, foams, cork, oil based paint, plastics, electrical equipment, floor finishes, caulking and adhesives.

Brominated flame retardants- BFRs (including Polybrominated Diphenyl Ethers -PBDEs) – insulation, electronics (computers, televisions), textiles, plastics, foams, furniture, window coverings, polyurethane materials, carpet, mattresses, cars

'Approximately 80 different types of brominated flame retardant are used commercially. The more widely used are the polybrominated diphenyl ethers (PBDEs). Polybrominated diphenyl ethers are a very common class of BFRs, and have attracted the most attention to date because of their potential to persist in the environment.

'Globally, the general trend in humans has been one of increasing PBDE levels in blood and breast milk samples.

'Studies have shown that people are mainly exposed to PBDEs through exposure to indoor dust at home and in the workplace. This is assumed to be due to the levels of PBDEs in products such as furniture and electronic equipment. Food is thought to be a minor exposure route, although this is still the subject of ongoing research.' (Australian Department of Environment Fact sheet, PBDE Fact Sheet, undated)

'PBDEs are not chemically bound to plastics, foam, fabrics, or other products in which they are used, making them more likely to leach out of these products.' (USA EPA, 2014)

According to the Pediatric Environmental Health Specialty Unit at Mount Sinai Hospital there are significant concerns about the effects of PBDEs on the developing nervous system, based on animal studies.

Some flame retardants are currently being reviewed due to concerns about their potential bio accumulative, environmentally persistent and endocrine disruptive properties.

Solvents – paints and coatings, glue, pesticides, resins, dry cleaning, cleaning products, nail polish.

'You can be exposed to solvents by breathing them, absorbing them through your skin, or swallowing them.

'Regular exposure to solvents can cause memory and hearing loss, mental illness, depression, fatigue, confusion, dizziness, feeling drunk or 'high,' lack of coordination, headache, nausea, stomach pains, skin rashes, cracking or bleeding skin, and irritated eyes, nose, and throat. Exposure to solvent vapours can cause hoarseness, coughing, lung congestion, chest tightness, and shortness of breath. If children are exposed to high levels of solvents at home, they may suffer from asthma.' (Tox Town, PERC 2013)

Toluene (used as a solvent) – paints, paint thinner, dyes, detergents, lacquers, rubber, spot remover products, leather.

'Because toluene is a common solvent and is found in many consumer products, you can be exposed to toluene at home and outdoors while using gasoline, nail polish, cosmetics, rubber cement, paints, paintbrush cleaners, stain removers, fabric dyes, inks, adhesives, carburettor cleaners, and lacquer thinners.

'A serious health concern is that toluene may have an effect on your brain. Toluene can cause headaches and sleepiness, and can impair your ability to think clearly. Whether or not toluene does this to you depends on the amount you take in, how long you are exposed, and your genetic susceptibility and age… The effects of toluene on children have not been studied very much, but toluene is likely to produce the same types of effects on the brain and nervous system in children as it does in adults.' (The Agency for Toxic Substances and Disease Registry, USA, 2000)

Volatile organic compounds (VOCs) – Indoor air from paints and coatings, flooring, cabinets, furniture, personal care products, cooking, personal care products, fragrances, pesticides, cleaners, cigarette smoke, dry-cleaned clothes, window coverings.

'Health effects from VOCs are usually temporary and improve once the source of the exposure is identified and removed. These health effects can include irritation of the eyes, nose, throat and skin. Headache, nausea and dizziness may occur, as well as fatigue and shortness of breath. Health effects vary depending on the chemicals involved and the duration of the exposure. Formaldehyde and pesticides are considered probable carcinogens.' (Mount Sinai Hospital – VOC Fact Sheet)

VOCs include a variety of chemicals, some of which may have short- and long-term adverse health effects. Concentrations of many VOCs are consistently higher indoors (up to ten times higher) than outdoors. VOCs are emitted by a wide array of products numbering in the thousands.

'Eye, nose, and throat irritation; headaches, loss of coordination, nausea; damage to liver, kidney, and central nervous system. Some organics can cause cancer in animals; some are suspected or known to cause cancer in humans. Key signs or symptoms associated with exposure to VOCs include conjunctival irritation, nose and throat discomfort, headache, allergic skin reaction, dyspnoea, declines in serum cholinesterase levels, nausea, emesis, epistaxis, fatigue, dizziness.

'The ability of organic chemicals to cause health effects varies greatly from those that are *highly toxic, to those with no known health effect. As with other pollutants, the extent and nature of the health effect will depend on many factors including level of exposure and length of time exposed.'* (USA EPA, 2012)

Triclosan – kitchenware, furniture, toys, bedding, clothing, toothpaste, cosmetics, soaps, pesticides, plastics, caulking compounds, sealants, rubber, carpet, textiles, polyethylene, polyurethane, polypropylene, paints, cleaning products, household dust, food boards.

Triclosan is a suspected endocrine disrupter.

'The antibacterial compound triclosan has been linked to numerous human health problems. Exposures come mainly by absorption through the skin or through the lining of the mouth. These exposures have resulted in contact dermatitis, or skin irritation, and an increase in allergic reactions, especially in children... Recent studies have also found that triclosan interferes with the body's thyroid hormone metabolism and may be a potential endocrine disruptor. Children exposed to antibacterial compounds at an early age also have an increased chance of developing allergies, asthma and eczema.' (Beyond Pesticides, 2014)

We cannot avoid all pollutants as we go about our day, however now you have this book you are well on your way to being an informed consumer. In the following sections we explore tips and resources that will help you make informed decisions in and around the home to minimise your exposure to toxic pollutants.

Read the following fact sheets listed in the resources section below to learn more about the pollutants listed above and their association with disease.

Further information

Mount Sinai Children's Environmental Health Center Fact Sheets:
www.mountsinai.org/patient-care/service-areas/children/areas-of-care/childrens-environmental-health-center/childrens-disease-and-the-environment/environmental-toxins

Fact Sheets:

- Acetone
- Ammonia
- Asbestos
- Benzene
- Bisphenol-A
- Carbon Monoxide
- Chlorine
- Endocrine Disruptors (BPA & Phthalates)
- Tobacco Smoke
- Flame Retardants (PBDEs or BFRs)
- Formaldehyde
- Lead
- Mercury
- Mould
- Particulate Matter (dust)
- Perchloroethylene
- Perfluorooctanoic Acid (PFOA)
- Pesticides
- Phthalates
- Polychlorinated Biphenyls (PCBs)
- Radon
- Solvents
- Toluene
- Volatile Organic Compounds (VOCs)

TOXNET - United States National Library of Medicine www.toxnet.nlm.nih.gov
Tox Town - United States National Library of Medicine toxtown.nlm.nih.gov
Agency for Toxic Substances & Disease Registry www.atsdr.cdc.gov
National Industrial Chemicals Notification and Assessment Scheme www.nicnas.gov.au
Safer Chemicals, Healthy Families www.saferchemicals.org

5 step approach to creating a healthy, sustainable home

BUILD/
RENOVATE

PRODUCTS &
FURNISHINGS

CONSUMER
CHOICE

LIFESTYLE
PRACTICES

MAINTAIN

Where we live, what we build with, what we use to decorate, our daily lifestyle practices, products we buy and how we maintain our home, all contribute to a home's overall health and efficiency.

As highlighted earlier, money makes the world go around – and we all have varying quantities of it, which impacts greatly on what we can or cannot do within our own home.

The following information is an overview of things to consider at different stages of homemaking. For most of us it is not possible to do it all or to have all the latest and best products, however there are many significant things you can do on a budget that contribute to a healthier home. It is not feasible or practical that we strive for perfection when creating a healthy, sustainable home. Given the complexities of buildings and people's lifestyles there is no 'one size fits all' solution for many of the issues explored in these chapters.

However, you will see demonstrated in many instances over the following pages that healthy and sustainable options around the home can save you money and that the ethos of healthy living values many of the simple things in life.

Learning about the types of pollutants in the home and their potential impacts on health can be overwhelming. It is important to understand that 'knowledge is power'. The following information is shared so that you can make small individual choices throughout your home that will culminate over time to significant reductions in pollutants and increased cost savings.

Step 1
Build it/renovate

What makes an energy efficient, sustainable, healthy building?

Answer: A structure that is designed, built, renovated, operated and reused in an ecological and resource efficient manner using products that do not compromise human health.

These days our homes need to cater for more than just keeping out the weather. With changing climates bringing extreme heat, health issues on the rise and the ever-increasing cost of resources (energy and water), our home is our sanctuary. With careful planning it can provide extremely comfortable shelter, contain interiors that promote health and wellbeing, while being highly resource efficient.

Green building does not have a 'one size fits all' solution. It's a carefully crafted consolidation of orientation, design, function, materials, appliances, landscaping and personal choices that works with local climate and caters for household needs.

It's worth knowing that up to 80 percent of a building's efficiency can be traced back to the design. If you get the design and orientation right, you're well on the way to an efficient, sustainable home.

However, before embarking on a home design, you need to understand your local climate. Knowing your climate enables you to create a home that works with, rather than against, the local climate for maximum efficiency (often referred to as 'passive solar design').

Finally, keep in mind that a house should work as a complete system which has a number of relations and interactions between the local climate, design, materials chosen, how it's constructed and how the occupants use it. The system needs to be crafted to work together to obtain maximum comfort and efficiency, while providing a healthy environment for those living within it.

TIP The NCC is updated annually. Be sure your builder is familiar with the latest requirements of the NCC, Volume 2, particularly in relation to Health and Amenity (Part 3.8) and Energy Efficiency (Part 3.12).

The following pages highlight a range of design considerations that are critical to achieving efficient, passive design. This section is not meant to be a comprehensive structural reference for sustainable design, it is an overview of comparable information and issues that significantly contribute to the operating costs of a home and the minimisation of pollutants within the interior.

The following topics are discussed:
- Site selection
- Know your climate
- Where the wind blows
- Design principles:
  - Passive Solar Design
  - Passive House
- Orientation
- Foundation considerations to minimise pollutants
- Passive heating and cooling
- Insulation and draught-proofing
- Condensation
- Windows and glazing
- Water
- Tips for a sustainable, healthy wet zone design
- Tips for a sustainable, healthy kitchen design
- Site health tips

For those new to the field of sustainable housing, a glossary of terms is available towards the back of the book.

General mantra for creating healthy, sustainable, efficient homes:

Choose materials that:
- Are sustainably sourced
- Are locally produced where possible
- Minimise VOCs (volatile organic compounds)
- Contain recycled products
- Are recyclable at end of life
- Have high quality and durable attributes
- Have minimal toxic chemical ingredients

And choose building methods that:
- Work with the local climate
- Optimise passive heating and cooling
- Minimise VOCs
- Minimise land disruption

Site considerations

Site selection overview

When choosing a site on which to build your new home there is a lot to consider. The lifestyle you are looking for will affect the amenities you will need nearby. Additionally, the time you intend to stay in the home will determine what changes may be required as you age, which impact on the future adaptability of the home.

The table below provides a guide to help clarify your requirements so you know what's important to you.

What	Considerations
Location Does it meet your needs?	• Is it near potential hazardous areas (mining, high voltage power lines, manufacturing or industry emissions and pollutants) • Is it prone to fire, flooding, or other risks? • Is it close to amenities you use regularly? • Is there public transport nearby? • Is it within walking distance to things you use most? • Are there any neighbouring sites that need to be considered (if so in what way)?
Orientation Does the site facilitate passive solar design?	• If in a climate that requires heating, does it provide good northerly access for solar gains? • If in a climate that needs lots of cooling, does it provide good access to cooling breezes? • If both heating and cooling is needed, can the site facilitate access to both sun and cooling breezes?
Size Appropriate for needs	• Is the land the right size for your needs? Too big and it becomes a maintenance issue, too small and you may not get that veggie patch you wanted • Do you need to allow for future expansion of the home? If so does it allow for it?
Site Suitable structure	• Is it on good soil for planting and food production? • Can building design be facilitated to minimise disruption to land and work with natural slopes? • If on a slope, is it susceptible to landslides or will this cause accessibility issues in later life? • Can you preserve any natural features? • What services are available (electricity, water, sewerage, data)

Table source © Green Moves Australia, 2014.

Know your climate

One of the most important things to understand is how your climate can be used to heat and/or cool the home. The Building Code of Australia defines eight primary climate zones, noted in the pages following.

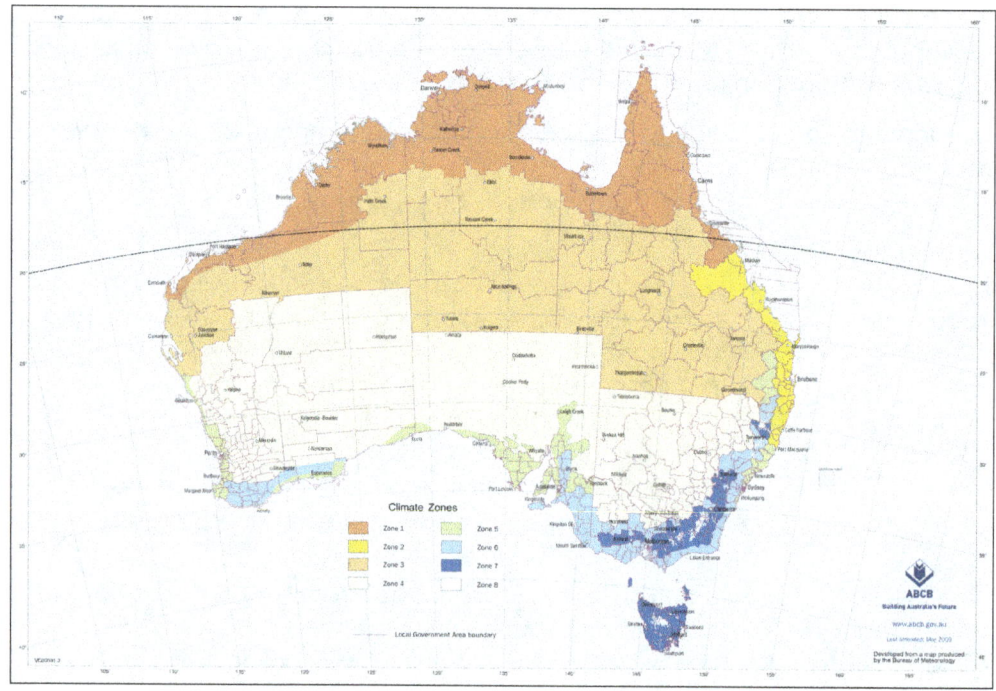

Image sourced from the Australian Building Codes Board (ABCB) www.abcb.gov.au

Zone 1 – Hot humid summer with warm winters

Primarily found along the northern coast of Australia including WA, NT and QLD

This climate is often referred to as 'tropical', with high humidity (wet season) and dry periods (dry season). Temperatures are moderate to high all year round and there is generally a low temperature variation between day and night.

Homes built in this zone should be constructed of lightweight, light coloured materials and be built to withstand tropical cyclones. They should be designed to maximise cooling breezes and cross-ventilation, provide building shading to all walls and windows, have ceiling fans in all living spaces and ideally be elevated for maximum air flow. Windows should be able to be fully opened; louvers are the most effective.

Light coloured buildings and roofs will help to reduce heat build-up.

This zone has excellent solar access. Use of solar hot water and solar PV systems is encouraged.

Zone 2 – Warm humid summer with mild winter

Primarily coastal areas of QLD and northern NSW.

This type of climate has high humidity in summer and has a definite 'dry season' during winter. Winters are generally mild while the summer is humid and hot to very hot.

Temperatures can vary significantly between coastal and inland regions and this area has moderate to low temperature variations between day and night.

Homes built in this zone should be lightweight and light-coloured and would not require heating. They should be designed to maximise cross ventilation, enable cooling breezes into the home and be well shaded (including outdoor living areas). Windows and walls, particularly west and east facing, should be permanently shaded.

Zone 3 – Hot dry summer with warm winter

Primarily central and northern Australia, including parts of WA, NT and QLD.

This climate zone has distinct wet and dry seasons with low rainfall and low-to-moderate humidity. It can be cool in winter and hot summers are common. There is generally a large variation between night and day temperatures.

Buildings in this zone should take advantage of north facing living spaces, include high levels of bulk and reflective insulation (walls and ceiling), with good thermal mass in the living area to take advantage of passive solar heating access. Ensure there is good cross-ventilation to bring in the cooling breezes and facilitate purging of hot air at night.

Compact floor plans and use of stack ventilation techniques are highly beneficial in this zone. Ceiling fans and well shaded walls and glazing will help to keep the home cool during the day. Ensure any shading on the north side is removable to take advantage of passive heating opportunities when needed. Light-coloured roof material and a construction type with high levels of thermal mass is beneficial.

Zone 4 – Hot dry summer with cool winter

Primarily the central inland areas of WA, SA, NSW and parts of Victoria.

This climate zone has distinct seasons with low humidity and low rainfall all year. Summers can be very hot and often come with hot dry winds. Winters are cool with very cold dry winds.

Homes in this zone should contain high levels of insulation and include thermal mass incorporated within a north facing living area to take best advantage of passive solar heating. Allow for cross ventilation and night purging of hot air, orientate openings to capture cooling breezes. Stack ventilation or solar chimneys would be beneficial in this zone. Aim for good ventilation in summer months and a well-sealed home in winter months.

Light coloured roofing material used with a structure containing high thermal mass and earth coupled slab would work well in this area. Insulation should contain bulk and reflective types in ceilings and walls. Double-glaze all windows and doors, ensuring frames are thermally efficient. Adjustable shading will allow the most flexible control of passive heating and cooling options.

Zone 5 – Warm temperate

Primarily along the southern coast of Australia including parts of WA, SA, and parts of southern QLD.

This zone has four distinct seasons, with summer and winter temperatures becoming more extreme. Winters are generally mild with low humidity, but summers can be hot to very hot. Day and night temperature range varies from moderate around coastal locations, to high further inland. Solar access and wind directions are highly variable creating a diverse range of conditions.

In this zone good simple designs can achieve high efficiencies that can minimise heating and cooling costs. Design should optimise passive heating and cooling opportunities and ensure cooling breezes can be directed through the home. Include ceiling fans in key areas (living areas and bedrooms).

Adjustable shading to the north, east and west, and glazing, provides for maximum flexibility and solar control. Insulation should consist of bulk and reflective types in both ceiling and walls. Insulate floors that are elevated and ensure the home is well sealed.

Light coloured roofing materials combined with composite thermal mass construction and earth coupled slabs are highly beneficial.

Zone 6 – Mild temperate

Primarily along the southern areas of WA, SA, Victoria and NSW.

This zone has four distinct seasons, with summer and winter temperatures becoming more extreme. Winters are generally mild to cool with low humidity, but summers can be hot to very hot. Day and night temperature range varies from low around coastal locations, to high further inland.

Very similar to Zone 5, homes in Zone 6 can achieve high efficiencies through good simple design. Each site is likely to offer different challenges which may need some adjustment depending on primary need for either heating or cooling. Appropriate windows and glazing is a key design consideration, as is providing for good cross-flow ventilation and use of adjustable shading.

Design the home to optimise passive heating and cooling opportunities and ensure cooling breezes can be directed through the home. Include ceiling fans in most areas.

Adjustable shading to the northern, east and west glazing provides for maximum flexibility. Insulation should consist of bulk and reflective types in the ceiling and bulk or reflective in the walls. Insulate floors that are elevated and ensure the home is well sealed. Ideally include main entrance air locks when possible.

Light coloured roofing materials combined with composite thermal mass construction and earth coupled slabs are highly beneficial.

Zone 7 – Cool temperate

Primarily Tasmania, Victoria, NSW and ACT

This zone has four distinct seasons, with summer and winter temperatures becoming more extreme and highly variable spring and autumn temperature ranges. Winters are cold to very cold with high rainfall; summers are hot and can be very dry.

Homes in this zone benefit from passive solar heating so maximise use of north-facing walls and glazing. Double glazing throughout with thermally efficient frames (i.e. wood) is recommended. Design living areas to the north, bedrooms and service areas to the south. Allow for good cross ventilation. Avoid high ceilings and provide for closing off of upper and lower floors.

The home should be well insulated with bulk insulation in ceiling, walls and flooring. Include a breathable sarking in the walls to allow for moisture removal from external wall cavities, and install reflective insulation on the underside of the roof. Ensure any elevated floors and slab edges are also insulated and that the building is well sealed.

Light coloured roofing materials combined with low thermal mass or lightweight construction and insulated earth coupled slabs can be highly beneficial.

Zone 8 – Alpine

Primarily the higher areas of Tasmania, Victoria and NSW.

This zone has four distinct seasons, with winter becoming cold to very cold with good rainfall and snow in some areas. Summers are generally warm to hot and dry with variable spring and autumn temperature ranges. This area has low humidity and highly variable temperature ranges from day to night.

Homes in this zone should optimise any solar access that is available to obtain benefit from passive solar heating. Design the home to maximise use of north facing walls and glazing and to protect from cold winter winds. Double glazing with thermally efficient frames is highly recommended in all areas. Design for compact living spaces that allow sunlight into all rooms with doors that can be used to close off upper and lower floors, and other areas when not in use. Avoid high ceilings.

The home should be well insulated with bulk insulation in ceiling, walls and flooring. Use the highest-rated insulation in the ceiling, install reflective insulation on the underside of the roof and ensure the roof space is well sealed. Include a breathable sarking in the walls to allow for moisture removal from external wall cavities. Ensure any elevated floors and slab edges are also insulated and that the building envelope is well sealed.

Select dark coloured roofing materials combined with highly insulated low thermal mass and insulate under slabs or floors.

Referenced from *Your Home*, 2013.

Where the wind blows

One of the key methods for enabling passive cooling is to know where your cooling breezes are coming from. The Bureau of Meteorology has wind roses at various locations around Australia that can provide very useful information for your local area (or close by).

To find the prevailing wind directions for your area go to the Bureau of Meteorology website **www.bom.gov.au** and search for 'Wind Roses'. Wind rose information is available for selected locations around Australia and can help you to identify where the winds are coming from, and whether it is in the mornings or afternoons.

An example from the Bureau of Meteorology website of Melbourne's prevailing winds is below showing 9am and 3pm wind strength and direction:

Below: Melbourne winds – 9am – prevailing from the north.

Below: Melbourne winds – 3pm – prevailing from the south

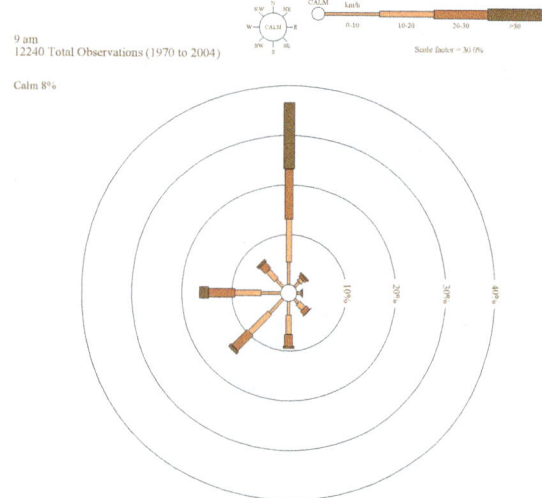
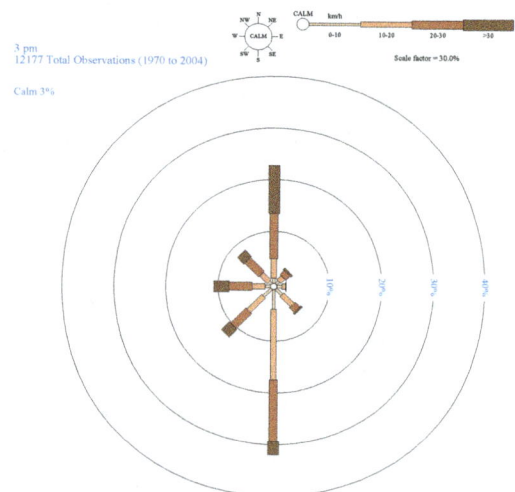

Image source: Australian Government, Bureau of Meteorology

To find your closest wind direction or for more information visit:

www.bom.gov.au/climate/averages/wind/selection_map.shtml

Further information

- Australian Building Codes Board (ABCB) website. www.abcb.gov.au
- Website of the Department of Industry. 2013. *Your Home: Australia's guide to Environmentally Sustainable Homes*. 5th edition. March 2014. www.yourhome.gov.au
- Bureau of Meteorology. Wind Roses for Selected Locations in Australia. www.bom.gov.au
- Passive design assistance for your climate, contact your local council, state or territory government. www.gov.au
- Nationwide House Energy Rating Scheme (NatHERS). www.nathers.gov.au

Design principles

Passive solar design is a methodology used to design buildings to use the local natural elements to assist with providing heating, cooling and natural light into a home. It enables the home to be more comfortable and use fewer resources in operation, leading to reduced operating costs. Maintaining a home's comfort and efficiency involves the right combination of design strategies to minimise energy, water, materials, waste and impact on land use. The local climate significantly impacts on how this can be achieved.

Local climate and aspects of passive solar design are now key considerations in meeting current (and future) national energy performance standards of a home.

There are two main methodologies for 'passive' homes. They are Passive Solar Design and Passive House. While both contain many of the same elements, there are differences.

Passive solar design

Passive design refers to a design approach that uses natural elements, such as sunlight and wind, to heat, cool, or bring light into a building. Incorporating passive solar design into our homes improves comfort, can significantly reduce heating and cooling requirements, minimises running costs and reduces greenhouse gas emissions.

A well designed passive building would require little, if any, mechanical heating or cooling to maintain internal comfort temperatures. In summer months the home would exclude the sun and maximise cooling air movement. In winter months the home would allow for good solar access, and the capture, store and reuse of heat energy.

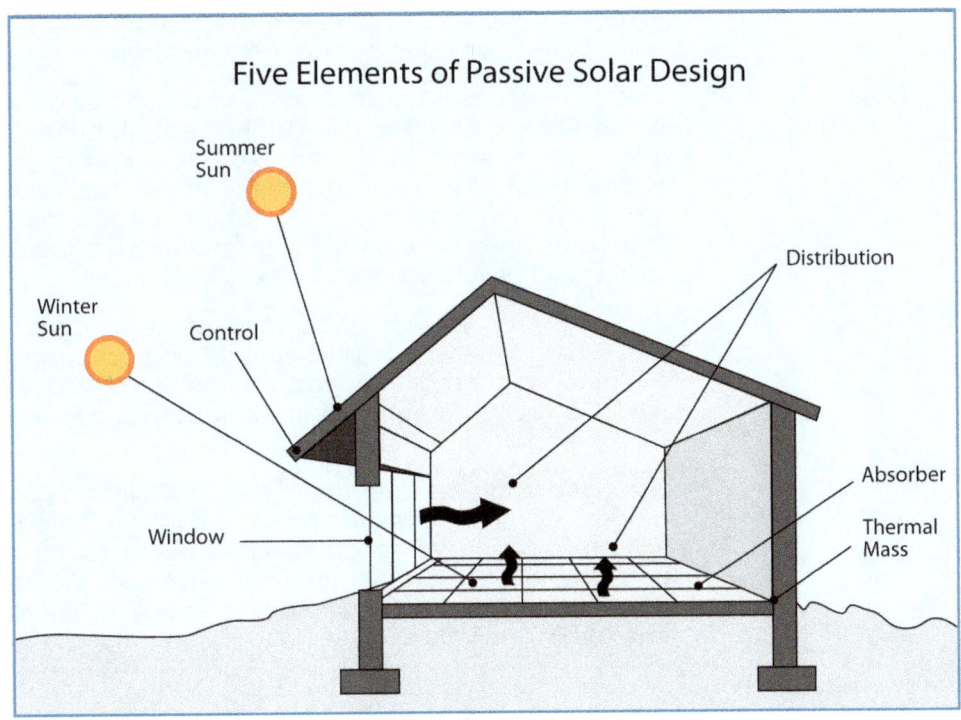

Image credit: Green Energy Times

The basic principles of passive design are relatively simple but must be considered in line with the local climatic conditions. Climate information is critical in designing for comfort and energy efficiency. The principles of passive solar design generally need to be incorporated into building design in order to meet the thermal performance requirements of the building code.

A combination of the following principles is applied according to climate.

Designing for local climate	Identify the local climate zone for the area and incorporate the relevant passive design responses for that climate.
Orientation	Maximises the benefit of any natural attributes of the site for comfort, economic and environmental benefit. Capturing breezes forces fresh air throughout a home, assisting with the removal of VOCs.
Passive heating	If applicable to the climate, passive heating allows the sun into the building during the day and stores the heat in a thermal mass structure for reuse later. This minimises the use of heating systems that blow air/dust around and helps to reduce operating costs.
Passive cooling	If applicable to the climate, passive cooling keeps the summer sun out of the building through shading and facilitates good air movement through cross ventilation. This contributes to comfort levels in the home and fresh air circulation assists with removal of VOCs.
Insulation	Essential component of good passive design. Provides protection against heat entering and leaving the building and assists with maintaining internal temperatures. Where low/no VOC insulation materials are used it can contribute to a healthier indoor environment.
Thermal Mass	This is a material's capacity to absorb, store and release heat (often called a heat sink). It helps to stabilise internal temperatures as part of a passive design. Examples of good thermal mass are concrete, solid bricks, dark slate and water. Materials with low toxicity attributes and low or no VOCs treatments are ideal for minimising pollutants around the home.
Glazing and windows	The weakest point in most buildings is the windows. Well placed windows with appropriate glazing contributes to maintaining internal temperatures and providing natural light. Good natural light promotes wellbeing and reduces reliance on other light sources.
Materials	Using materials appropriate to the local climate can have a significant effect on how the building performs. For example light materials release heat faster than heavier materials and are more suited to hot climates. Again, check treatments and opt for those with minimal chemicals and VOCs.

Table source © Green Moves Australia 2014.

Health aspects of passive solar design include maximising natural lighting, natural ventilation and natural temperature control. The materials and appliance choices in the home also have a significant role. Opting for non-toxic building materials/finishes and ensuring all exhaust fans vent externally can greatly assist in minimising pollutants in the home. Some 'whole of house' ventilation systems (such as noted below in Passive House), provide well filtered fresh air and can help improve indoor air quality.

Ensure any heating/cooling or ventilation system obtains its input air from the outside (fresh air). This is particularly important in a well-sealed building.

Passive house

The Passive House standard is based on the ideas of passive solar design, but takes it further by including superior air tight construction, higher levels of insulation, highly energy efficient windows and carefully controlled mechanical ventilation. It does not rely on the sun to heat thermal mass; instead it relies on the heat generated from the occupants in the building and the appliances (i.e. the fridge) that produce heat. Passive house is still a niche market in Australia, however interest in it is growing.

A passive house is a building where thermal comfort is provided through good design, and where heating or cooling of the fresh air flow (which is required for good indoor air quality) is provided without bringing recirculated air back into the building. In a passive house, no additional heating or cooling systems should be required because the ventilation system, which is also a heat recovery unit, provides all that is necessary.

Known as Passivhaus in Germany, where they are very popular, passive homes are built to a rigorous, voluntary building standard that is energy efficient and comfortable. It is a tried and true construction method that can be applied by anyone, anywhere.

In terms of healthy homes, a true passive house will assist to provide excellent indoor air quality by providing constant, filtered air to the indoor environment. It does this through a highly efficient, controlled mechanical ventilation system which continuously replaces the indoor air with filtered, fresh outdoor air.

This is an excellent system for balancing humidity, dust and allergens inside the home. Windows in these homes can be opened like any other window, however if anyone living in the home has severe allergies, the householder may choose to keep them closed to ensure all fresh air is filtered.

Passive houses allow for space heating and cooling related energy savings of up to 90 percent compared with typical building stock and over 75 percent compared to average new builds. Vast energy savings have been demonstrated in warm climates where typical buildings also require active cooling.

During warmer months, passive houses make use of passive cooling techniques such as strategic shading to keep comfortably cool. Passive houses make efficient use of the sun, internal heat sources and heat recovery, rendering conventional heating systems unnecessary throughout even the coldest of winters.

These homes can provide a high level of comfort. Internal surface temperatures vary little from indoor air temperatures, even in the face of extreme outdoor temperatures. Triple-glazed highly efficient windows and a well-sealed building envelope consisting of a highly insulated roof and floor slab as well as highly insulated exterior walls keep the desired warmth in the house, or undesirable heat out.

A ventilation system imperceptibly supplies constant fresh air, making for superior air quality without unpleasant draughts. A highly efficient heat recovery unit allows for the heat contained in the exhaust air to be re-used.

Further information

- Hollo, N. *Warm house, cool house – Inspirational designs for low-energy housing* (Choice, 2012)
- Wrigley, D. *Making your home sustainable: a guide to retrofitting* (Scribe, 2012)
- Passive House Institute **www.passive.de**
- Passive House Australia Institute – **www.passivehouseaustralia.org**

Design considerations – for sustainable lifestyle outcomes

Orientation considerations

Orientation is a key principle of passive designed homes. Orientating the home on the land to maximise solar access and cooling breezes provides for a variety of efficiencies, which can make the home more comfortable and cost efficient. Orientation works hand in hand with passive design to maximise performance of the home.

Consideration of roof design during this process can also provide for any solar systems that may be incorporated either during the build process or in the future.

As Australia is in the southern hemisphere the sun is predominantly to the north. During summer the sun is higher in the sky; in winter it is lower. This allows eaves and shading devices to be calculated and appropriately angled to cater for both seasons. Refer to the diagram on page 37.

In terms of building material costs and energy efficiency, the most ideal building shape is a simple rectangle. This shape is also cheaper to build (refer to the CSIRO report 'The Evaluation of the 5-Star Energy Efficiency Standard for Residential Buildings', December 2013) which states:

'The higher-rated houses cost at least $5000 less in Adelaide and Melbourne for those elements of the building related to energy efficiency than lower-rated houses, and up to $7000 less in Brisbane. Increases in the amount of insulation and an apparent shift to more rectangular house design were the most influential aspects observed in the shift to higher-rated houses.'

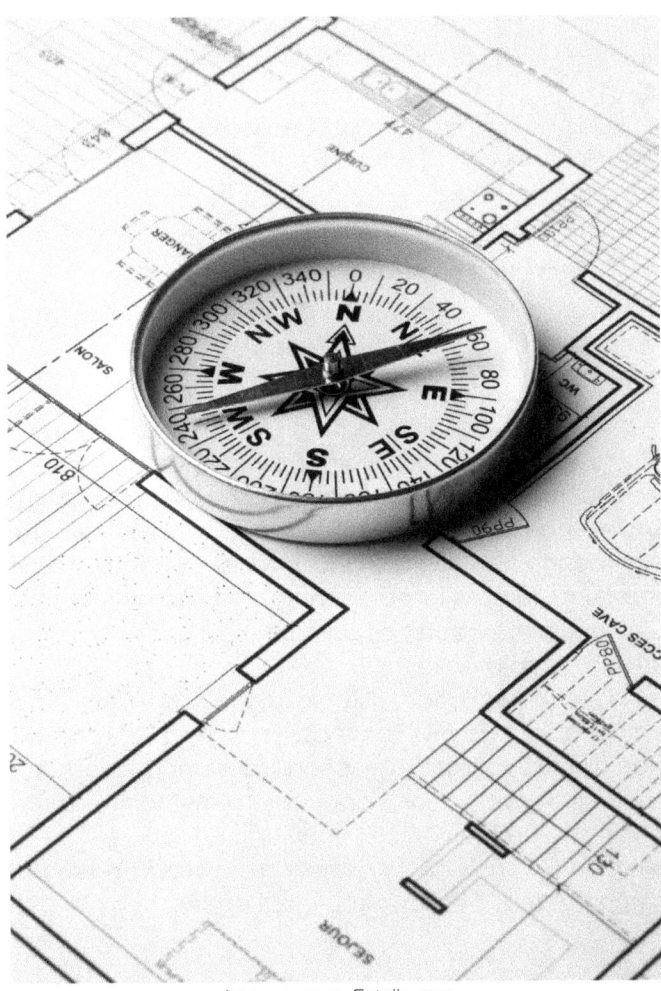

Image source: Fotolia.com

The idea is to take advantage of the sun's warmth in winter, and shield the home from the sun's heat in summer to help maintain comfort levels in the home. The best orientation for a home will depend on the location and local climate and should take into account prevailing winds and cooling breezes.

In climate zones that are hot and humid (such as Zone 1) the main focus should be on facilitating cross-ventilation and shading the home from the sun all year round. However in the cooler areas, such as zones 7 and 8, opportunities to maximise any available benefit from passive solar heating during winter should be included, along with consideration for facilitating cooling breezes through the home, and shading in summer.

To gain benefit from passive solar heating during winter months, design should have:

- Living rooms to the north (ensure adjustable shading is available for summer months)
- Bedrooms to the south and/or east
- Service areas to the east, south or west
- Garage and carports ideally to the west
- Maximised glazing to the northern living spaces
- Minimised glazing to south, east and west sides (unless needed to bring cooling breezes into the home)
- Use of thermal mass to maximise passive heating opportunities

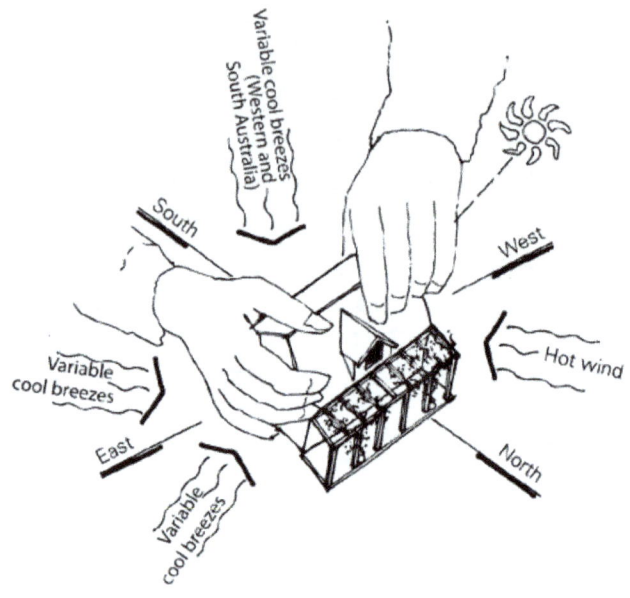

Image source: Your Home

To facilitate cross ventilation and passive cooling, check the local prevailing wind directions, focusing on the direction of cooling breezes, and:

- Ensure openable windows and/or doors are allocated to catch the cool breezes and direct it into the home (does not need to be a large opening). Casement windows and louvers provide for better ventilation than awning window types
- Design openable windows and/or doors on the alternate side to facilitate exit of the breeze (should be a large opening)
- Design internal layouts to facilitate 'straight through' path for breezes (ideally no obstructions to breeze flow)
- If using stack ventilation, use glazing (e.g. skylight, windows placed high in the building) to warm air at high points to create a draught and draw air through the home
- Shade all glazing from direct sunlight during summer months
- Use eaves or overhangs, especially to the north, east and west sides to reduce heat gain on the structure
- Use plants for shading, to protect from wind and to direct breeze flow when necessary (i.e. if the home does not have the ideal orientation)

TIP — Check the local climate and prevailing winds before design work starts so you can design accordingly. If renovating, there are ways to include these features. Careful planning with a good building designer, architect or sustainability consultant should find ways to make almost any home more comfortable and work more efficiently.

Remember to aim to place living areas to the north, optimise use of glazing and align roof lines to facilitate future inclusion of solar.

Foundation considerations to minimise pollutants

Solid structural foundations are essential for a durable, quality home. At the beginning of a project it is important to consider the longevity of the structure. A home is an expensive investment and although avoiding chemicals is a priority so too is keeping your home from being eaten out from under you. Where insecticides need to be used for termites (or other pests) at the foundation stage of building or renovating, opt for treatments that provide a physical barrier in a contained, concealed form rather than treatments such as sprays and powders that have the potential to be carried to different surfaces.

Refer to the Shop Wise – Pesticides in and around the Home section for further information on types of pesticides.

Fire protection consideration

Sustainable design and construction has come a long way over the past 10 years. Good design and smarter construction is bringing reduced carbon footprints, more efficient energy use, better natural light and ventilation, water recycling, harvesting of renewable energy supplies and reductions in equipment demands. All of these contribute towards more sustainable 'greener' homes and buildings.

What is often forgotten, however, is the importance of creating a home that is as safe as it can be from fire. Many building materials these days contain fire retardant chemicals (which are generally not good for human health) and which simply slows the burn rate. Smoke detectors which are a legal requirement as part of the NCC of Australia (Volume 2, Part 3.7 Fire Safety), are often poorly maintained and batteries often left to go flat without being replaced. When smoke detectors are maintained properly they do go some way to providing a degree of fire protection, but it could be better.

Ask anyone in the fire industry and you'll find most deaths occur in residential fires. The reason is that homes don't have to have the same level of fire protection we see in commercial buildings and multi-unit residential apartments. The difference is regular smoke alarm maintenance, sprinkler systems and fire extinguishers.

Ensuring suitable fire protection is designed into a building means that traditional objectives as well as progressive sustainable design concepts can be met. Protecting a home from fire through the inclusion of fire detection and suppression systems and extinguishing equipment helps the property, its occupants and the building to survive much better in the event of a fire.

Current and emerging fire protection technologies can assist by reducing the environmental, economic and social cost of fire. Fire protection systems support sustainable properties by ensuring the design and construction includes effective fire prevention and control. These can significantly reduce the environmental impact of fire through repair and re-building, pollution from combustion and the costs associated with the major disruption of losing a home to fire.

Maintained smoke alarms are only part of the picture. The inclusion of sprinkler systems (which can be flush to the ceiling and hardly noticeable) and fire extinguishers around a home could not only prevent significant loss of property, it could save a life if included in the initial design and build process.

There are also new requirements in the NCC for homes that are in bushfire prone areas. The new Bushfire Attack Level (BAL) standard 3959-2009 now includes evaporative coolers (covered in more detail later). This standard requires that evaporative cooler units are fitted with 'non-combustible covers' or butterfly covers at (or near) ceiling level, designed to stop the entry of fire embers during bushfire attacks.

There have been cases where houses have burned down during bush fires because embers have been sucked into the house due to large pressure differences. Properly sealing the building envelope (and closing off evaporative cooler vents) also creates an additional level of fire protection.

Refer to the NCC of Australia (Volume 2 Part 3.7) and the Fire Protection Association of Australia at **www.fpaa.com.au** for further information.

Passive heating and cooling

Designing for passive heating and cooling can be achieved using a broad range of construction systems incorporated into a home (or plan) through correct orientation, good solar and cooling breeze access and design considerations addressed at the project design phase.

Heating and cooling a home passively (without use of mechanical systems) is about keeping the home at a comfortable temperature in the least expensive manner. How this is achieved will depend on the local climate. For example if you are in Zone 1, the tropical zone, the focus will be on cooling the home. If you are in Zone 8, alpine zone, the focus will be on keeping the home warm.

Essentially, passive heating or cooling is achieved by letting the sun into the home during winter, and keeping it out in summer. This image shows the average amount of solar radiation on a vertical surface during summer and winter seasons. It's easy to see that during winter months the majority of the sun is from

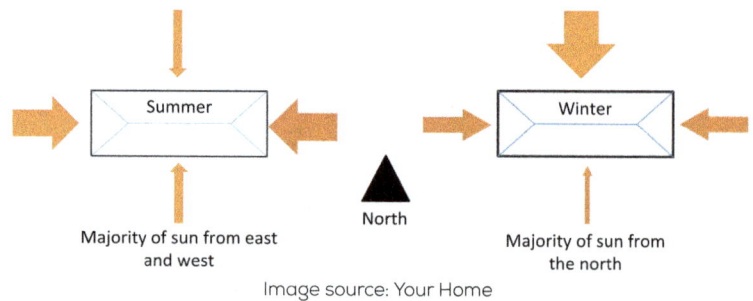

Image source: Your Home

the north, during summer it's on the east and west sides. Homes can be designed to use the winter sun and exclude or minimise the effects of the summer sun.

Refer to the image in the overview Five Elements of Passive Solar Design in the Design Principles section to see a cross section of solar radiation entering the home (winter sun), and being shaded from entering (summer sun).

Thermal mass

Thermal mass is a term used in passive building design that describes how the 'mass' of a construction material can be used to store heat (thermal energy). It is generally used to help stabilise internal temperatures and can work for, or against a building, depending on the local climate and how and where it is included.

The use of thermal mass to assist with passive heating and cooling usually requires consideration at the design phase of a project as thermal mass is difficult to retrofit later.

The diagram below demonstrates how a thermal mass can stabilise internal temperatures.

Image credit: New4Old, Guidelines for Building Designers

Thermal mass is the ability of a material to absorb and release heat energy. Where a lot of energy is needed to change the temperature of a material it is considered to have a high thermal mass. Building material examples include concrete, bricks, natural stone, insulated concrete fibre sheeting and tiles. Lightweight materials such as timber and insulation have a low thermal mass.

Materials that are ideal to use as a thermal mass are those that have a high specific heat capacity and high density. The following table is an extract from the Your Home manual and shows the thermal mass performance of common materials (the higher the number, the higher the thermal storage capacity).

Thermal mass for various materials	
Material	Thermal mass (volumetric heat capacity, KJ/m3.k)
Water	4186
Conctrete	2060
Sandstone	1800
Compressed earth blocks	1740
Rammed earth	1673
Fibre cement sheet (compressed)	1530
Brick	1360
Earth wall (adobe)	1300
Austoclaved aerated concrete	550

Source: Baggs and Mortensen 2006. Image source: Your Home

Objects with high thermal mass are good at absorbing, storing and re-releasing the stored heat back into the room when the ambient temperature drops.

Phase change materials

Newer products such as phase change materials offer an alternative way to include thermal mass heat storage capacity without adding significant additional weight to the structure. Phase change materials do not store heat or coolness; they change their state depending on the temperature from a solid to liquid and vice versa, in the process of which they either absorb or release heat.

The phase change point depends on the type of material used. If this temperature is too low, the heat storage capacity is exhausted too early; if it is high, it starts too late and the influence is small.

Temperatures at which the 'phase change' occurs differs significantly so be sure to obtain professional advice on the type, use and location of these materials before installing them.

For more information on passive heating and cooling refer to the Heating and Cooling section in the Products and Furnishings chapter.

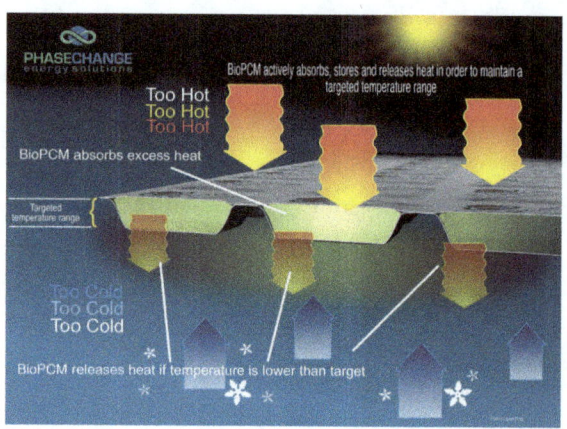

Image credit: Phase Change Energy Solutions

Insulation and draught-proofing

When trying to maintain a comfortable indoor temperature it comes down to good design, good building envelope and good practices. The building envelope is a key consideration and needs both thermal and vapour barriers. The thermal barrier (created by good insulation) provides protection from temperature differences. The vapour or air barrier, is facilitated by good draught-proofing, which reduces the flow of air between the inside and outside. The NCC of Australia (Part 3.12) states the minimum insulation requirements for each climate zone and draught-proofing requirements. Note that stated minimum insulation levels may need to be increased to meet the minimum thermal performance standard levels (i.e. 6 star energy efficiency rating) of your particular design.

Insulation offers the best value for money in relation to maintaining internal comfort. In short, it helps to keep your home at a comfortable temperature, helps to reduce heating and cooling costs and can contribute to a healthy home if non-toxic product options are chosen. Without good insulation and draught-proofing a home can lose and gain heat very quickly.

What's a building envelope? It is the external walls, floors and ceiling of a building, which separate the inside and outside environments. The building envelope includes a thermal barrier (insulation) and a vapour barrier (draught sealing). The outside skin of a building envelope provides protection against wind and rain. The image on the following page shows the building envelope outlined in bold.

Most insulation, if kept dry and in place, should remain effective for at least 20 years.

TIP If you're in a home where the ceiling insulation is older than 20 years, consider getting it inspected as it may need to be replaced. If it does need replacing, it's better to remove the old insulation first (not to install new insulation over the top).

Insulation of walls, roof cavity and floors is a major contributor the comfort of a home and should be installed at the build (or renovating) stages. Trying to retrofit later, particularly into walls, is very difficult and can be expensive. The appropriate level and type of insulation will depend on your local climate and where the insulation is going. Consult your architect, building designer, thermal performance assessor or sustainability advisor to determine the most appropriate type and levels for your situation.

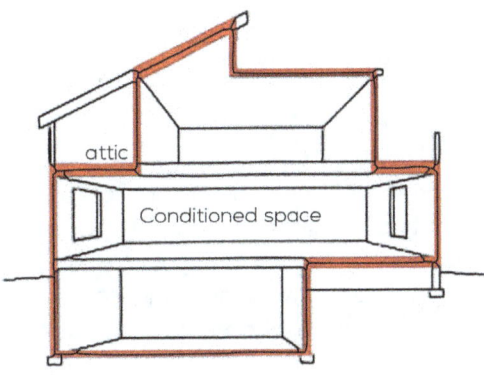

Image credit: AIM Specialty Services

The NCC includes requirements for residential buildings that cover thermal performance (energy efficiency) of the building fabric. Currently most states and territories must meet the 6 star energy efficiency rating. Whether building or renovating, check the requirements in your local area and ensure you comply. If the opportunity is available to improve the rating to 7, 8 or even 9 stars, it would be well worth it and cost justifiable within a relatively short time.

So how does it work? Heat will always move towards cold. If it's warm inside the home, and cold outside, the heat will travel towards the cold and through any materials, such as windows, walls and particularly ceilings. Similarly, if it's hot outside and cooler inside, the heat will move towards the inside of the home. Insulation effectively places a barrier between the cold and the warm to reduce the heat transfer to the cold.

Heat rises, so the majority of heat transfer (loss) in winter months is through the ceiling and roof areas. This is why in the cooler climates, ceiling insulation is the most important of all areas to be insulated.

There are three main types of heat transfer:

- **Radiant** – the transfer of heat through electromagnetic waves (mainly infrared). An example is the warmth from the sun, a fire or bar radiator heater
- **Convection** – the transfer of heat through movement of a substance (air, water currents), i.e. warm air rising from the ground floor to the upper floors of a two storey home
- **Conduction** – heat transfer through a molecular motion from warm to cold. i.e. a metal bar which conducts heat quickly. For example, if you hold one end in your hand and put the other end in a fire, heat will be conducted to the cold end and eventually you'll have to put it down before your hand burns

When looking to insulate a home all three types of heat transfer should be considered. Reflective insulation is good at reducing the radiant heat transfer, whereas bulk insulation is good at reducing convection. The conduction of heat is controlled through the use of insulation or isolating strips on framing materials (i.e. steel frames) that allows transfer of heat or cold within the building structure, often called thermal bridging.

Choosing the right insulation is the first important step, the second is ensuring it is installed correctly.

Thermal bridging

This is where heat can transfer through building materials that have a lower thermal resistance value than the installed insulation (through conduction). This is very important in buildings with steel framing. Thermal bridging can be reduced by installing the bulk insulation over the top of the frame, or alternatively installing isolating strips. For more information on this refer to the Your Home Guide. www.yourhome.gov.au/passive-design/insulation-installation

What's an R-value?

Insulation is measured in 'R-value'. The R stands for Resistance. The 'R-value' of a material is describing how much thermal resistance the material has to the transfer of heat. The higher the R-value, the better it is at inhibiting the transfer of heat and the more effective the insulation. In Australia, R-values on insulation products range from zero (not effective at all) to six (very effective).

'Up R-values' refer to the resistance of heat flowing up (sometimes called winter R-values as they refer to keeping heat in the home).

'Down R-values' refer to heat coming downward in to the home (sometimes called summer R-values as they refer to keeping the home cool).

There are product R-values (for example the resistance value of an insulation batt on its own), and system R-values (that is the total value of the materials working together). When building or renovating a home, the total or system R-value is calculated by including the entirety of the materials, including the air gaps. System R-values are used as input into a thermal performance assessment (TPA) of a home and contribute to the home's final energy performance rating. Architects, building designers, thermal performance assessor or a sustainability consultant should be able to assist in identifying the most suitable products for your project.

Types of insulation

There are two main types of insulation commonly used. They are Bulk and Reflective insulation, available as separate products, or as a combined insulation product.

Bulk insulation

Bulk insulation usually comes in rectangular batts or blanket rolls and is made out of a variety of materials that includes recycled glass or paper, wool, mineral wool, polyester or even polystyrene. Bulk insulation contains lots of tiny pockets of still

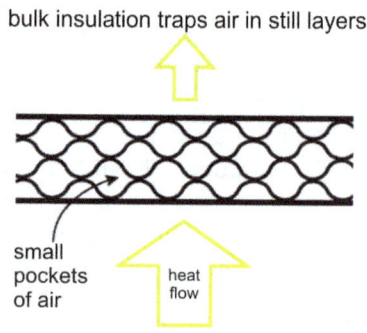

Image source: Your Home

air within the batts. The still air is a poor conductor of heat and is what provides resistance of the heat flow. It is very important not to compress insulation batts as this removes the air pockets and reduces the effectiveness of the insulation.

Bulk insulation can also come in loose fill types that is 'blown' into a space. This type is good for some situations (retrofitting into walls for example), but don't use it in areas where there are draughts. For example installing loose fill insulation into a draughty loft will result in the fill being blown around and settling in corners and becoming ineffective very quickly.

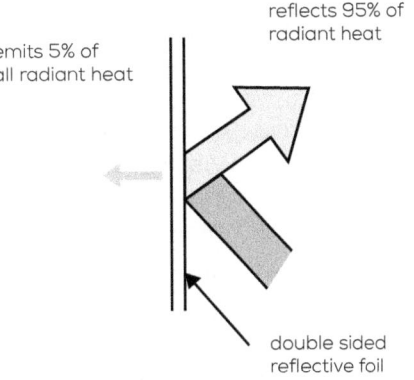

Reflective insulation

Reflective insulation is a foil that can be single or double sided and stops up to 95 percent of radiant heat through reflection. It's a very good material for reducing heat build-up in homes in hot climates. It looks like a tough aluminium foil and comes in sheets or rolls; it can be multi-cell and concertina type foil batt types. Double sided foils generally have one side more reflective (shiny) than the other, and the most reflective (shiny) surface should always be facing down.

Image source: SEAV 2002, Your Home

The foil itself has a very low R-value. Its effectiveness comes from the surrounding air gaps which must be a minimum of 25mm in order to be efficient. Bear in mind that if the foil contacts another surface, is torn or gets too dirty it can become ineffective. Foil sarking under roof tiles can also protect from condensation issues.

Composite

Composite products simply combine both bulk and reflective insulation together into one product. They tend to come as polystyrene or insulating boards with foil outers, or batts or blanket type rolls with foil on the outside.

The ideal healthy home insulation is a product that is functional while being naturally flame resistant (no chemical treatments), made from nontoxic materials, safe to install, long lasting, pest proof (without the use of pesticides), free from VOCs and can be reused or recycled after it is no longer needed. Currently there is no one product (that we know of) that offers all these golden attributes; therefore deciding on a priority of attributes is needed when choosing an insulating product for the home.

Insulation comes in a variety of types and materials. The right solution for you will depend on your situation, climate zone, functional need, area being insulated, price, ease of use and product attribute priorities.

Product considerations

- Opt for insulation that is made from materials with low toxicity e.g. avoid insulation containing formaldehyde
- Consider what the insulation material is made from – opt for a product that is considered safe to install and cut (if the installer has to wear protective clothing, question why)
- Opt for an insulation product that meets Australian Standards (not all do)
- Does this product need to be suitable for bushfire prone areas?
- Is the product considered non allergenic?

- Does it contain recycled content? Products such as polyester batts (made from recycled PET bottles) is an exciting reuse of plastics
- Is it from a sustainable source or made from renewable natural material?
- Can it be recycled when no longer needed?
- Do you require acoustic (noise reduction) qualities to the insulation?
- Does the material have long term stability (prevent collapse)?
- Is the material considered an irritant (non-irritant preferred)?
- Does the material have an odour (low emission preferred)?
- Is the material subject to dust release?
- Has a sealant been applied to prevent dust movement? If so, what is the sealant made from?
- Is the material naturally pest resistant? If not, has it been treated with insecticide? What type of insecticide has been used? (if necessary, the one with the least toxicity is preferred. Refer to the Shop Wise resources section to investigate pesticides)
- Is the material subject to mould growth (conditions permitting, such as condensation)?
- Does the product have any independent certification?

Ideally opt for an insulation that has both non-toxic and sustainably sourced attributes and check for independent certifications.

Installation health considerations

- Wear protective clothing including glasses and gloves when working in the roof space, under floor or other areas prone to significant dust
- Use eye protection if installing reflective insulation
- Reflective foil insulation must be clear of any electrical appliances and wiring and must not be secured using metal staples due to the electrocution risk
- To reduce fire risk, be sure to allow the recommended clearance around downlight fittings, exhaust fans, fire chimneys/flues or appliance fittings that penetrate the ceiling. Ideally keep ceiling penetrations to a minimum
- To assist with good internal air quality opt for non-toxic insulation products that do not off-gas

Insulation zones

Vapour (Air) Barriers

Vapour (air) barriers are needed to protect the home's external wall cavities and the insulation. If insulation gets damp it can become ineffective and become a breeding ground for mould and other issues. The intent of an air barrier is to restrict air flow from inside to outside to reduce energy loss and it also protects the wall cavity from moisture. Vapour/air barriers (or airtight plaster approach) is a building methodology. A proper vapour barrier is considered plaster board sealed with two coats of paint. Attention needs to be made to any penetrations through the plaster which includes windows, doors, plumbing, electrical or any service that goes through the barrier. These should be well sealed to prevent moisture from traveling from the inside of the building into the wall cavity.

The Australian Building Codes Board has a good free condensation in buildings handbook; links are in the Online Resource Summary section.

Where does all the heat go?

The images on the following page show typical heat loss and gains during the winter and summer seasons.

Ceiling and roof insulation

Insulation in the ceiling is the most important as this is where the majority of heat can leave and enter the home. According to Sustainability Victoria, installing roof and ceiling insulation can save up to 45 percent on heating and cooling energy costs.

The right insulation will depend on the roof structure you are insulating. Standard pitched roofs with flat ceilings are the most common. Insulation generally comprises bulk insulation batts between the ceiling joists and reflective foil (or sarking) under the roof structure (the tiles, Colorbond), between the battens and rafters.

Sloping ceilings where the ceiling is in line with the roof and there is no ceiling space can be more difficult and should be designed to allow the appropriate insulation for the climate zone. The right type will depend on the designed structure and the amount of insulation required.

Avoid ceiling penetrations where possible (e.g. downlights) as the clearance required around them will reduce the effectiveness of your insulation.

Roof spaces should allow for ventilation, particularly during summer months to enable removal of heat build-up during the day. Where there are 'holes' in the ceiling (i.e. downlights penetrating the ceiling to the roof space), this could allow moisture to get into the roof space which could possibly cause condensation. Venting a roof space during both winter and summer is important in order to keep the attic space dry.

Wall insulation

Insulating external walls can reduce heat loss and save up to 15 percent on heating and cooling bills. Bulk and reflective insulation can be used in walls. Be sure to include the 25mm air gap for reflective insulation; do not compress bulk insulation and include a vapour protection barrier to protect against condensation issues if you are in a condensation-prone area.

Vapour barriers are needed in areas where there is a large difference between indoor and outdoor temperatures, or in hot humid climates.

Be careful of services running through walls and to avoid fire risk keep bulk insulation away from wall penetrations that may get hot.

Internal walls tend not to be insulated. However if you have the budget and would appreciate the acoustic benefits, it can assist with temperature control of internal areas and reduce noise transfer

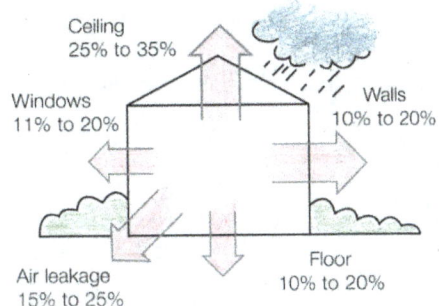

Winter Heat Loss

Ceiling 25% to 35%
Windows 11% to 20%
Walls 10% to 20%
Air leakage 15% to 25%
Floor 10% to 20%

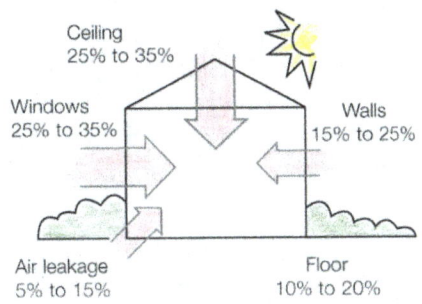

Summer Heat Gain

Ceiling 25% to 35%
Windows 25% to 35%
Walls 15% to 25%
Air leakage 5% to 15%
Floor 10% to 20%

Image source: SEAV 2002 and Your Home

between rooms. Alternatively, should you have areas of a home that are rarely used, having them insulated between the main areas and keeping them closed off could provide a buffer zone and assist with maintaining temperatures in the areas highly used.

Floor insulation

Insulating the floor is very effective in homes where ground temperatures can get very cold or where it is ideal to prevent draughts and heat loss through the floor. It can be applied to suspended floors (timber or concrete) and can be included in slabs on the ground. Note that if insulating a slab on the ground, the edge should also be insulated if you are in the alpine climate zone (Zone 8) or if you are installing in-slab heating.

Floor insulation would not be required in suspended floors in hot climates as the suspended floor itself would assist with promoting natural cooling.

Installing insulation

Most climate zones in Australia would benefit from a combination of both bulk and reflective insulation. Bulk insulation is most effective when installed directly above the ceiling.

When it comes to insulation think 'blanket on the bed', any holes or gaps in it and it won't keep you as warm as it could. Insulation is literally a blanket around the house to reflect heat out and keep heat in. To ensure it is as effective as possible it is important to:

- Make sure there are no gaps (but you'll need to allow a minimal clearance around halogen down-lights and chimney flues – best to avoid these in the first place)
- Be aware of any thermal bridging issues and minimise them where possible
- Ensure the insulation does not come into contact with moisture
- To stop any condensation issues be sure to include vapour barriers in appropriate areas
- Do not compress bulk insulation because it compresses the air gaps and can render it ineffective
- Make sure you include suitable air space around reflective insulation

TIP If you can be on-site when the insulation is installed, check it is installed correctly. Once the walls are up it will be very difficult and costly to rectify any gaps.

Draught-proofing and air leakage

Having good insulation is only part of the story. Ensuring the home is draught-proofed assists with retention of heating and cooling and can save up to 25 percent of heating and cooling costs. Studies have found that in a typical home, if you combined all the gaps and cracks together you would have a hole approximately 1.5 m2 in your home (source: Brandjes Environmental Building Consulting).

TIP Why invest thousands of dollars in double glazing and insulation, and then effectively leave the front door wide open year round? Sealing gaps should always be the first step because it's difficult to keep a home comfortable with a large hole in it!

The diagram below shows the most common air leakage points. Good insulation combined with effective draught-proofing contributes significantly to a more comfortable, cost effective home.

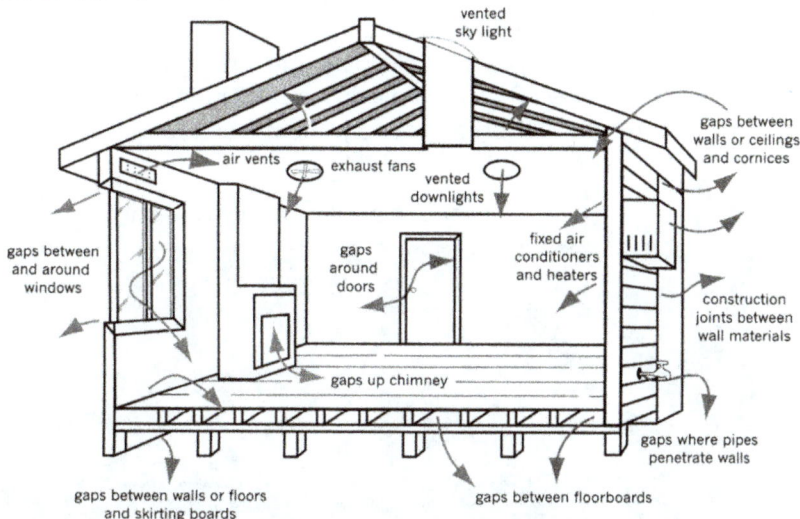

Image source: SEAV and Your Home

In climates where heating is required, draught-proofing is particularly important. The graph below shows the most common areas of air leakage by percentage in a typical Australian home.

It's easy to see that the most common area is through floors, walls and ceiling. Recent research on new build homes has found that even in a well-insulated home, leaks can be caused by construction gaps between walls and window/door frames and corner joins.

There are several ways to identify the sources of air leakage in a home.

DIY – You can do it yourself by looking carefully around doors, windows, and other areas for gaps in the construction and closing them with appropriate fillers and seals. Using an incense stick on a windy day also helps

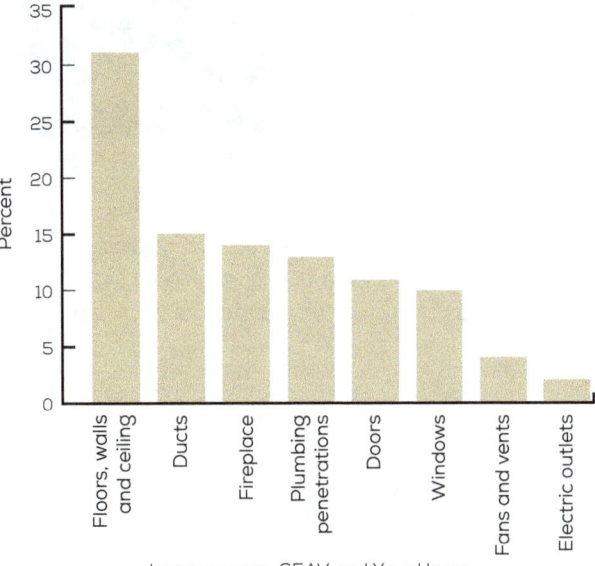

Image source: SEAV and Your Home

to track where some of the more difficult draughts are coming from. There is a DIY Draught-Proofing checklist in the back of this book to work through when you're on your draught hunt.

Draught-proofing professionals are also available to conduct an air leakage assessment and many will also install the draught-proofing for you. They are likely to use thermal imaging equipment and/or conduct a blower door test to identify the sources of leaks before fixing them.

Thermal image cameras are very effective at identifying temperature differentials and can be used to spot air leakage in a home. They are most useful when there is at least a three degree temperature differential between inside and out. The bigger the temperature difference, the more obvious the air leakage will be.

Blower door testing is a tool that is used to measure how airtight a building is. It works by closing up the home and installing the 'blower door' on an exterior door. This is a flexible frame that fits into an exterior door opening with a strong fan connected to air pressure gauges. The gauges measure the air flow and air pressure. The fan pulls air out of the home which lowers the air pressure, which then effectively sucks outside air through all unsealed openings. Smoke pencils are used to detect the leaks.

Blower door　　　　　　　　Smoke showing air leakage through downlights

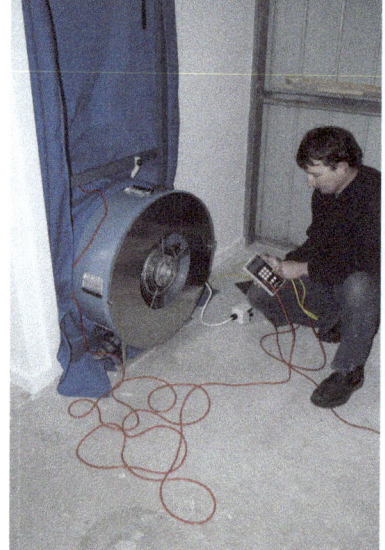

Images courtesy of Brandjes Environmental Building Consultancy, 2014

Draught-proofing your home is one of the simplest undertakings that can be done to reduce heat loss and draughts. It is also now a requirement of the NCC. There are a variety of draught seals available and there is one to suit almost every situation. The table on the next page summarises the key items and how to draught-proof.

Draught source	How to fix
Gaps between door and window frames	There are many draught seals including brush seals, rubber and foam varieties available at most hardware stores. Find the one that best suits your situation. Most are easy to fit. Quality seals will last longer.
Gaps between door and window frames and the walls	Options include expanding foam, using thin cut strips of insulation, polyfil and gap fillers. The right option will depend on the situation. Opt for low emission products where available.
Gaps between floor boards	These can often be stopped with underfloor insulation (if accessible) or by filling the gaps with an appropriate filler. Alternatively cover the floor with rugs in winter months to reduce the draughts.
Around the manhole in the ceiling	Insulate the manhole cover with the material used in the ceiling and draught-proof where the frame meets the access door.
Plumbing penetrations through walls	These can be repaired by using the appropriate filler to close of the gap. Opt for low emission products.
Exhaust fans	Install exhaust fans that have a damper, are self-closing and externally vented. Where retrofitting, use a draught stopper exhaust fan cover to minimise draughts.
Evaporative cooling ducts	Many systems have dampers that should close, but if not, evaporative cooling vent covers are available that allow vents to be sealed in winter months, and removed again for use during summer.
Lighting that penetrates and vents into ceiling space (e.g. downlights)	Replace the lighting by fitting pendant or track lighting internally. Alternatively use sealed downlight covers (be sure to check fire ratings and keep insulation away) or replace with sealed LED units.
Chimney flues and open fireplaces	If there is a damper available close it when the fire place is not in use. Otherwise use a chimney sealing product that is easily removable, these fit into the chimney flue. If permanent sealing is needed, close it off at both the top and the bottom and stuff some bulk insulation into the chimney cavity to stop draughts.
Sky lights	These can be the source of significant heat loss. Options include installing a 'double glazed' unit at ceiling level (could be glass or acrylic and should be openable in case of maintenance), or replace the skylight glazing with a double or triple glazed unit.

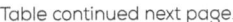
Table continued next page.

Draught source	How to fix
Air vent bricks	In some homes air bricks are in the structure and on both inside and outside of the wall. The wall will need to be ventilated so the external vents should remain open, however the internal vents are a source of heat loss and should be plastered over or sealed. Take caution with vents in wet areas – if these are sealed over and there are no exhaust fans, condensation issues may occur.
Windows – particularly single glazed windows	Use good thermally lined curtains, Roman blinds or honeycomb blinds to reduce draughts through single glazing. See Windows section for more information.
Pet flaps/doors	High quality brush seals are a good option to minimise heat loss through pet doors.

Table source © Green Moves Australia 2014.

Draught-proofing maintenance

- Check and replace door and window seals when necessary
- Inspect ceiling insulation after work has been done in the ceiling space (it is often not replaced again) or every few years to see if it needs topping up or gaps repaired

Condensation - a cautionary word

While insulation and draught-proofing can provide good levels of comfort and reduced energy bills, it can sometimes cause condensation issues leading to mould or mildew. Areas of the building that are at high risk are bathrooms, laundries and kitchens; anywhere moisture can accumulate.

To minimise issues from occurring these rooms should be externally vented with self-closing exhaust fans. Homes that are particularly airtight, such as those built to passive house standards, should include heat recovery ventilation systems and have adequate vapour barriers.

The Australian Building Codes Board has a good free Guide to Condensation; links are in the Online Resource Summary section.

Windows and glazing

Windows are a key feature in a home, a prominent component of a home's style. They allow natural light into a space, provide for views outside and can be used for providing ventilation and fresh air into the home. Windows give a home that 'feel good' factor. However, windows and their glazing can also be a major contributor to heat loss in winter and heat gain in summer which is why window selection, location and glazing type are essential design considerations to achieve a sustainable, healthy home.

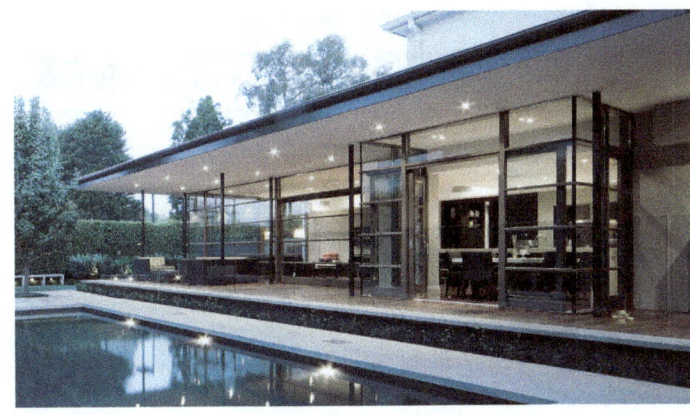
Image: Paarhammer

The *Your Home* technical manual states that 'up to 40 percent of a home's heating energy can be lost and up to 87 percent of its heat gained through glazing'. This is a significant amount and is why windows (glazing and the frame) are an important contributor to the comfort of a home.

The type of glazing, frame, the direction it faces and surroundings (eaves, buildings etc.) determines how well a window can operate. Windows should be chosen to work with the local climate. For example, in hot humid areas louver windows are an excellent choice as they maximise ventilation opportunities, where in colder climates double glazing is ideal to reduce heat loss. The Australian Window Association (AWA) in conjunction with the Window Energy Rating Scheme (WERS) has created some useful climate zone based guides on choosing windows. To see the guides or obtain further information visit the Windows Energy Rating Scheme website: **www.wers.net/werscontent/how-to-select-windows**

Window Energy Rating Scheme (WERS)

When looking for windows check the WERS label which provides a heating and cooling rating for energy efficiency. This rating scheme is managed by the Australian Window Association (AWA) and is independent of manufacturers. The scheme provides rigorous testing to confirm performance claims and ensure windows meet relevant Australian Standards. WERS ratings have been designed to easily 'plug in' to the National House Energy Rating software to assist with providing thermal performance star ratings for homes. To the right is a sample WERS rating label.

Heating Band: Where windows are required to keep warmth in.

Cooling Band: Where windows are required to keep heat out.

Image: AWA

Use of appropriate glazing can significantly help with heat reflection, absorption and transmittance through the glazing. All glass types perform at different levels of reflection, absorption and transmittance (the RAT equation).

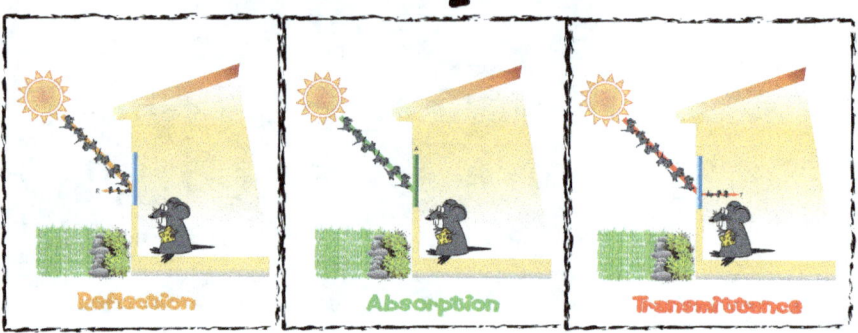

Image: AWA

Windows gain and lose heat through conduction which is expressed as 'U-value', and solar heat gain which is expressed as SHGC (Solar Heat Gain Co-efficient).

The U value measures how well a window (in its entirety) prevents heat escaping and entering the home. Usually specified in watts per m2, ratings are between 0.0 and 10.0 w/m2. A low U value number means that the window is resistant to heat flow and has a good insulating value.

Can be used to keep heat out

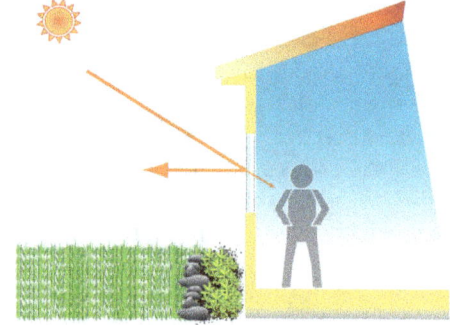

And to keep heat in

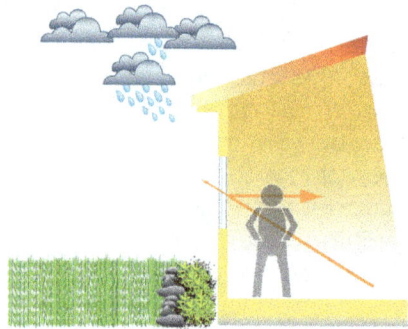

Images: AWA

SHGC measures how easily solar heat flows through the window (see image below). It is specified as a number in the range 0 to 1. The lower a window's SHGC number, the less solar heat it transmits into the home, helping to keep it cool.

Solar heat gain through direct contact

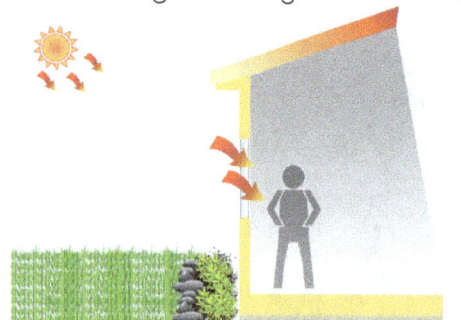

And through reflection

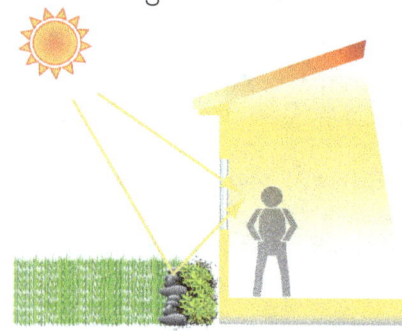

Images: AWA

Other heat loss and gain issues

There are four main ways that windows and doors gain and lose heat.

They are:

- Air leakage through gaps and around fittings
- Radiation through the glass
- Convection through air affecting the glass
- Conduction transfer through materials

TIP: Your climate is key. If you are living in a hot climate, windows with a high number of stars indicating the cooling efficiencies are ideal (keeping heat out), as heating attributes won't be important. If you are living in a cool climate where you use heating, the heating efficiency rating indicated by the stars on the label (how good it is at keeping heat in) will be very important.

Window compliance

All residential windows and doors should be marked with a performance label confirming that they are certified to comply with Australian Standard 2047. Products purchased from an accredited AWA member have a compliance certificate that supports a minimum six year warranty. This should be provided with the window.

Manufacturers participating in the WER scheme can provide energy efficiency rating certification. Obtain the relevant compliance certification documents where you can and keep them for future information and reference.

You can also search and check the ratings of any window type and configuration by supplier on the WERS website. This is a free resource and can be found at **www.wers.net/wers-home**

TIP: Always check for the compliance sticker. Stickers are generally applied to the window frame and sometimes they can be found on the glazing. Below is an example of what they look like.

 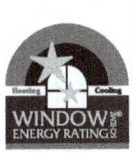

Image: AWA

Further information

Window Energy Rating Scheme – www.wers.net
Australian Window Association – www.awa.org.au

Types of window frames

There is a wide variety of frame types and glazing available, you can mix almost any frame with any glazing type.

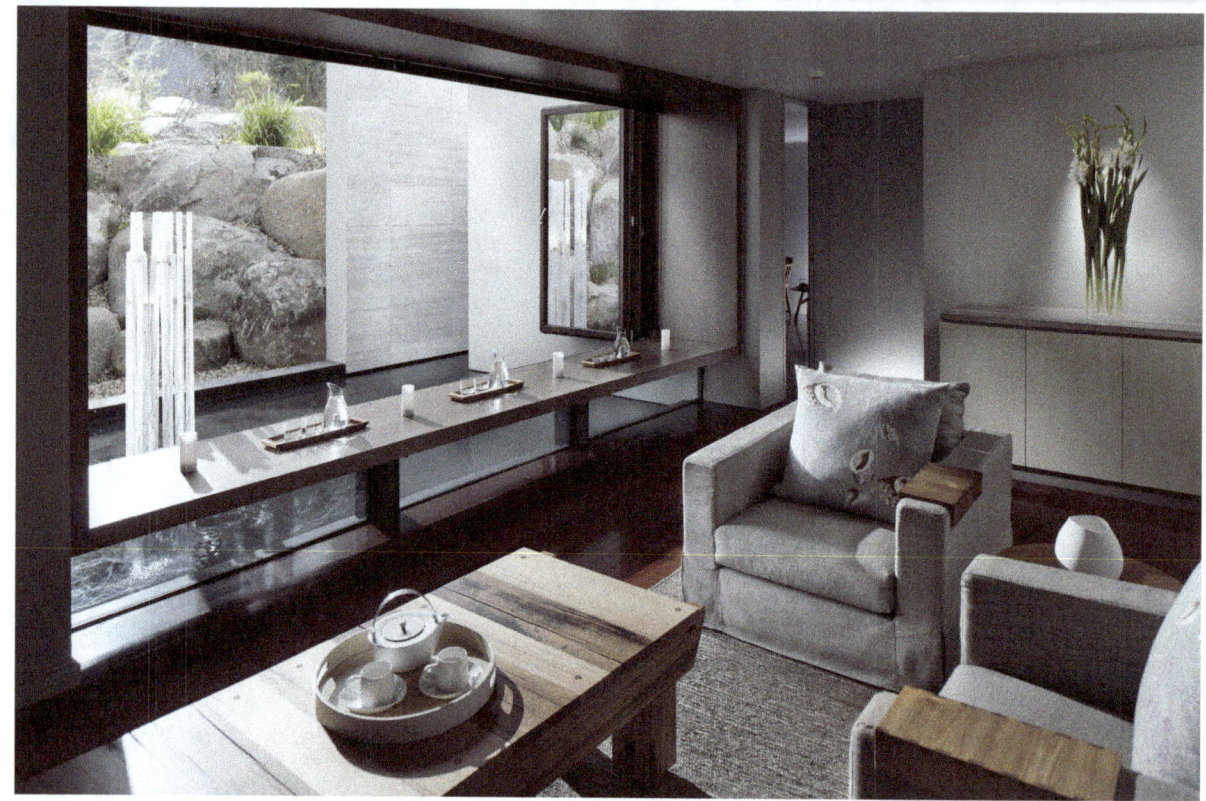

Image credit: Paarhammer (Saffire Freycinet)

Common frame types

Frame type	Pros	Cons
Timber	• Thermally efficient • Renewable source • Recyclable product • Long lifespan if maintained correctly	• Requires regular maintenance • Can expand and contract due to weather conditions
uPVC (Vinyl) uPVC is 'unplasticized polyvinyl chloride'	• Thermally very efficient • Very low maintenance • Strong and durable • Long lifespan • Supports various glazing combinations and styles	• Can be expensive • Manufacturing process is greenhouse gas and resource intensive • Manufacturing of PVC is controversial. PVC is not biodegradable and if incinerated at end of life releases carcinogenic dioxins into the atmosphere
Aluminium	• Lightweight • Strong and durable • Powder coat finishes provide low maintenance • Low cost • Recyclable product	• Thermally inefficient • Regular washing is necessary to preserve appearance • Manufacturing process is greenhouse gas and resource intensive
Thermally broken aluminium	• As above but with improved thermal efficiency.	• As above, but provides better thermal efficiency. • More expensive than standard aluminium
Steel	• Very strong and durable • Recyclable product • Long life expectancy • Galvanised products are considered nontoxic and have neutral impact to indoor air quality • Does not attract vermin, insects or termites • Can be load bearing	• Thermally inefficient • Made from non-renewable resources • Process is greenhouse gas intensive • Potential for rust

Table continued next page.

Frame type	Pros	Cons
Composite wood and aluminium	• Thermally efficient • Made of composite wood products • Stable and durable • Good moisture and decay resistance • Aluminium section can be recycled at end of life	• Will need cleaning occasionally • Manufacturing process is greenhouse gas intensive for aluminium section
Fibreglass	• High thermal performance • Very strong and versatile • Long life expectancy • Allows for high glass to frame ratios • No maintenance if not painted • Does not swell, warp or rot	• Made from non-renewable resources • Process is greenhouse gas intensive

Table source © Green Moves Australia 2014.

Common types of glazing

Type	Comments	Good for
Float glass	Used as the base material for many glazing types. Can break easily into large jagged shards.	• Base product for other glazing products
Toughened	Treated with a thermal tempering process that strengthens the glass. When it does break it breaks into small square shaped fragments that are less likely to cause injury.	• Windows and doors (especially sliding doors) • Building facades • Partitions
Laminated	Made of two or more layers of glass with an interlayer of polymeric material bonded between the layers. Other technologies such as colouring, fire resistance, ultraviolet filtering can be embedded.	• Windows and doors • Skylights • Very safe and secure as it does not shatter • Building facades • Car windscreens
Coated	Surface coatings can be applied to increase solar reflection, heat transmission, absorption, and provide scratch and corrosion resistance. Can be toughened, laminated or incorporated into a double glazed unit. Usually applied at manufacturing stage.	• Windows and doors • Skylights • Building facades

Table continued next page.

Type	Comments	Good for
Reflective coatings/tints	Can be applied after installation and can assist in reflecting heat. Plasticised films may contain phthalate chemicals. Ask the supplier if any phthalate migration testing has been done to ascertain if phthalates chemicals from their product migrate into household dust.	• Windows and doors • Skylights
Mirrored	Involves a metal reflective coating applied to one side of the glass and can include vinyl backing for safety. One way mirrors and mirrored glass are gaining popularity and architectural appeal.	• Specific situations
Patterned	Flat glass that contains a regular pattern, usually applied at manufacture. Also includes opaque glass.	• Windows and doors • Design feature • Provide light but not view (e.g. bathrooms)
Low E	Low emissivity glass has a spectrally selective coating that can reflect infrared (heat) and ultraviolet light while retaining visible light. In cooler climates it is useful to reflect heat back into the room to help keep it warm. In hot climates it can help to keep a home cool. Requires special cleaning attention. May block mobile phone and radio signals but no scientific evidence found (yet) to support this claim.	• Windows and doors • Retaining or rejecting heat into the home (dependent on which way the coating is facing).
Double glazing (Insulated glass units)	Two panes of glass sealed in a frame with an air gap to reduce heat flow. Some have argon or krypton gas between the panes that provides higher resistance to heat flow. Note – depending on the situation, single glazing can be removed and a double glazed unit installed. This provides an upgrade option.	• Windows, doors and skylights • Retaining heating inside • Reducing noise levels from outside

Table continued next page.

Type	Comments	Good for
Triple Glazing (Insulated Glass Units)	Three panes of glass sealed in a frame with air gaps between each pane to reduce heat flow. Can have argon or krypton gas, contain low E coatings or other treatments.	• Windows, doors and skylights • Retains heating inside • Reducing noise levels from outside
Secondary Glazing	This is where a secondary pane of glass or acrylic sheet is retrofitted onto a single glazed area with a gap (approx. 1cm) and sealed. This improves the glazing performance and reduces heat loss and noise. It is not as good as double glazed units but can be quite effective. The main methods are installing a second pane using magnets to secure and seal. There is also a DIY solution using a clear heat shrinkable membrane that can be fitted to the frame using double sided tape.	• Reducing heat loss through skylights • Improving the performance of single glazed windows and doors • Reduces heat loss and gain • Reduces noise from outside
Security glass	Can resist physical attack, ballistic and bomb blasts. Uses a specialised laminate and multiple layers of glazing, built to required resistance.	• High risk windows and doors that need to be very strong
Self-cleaning glass	There are several types of self-cleaning coatings that enable a glass surface to keep itself free of dirt. They are applied during manufacture and work by using sunlight to break down organic dirt and grime. When water hits the glass the coating assists to wash the glass without leaving marks.	• Exteriors that are difficult to reach.

Table source © Green Moves Australia 2014.

When looking at window systems (glazing and framing) it can get quite confusing. To help identify and compare window systems, the AWA has created an Efficient Glazing Calculator and Window Comparison tool. This is available from the AWA website at **www.efficientglazing.net**

Product considerations

- Design glazing to maximise passive heating/cooling techniques and to capture cooling breezes

- Choose window types (louvers, casement, sliding) that are suited to the local climate, purpose and site
- Choose thermally efficient window frames, ideally with sustainable features that do not off-gas
- Opt for high performance glazing that is suitable for the particular climate and space
- Provide adjustable shading devices for glazing during hot periods
- Use the WERS website and check the ratings on the glazing
- Look for independent certifications (e.g. Ecospecifier, FSC® timber etc).
- Choose frames that are from a renewable source and coatings that are low/no VOC

Other considerations

If you are building new or renovating, identifying the right window system for your home will depend on a number of factors including your local climate, location, size of the windows, budget and aesthetics. Ensure the person designing the building or renovation is familiar with passive solar design techniques to maximise performance as much as possible. Where glazing is well planned, windows can assist in maintaining year-round comfort and contribute to the thermal performance assessment rating of your home.

Carefully consider where operable windows are required in the home. Often too many operable windows are placed into one room. Building costs can be better managed by ensuring operable windows are in necessary positions and use fixed windows to assist with additional natural light. This is a cost saving tip because operable windows tend to be more expensive than fixed windows.

Your architect, building designer or thermal performance assessor should be able to advise on the most appropriate windows for your project. If not, contact a sustainability consultant.

Check the windows when they arrive onsite and ensure they are what was ordered. Make sure the builder installs the right window in the right place. Errors can occur where the wrong glazing is delivered on site and the wrong window is installed, or in an area where a different window was intended.

Improving what you have

If you want to make the best use of what you have, there are a number of ways you can reduce heat loss and gains to the home without having to replace your windows. Large windows, particularly those facing north, east and west, can contribute significantly to heat loss and gain over the seasons.

TIP Focus on the areas you use the most or that are problematic first.

Many older homes have wooden window and door frames. These are good because they are a slow conductor of heat and cool and come from a renewable source. They also generally facilitate easy installation of secondary glazing or replacement of the panes with double glazed units. However they do require regular maintenance to keep them in good condition. If your home has wooden frames, look after them, they are an asset.

Regardless of the frames in your home, you can improve your windows' performance through the use of window treatments. This is done through appropriate use of blinds, window films, window coverings and other related products. Remember, heat travels towards cold.

Keeping warm with existing windows

Window treatment options for keeping warmer in winter include:

- Draught seal around the framing and the wall if any gaps, and draught seal the window itself to stop air leaks and prevent heat loss
- Let the sun in if it's shining on the glass, close the curtains at night
- Use close fitting thermally lined curtains to cover the area and create a barrier between the glazing and internal air
- Some curtain track systems have a built-in return to the wall providing a pelmet effect. Choose your tracking system to take advantage of this if you can
- Use close fitting, thermally lined curtains with pelmets (the pelmet is important as it facilitates a still air barrier behind the curtain, stops air flow and reduces draughts). Close the curtains when the heating is on to produce a barrier to the heat being drawn to the cold
- If you already have curtains that aren't lined, have a thermal lining added.
- Use pelmets. A pelmet doesn't have to be big and bulky. The point is to deflect the air moving down the wall, to the room side of the curtains, not the window side. It can be a clear bit of Perspex, acrylic or recycled boards. Ensure you use a pelmet (or similar air deflector) to direct heat away from the window and to the room side of the curtain
- Consider close fitting, thermally lined Roman blinds. They are a good alternative to curtains and pelmets and do the same job while capturing less dust
- Honeycomb or cellular blinds fitted into the window rebate. These have a honeycomb structure and create still air pockets. They are available in opaque and transmit some natural light but protect from heat loss. Some are even rated with an R-Value
- Highly effective window coatings can help reflect heat back into the room (and reflect the heat out in summer). Query the supplier for information to confirm the product does not release phthalates (plastic softeners) into interior dust
- One of the DIY solutions is to use a form of secondary glazing that uses a heat shrinkable film fixed with double sided sticky tape. This is a good option in places that won't get damaged by children or pets, but is not good in wet areas or as a long term solution (more than a year or two). It is useful to see if double glazing will actually make a difference to a room as it's a cheap way to test the theory

- Replace the single glazing unit with a custom-made double glazed unit. This can be a DIY job as well if you're handy. It simply involves measuring the glazing, having a double glazed unit made up to fit, and fitting it yourself. If you DIY, this option can be cheaper than secondary glazing
- Apply secondary glazing. The acrylic and glass types are usually made to order and fitted with magnetic strips. These can be very effective
- For skylights, to reduce heat loss without losing too much light, retrofitting secondary glazing is an option, or the installation of opaque honeycomb type blinds (with reflective backing)

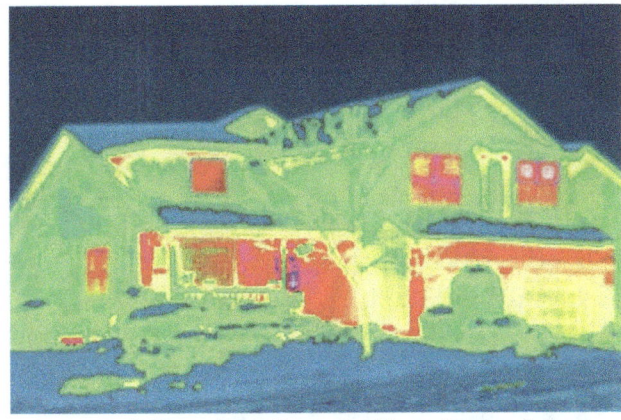

Image credit: Bazaar Home Decorating. Thermal image of a home. Red shows heat coming through the windows (heat loss). Green/blue is cool to these areas and is retaining heat in the home.

Keeping cool with existing windows

In the hotter months, every square metre of single glazed glass the sun hits directly can radiate the same amount of heat as a single bar radiator (McGee, 2013). It makes sense to shade the glazing.

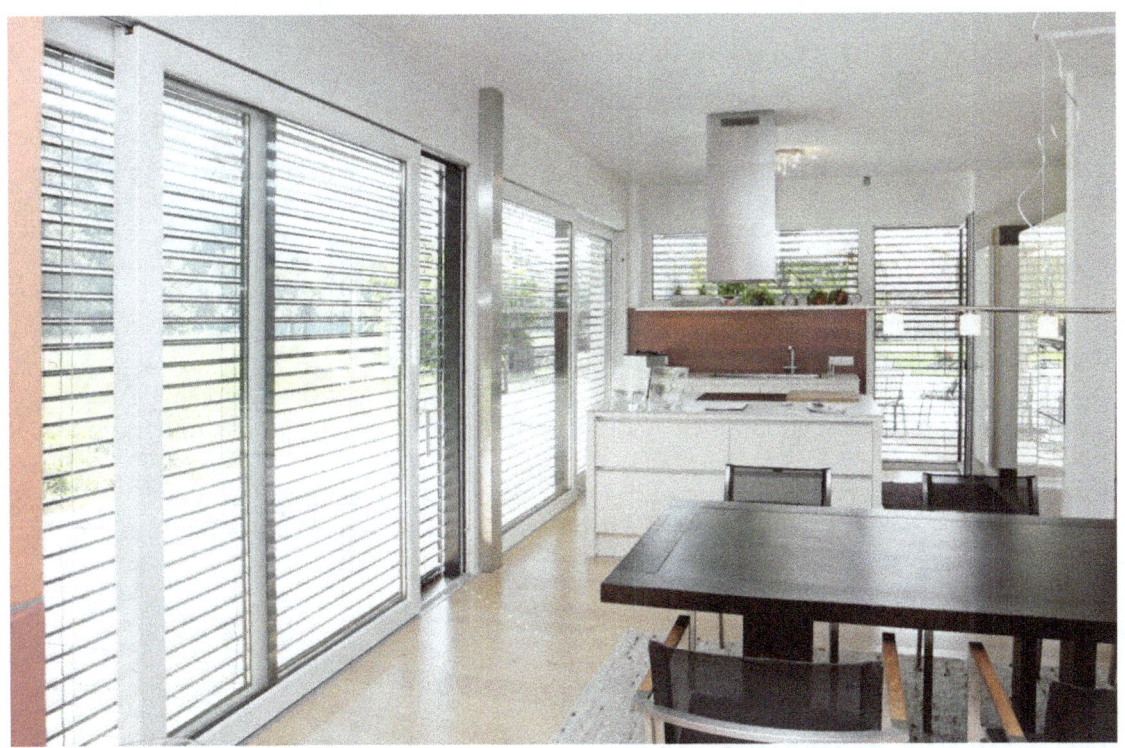

Image: Paarhammer External Ventilation Blinds

Window treatments for keeping cool in summer include:

- Externally shading glazing from direct sun is always the most effective method and can reduce heat gains in the home by up to 90 percent (McGee, 2013). External shading should be adjustable and well designed to cater for the change in sun angles during winter and summer. Ideally you want to allow the winter sun through, but stop the summer sun from reaching the window. Fixed options include eaves and pergolas. Adjustable solutions include awnings, blinds and shutters. Deciduous trees are also a good solution where gardens are available
- Internal shading can also be effective, but only reduces heat gain by up to 15 percent (McGee, 2013). Where internal shading is used, opt for reflective backings on curtains and blinds, or honeycomb type. If the situation is particularly bad and other options are not suitable, Renshade is a good alternative. It can be fitted against the inside of the glass to reflect heat back out. Renshade is a strong, perforated, reflective foil material that can be constructed into blinds or used as a covering installed on the inside of glazing. It has significant reflective abilities (up to 85 percent heat reflection) and can be seen through (although view is restricted)
- Apply a heat reflective window film to the glazing. There are several on the market that are particularly good at reflecting heat and keeping views. Note that this can reduce your solar heat gain in winter months
- If you have skylights these can also be problematic. Ideally shade them externally with shade cloth in hotter months. Alternatively install a honeycomb type blind with a reflective coating that fits into or just under the glazing to reduce heat loss and heat gain. Another option is to fit some Renshade during summer months to reflect heat and maintain some light

Window operational considerations

- In winter, keep windows and doors closed to minimise heat loss
- In summer open windows to encourage cross flow ventilation and cooling breezes to enter the home. Note that casement window types are more effective at directing breezes into the home

Window maintenance

- Clean window coverings regularly using a HEPA vacuum cleaner
- Dust pelmets regularly to prevent dust build up
- Clean windows as needed with non-toxic solutions (vinegar and water works well)
- For sliding windows/doors, vacuum slider tracks regularly to maintain ease of movement and prevent damage
- Check draught seals regularly to maintain optimal draught-proofing
- Clean external windows' awnings before use to prevent excess dust from entering the home when windows are open

Window health considerations

- Ensure windows have flyscreens fitted to prevent pests from entering the home when the window is open
- Ensure windows are maintained in working order and open them regularly - good ventilation of the home prevents mould and mildew problems and provides fresh air to

flush out VOCs and any smells or fumes
- Window coverings collect dust which may trigger allergy and respiratory conditions. Clean window coverings regularly. Keep sufferers out of the room for a couple of hours after cleaning has occurred
- Windows with 'green' or interesting views contribute to overall wellbeing, if you have a window with an uninspiring view try improving the appeal with screening, painted surfaces or exterior vertical gardens
- Choose pre-made window coverings or custom fabrics that are Oeko-Tex certified (certified as free from harmful textile substances). For more information on this refer to the Window Coverings section of this book

Further information

Department of Industry, Your Home - Passive Heating and Cooling – www.yourhome.gov.au

Window Energy Rating System (WERS) – www.wers.net

Australian Window Association (AWA) – www.awa.org.au

Guides to complying with the National Construction Code (NCC)

Guide to Window and Door Performance Accreditation

Australian Window Association – www.efficientglazing.net

Efficient Glazing Calculator and Window Comparison tools

Glass and Glazing Association of Australia – www.agga.org.au

Choice website – Household section – www.choice.com.au

Nationwide House Energy Rating Scheme (NatHERS) – www.nathers.gov.au

Australian Building Codes Board at www.abcb.gov.au. The ABCB has some very useful free booklets online. These include:

- Condensation in Buildings (2011)
- Construction of buildings in Flood Hazard areas (2012)
- Using on-site renewable and reclaimed energy sources (2011)
- Sound Insulation (2004)
- Various Energy Efficiency Provisions

You can find these and other ABCB ebooks at www.abcb.gov.au/education-events-resources/publications/abcb-handbooks

Commonwealth of Australia, Bureau of Meteorology –www.bom.gov.au

United Nations Centre for Human Settlements (Habitant), Nairobi 1990, National Design Handbook Prototype on Passive Solar Heating and Natural Cooling of Buildings. Available: www.unhabitat.org/pmss/getElectronicVersion.aspx?nr=1230&alt=1

Passive House Institute Germany, 2012 – http://passiv.de/en

Australian Passive House Association – http://passivehouseaustralia.org

CSIRO, The Evaluation of the 5-Star Energy Efficiency Standard for Residential Buildings, 2014 – www.industry.gov.au/Energy/Pages/Evaluation5StarEEfficiencyStandardResidentialBuildings.aspx

Phase Change Energy Solutions – http://phasechange.com/index.php/en

Brindle, Beth, 2011. '10 Benefits of a Passive House' HowStuffWorks.com. Available: http://home.howstuffworks.com/home-improvement/construction/green/10-benefits-of-a-passive-house.htm – 28 March 2011.

Water

Less than two percent of the world's water is potable (fresh water that is suitable for drinking). Fresh water is essential to support human, animal and plant life and is needed for food production and manufacturing. Changes in climate and rainfall patterns have already caused significant water shortages across Australia. This has resulted in water restrictions, crops failing and alternative water supply options (such as desalination plants) being built at great taxpayer expense. Globally approximately one third of the world's population is already suffering from fresh water shortages (source: SaveWater, 2013).

Australia is one of the driest continents on earth, yet we use on average 100,000L per person per year, globally the highest water use per person (source: SaveWater, 2013). As our population continues to grow, so does the demand on our water.

Every individual in Australia is responsible for conserving water resources. Not just at home, but everywhere we go and in everything we do. Our future depends on it.

This section is dedicated to how you can reduce water consumption in and around the home. Water services, delivery and storage products can be costly additions to a home and are worthy of consideration at the design phase of a project.

Note that water filtration is not covered in this section. Refer to water filtration in the Products and Furnishings chapter.

General considerations:

- Design in water capture and storage at initial build stage where possible
- Check taps and toilets regularly and fix leaks quickly
- Buy water efficient appliances and tapware (check the WELS ratings)
- Use nontoxic cleaners to minimise toxic waste that finds its way down the drain, healthier for you and the planet

Reducing water use at home

The key items to remember in relation to appliances are:

- Select the right-sized appliance for the job
- Choose the most water efficient model you can, and
- Opt for quality where you can

There are many ways we can reduce water usage in and around the home. Here is a summary of where, what and how.

Where	What	How
In the kitchen	Kitchen sink taps	• Fit a water efficient tap (or install flow restrictors, or aerators) to minimise water flow • Collect water from washing vegetables and use it to water plants • When rinsing dishes, put some water in the sink and rinse in that before stacking in the dishwasher or washing properly • Don't use running water to defrost food (use the fridge, bench or microwave) • Use a bowl or jug to catch any cold water when waiting for the hot water to come through. Use it for drinking, cooking or plant watering
	Dishwasher	• Choose a water efficient dishwasher, ideally one that is 6 stars • Use short or eco run cycles as often as possible • Only run the dishwasher when it is full • Look for a biodegradable dishwasher detergent
	Garbage disposals	• Can use up to six litres of water per day. Put food scraps into compost or worm farms rather than use the garbage disposal. Saves energy, water and provides fertiliser for your garden
	Cooking	• When boiling vegetables, use enough water to cover the vegetables and use the lid. They will cook faster and it saves water and energy • Let cooking water cool and put onto the garden
In the laundry	Sink and taps	• Don't use flow restrictors in the laundry because they reduce the water flow which slows down filling of buckets for washing etc. • When hand washing clothes, use enough water to cover the clothes and allow movement, no more • When hand washing, use grey water or eco-friendly detergents so when hand washing is finished the water can be poured onto the garden (not on edible plants) • If subject to eczema, use sensitive washing products free from artificial fragrances, optical brighteners and enzymes

Table continued next page.

Where	What	How
	Washing machine	• Choose a washing machine with a four star or higher water rating, and a high energy rating • Front loaders are generally more water and energy efficient than top loaders. They also save laundry space, use less detergent and are gentler on clothes • Use the cold wash program in preference to hot wash as this saves energy • Use a high spin cycle to reduce wetness of clothes, this helps them to dry faster • Try out the 'short' cycles for lightly soiled clothes • Only wash when there is a full load • If your machine has a 'sud saver' option, use it. Wash cleaner clothes first, then the dirtiest ones last • Use 'grey water' safe or eco-friendly detergents. This keeps the water suitable for reuse through grey water systems on gardens • If subject to eczema, use sensitive washing products free from artificial fragrances, optical brighteners and enzymes
In the bathroom	Basin taps	• Use water efficient tapware or install a flow restrictor or aerators • If using a mixer tap use the cold side as much as possible. When the tap is positioned in the middle, the water is usually warm which is often not needed when brushing teeth etc. • Use a glass of water to brush teeth rather than run the tap • When shaving put a little warm water in the basin and use that to rinse the razor rather than run the tap
	Shower	• Use water efficient shower heads, a three star model usually provides good water flow • Take shorter showers, keep to three minutes if you can. Use a timer that beeps • Turn the tap off when soaping up and washing hair, turn it on again when rinsing off • Collect water in a bucket when waiting for temperature to be reached and put into the garden afterwards
	Bath	• Minimise the use of the bath (showers are more water efficient when kept to a few minutes) • Do not use flow restrictors here, you'll want a bath to fill up quickly. Only use as much water as you need • Occasionally check the plug isn't leaking • Maximise use of the bath water if you can (if you have young children they could possibly share it) • If using grey water-safe soaps, the water can be reused in the garden (via grey water systems or bucketing it out)

Table continued next page.

Where	What	How

	Toilets	• Install dual flush toilets with a high WELS rating. Opt for four star rating if you can - just 4.5L for a full flush and 3L for a half flush
		• Alternatives to reduce water wastage in toilets that are not dual flush are
		   – Get an empty 1.5L (or similar) plastic drink bottle, fill it with water and place in the cistern. This displaces water and reduces the amount flushed each time
		   – There are products that fit to the button on the toilet to reduce the amount of water released when flushing
		• Check the toilet regularly for leaks. You can do this by putting a drop of food dye into the cistern, which will be visible in the bowl if it's leaking
		• Consider waterless, composting toilets if your council allows them to be installed

Outside	Pools and spas	• Use a cover when not in use. This significantly reduces evaporation, helps keep the pool/spa clean, can reduce chemical needs and saves on filtering • Minimise backwashing on filters and stop as soon as the water is clear • Minimise splashing in the pool to reduce water loss • Use rain water to top up the pool if you can • Check regularly for any leaks • Keep filters clean
	Gardens	• Fix any leaky taps quickly • Install a drip system and water from under the ground. This reduces evaporation losses • Use rain water, recycled water or grey water where you can (see notes on grey water below) • Plant drought tolerant plants • Mulch well to reduce moisture loss from the soil
	Car washing	• Use a bucket and sponge to wash the car and rinse off with a hand held trigger nozzle • Wash vehicles on the lawn if possible • Use a waterless car wash or a commercial car wash that minimises/recycles water use • Don't hose down the driveway, sweep or blow it off instead • If you must use water to wash paving, use a water efficient pressure washer to get it done quickly (don't use this on exposed aggregate)

Table source © Green Moves Australia 2014.

Capture and reuse of water

Here are the systems available for capture and reuse and what you will need to know.

What	About	Comments
Rain water tanks	Can be made from steel, plastic, concrete, flexible plastic bladders. There is a variety of sizes and shapes: round, rectangle, square, fence tanks, barrel, etc. Can be installed above or below ground. Tank plumbing can be 'dry' or 'wet' systems. Tank water can be used for garden watering, pool filling, washing cars, toilet flushing, clothes washing, showering and bathing, drinking (if correctly filtered and safe healthy pH levels are ascertained). **Potential issues:** • Contamination from bird droppings, local pollution and pollutants on roof and in pipes • Breeding of mosquitos in water • If in a bushfire prone area, ash and soot can accumulate on the roof and be washed into the water tanks	**Benefits:** • Provides free water • Can save lots of water in the home • Simple to install and maintain **Install considerations:** • Tanks need to be on a stable base • May need a pump and tap connected • Use a first flush diverter • Use strainers on the inlets to provide additional filtering • Use mosquito proof mesh on all openings • Must have overflows connected to storm water in urban areas • Collection source (e.g. roof, guttering) must be free from lead flashing or soldering **Maintenance:** • Clean filters and guttering regularly • Check for leaks regularly • Sludge build up should be checked every few years. Use a professional for this • If contaminated (through fire ash or similar), completely drain and clean before re-using water, especially if water is used internally in the home

Table continued next page.

What	About	Comments
Grey water systems	Grey water is water collected from laundry, bathroom showers and basins for reuse. Systems can be above or below ground, and can be direct reuse (diversion) or treatment systems. Reused water is suitable for garden watering. If appropriately treated it can be reused for toilet flushing and laundry. **Potential issues:** - High maintenance system that needs regular cleaning - Do not use grey water on food producing plants (unless properly treated) - Grey water reused in the home (toilet/laundry) must be well filtered and disinfected to prevent disease - Don't use grey water if someone in the home is sick Note: there are regulations around the installation and use of grey water systems. Check with your local council to find out what they are and ensure you can comply before you install a grey water unit.	**Benefits:** - Reuses water - Can reduce water bills - Reduces pollution into waterways **Install considerations:** - Size the unit correctly and place close to the outlets being collected - Ensure filters are easy to clean - Plumb into sub surface irrigation (purple piping is used for grey water systems) - If water is going to the garden, use on lawn and flowering plants (not edible plants) **Operational considerations:** - Use grey water safe cleaning products in areas where water is routed to grey water - Use natural cleaning products where you can - Don't dispose of chemicals down the sink, check the Detox Your Home website or local council for disposal information - Grey water must not be stored for more than 24 hours unless appropriately treated - Only use on gardens in dry conditions. Too much grey water can affect plant health - UV or ozone disinfection systems should be used where possible (as opposed to chemical chlorine systems) **Maintenance:** - Clean filters regularly - Clean unit regularly - Check irrigation water outlets regularly to ensure they are not blocked

Table continued next page.

What	About	Comments
Black water systems	Black water is the term used for water from toilets, kitchens, and any other areas that could produce high potential for contamination by pathogens and grease. Systems are generally underground. Black water must be appropriately treated and can only be used outdoors with sub surface irrigation. Note: there are regulations around the installation and use of black water treatment systems. Check with your local council to find out what they are and ensure you can comply with requirements.	**Benefits:** • Reuses all water • Can reduce water bills • Reduces pollution into waterways • If treated by a worm farm, can provide food/water to plants **Operational considerations:** • Use grey water safe cleaning products • Use natural cleaning products where you can • Don't dispose of chemicals down the sinks, toilets or drains feeding the black water system **Maintenance (will depend on system used):** • Check regularly • Maintain in line with suppliers recommendations

Table continued next page.

What	About	Comments
Storm water	Stormwater is rain water or melting snow runoff from a site. It flows into water ways through storm water drains and brings with it harmful pollutants such as oil, rubbish, garden fertilisers, and various sediment that contaminates water ways and damages ecosystems. If building or redesigning your home and landscape consider a Water Sensitive Urban Design (WSUD) which contributes to reducing and filtering water before it reaches the end water way. Note: there are regulations around storm water runoff. Check with your local council to find out what they are and ensure you can comply with requirements.	Ways to reduce the effects of stormwater runoff are: - Capture and store rain water from roof run off - Bin all your litter and ensure bins are securely closed - Pick up after your pets - Put dirty water onto the lawn, garden or down the sink, not into street gutters/drains - Utilise landscaping to encourage more water absorption into the ground by planting more trees and ensure the garden slopes to move the water to storage or filtration areas. - Use berms and vegetated swales to direct and minimise water runoff - Add compost or mulch to help reduce runoff and increase absorption of water - Use organic alternatives to chemical fertilisers and pest control - Use permeable paving on patios or driveways to allow water to soak into the ground - Line impervious surfaces with gravel trenches to catch water and allow it to seep into the ground - Consider a green roof or wall (if appropriate) to capture and filter water - Install a rain garden - Keep pool/spa water away from storm water drains

Table source © Green Moves Australia 2014.

Working towards better onsite water management and water conservation is the responsibility of every individual. By being smarter with our use we can reduce our consumption considerably with little loss of amenity.

A Water Smart Checklist is at the rear of this book. Copy and use it to review your home and start saving water now.

It's quite simple: no fresh water, no food, no life. Our future really is in our hands when it comes to fresh water.

Further information

Australian Water Association (AWA) – **www.awa.asn.au**
Environmental Protection Authority (EPA) – **www.epa.vic.gov.au**
Detox Your Home – **www.sustainability.vic.gov.au/detoxyourhome**
Save Water – **www.savewater.com.au**
Water Rating – **www.waterrating.gov.au**
Website of the Department of Industry. 2013. *Your Home: Australia's guide to environmentally sustainable homes*. 5th edition. March 2014 – **www.yourhome.gov.au**

Renewable energy for the home

There is a growing amount of options - varying in suitability, effectiveness and cost - for those who are looking to generate some, or all, of a home's energy needs. In this section we discuss the four main types of renewable energy available for residential homes. They are solar photovoltaic (PV), wind power, geothermal and micro hydro systems.

Why is it important to consider renewable energy?

Generating your own renewable energy on-site provides many benefits to the home and the environment. These include:

- Reduced energy bills - or no energy bills - depending on the home and size of system installed
- Zero greenhouse gas emissions (less pollution) from energy generated
- Minimal operational costs
- Opportunity to sell energy back to the mains grid (depending on location and connections)
- Opportunity to be totally off grid and independent of energy providers
- Potential to gain immunity from blackouts (dependent on renewable energy system and set up)
- Protection from ongoing energy price rises (risk reduction)
- Increased value of the home
- Feel-good factor that you're doing your bit

What's the down side?

- Initial installation costs can be high with long return on investment

Note that as you progress down this list below, the implementation cost increases. Consider carefully what you want to achieve.

- Reduce your current energy bills by generating some of your energy needs
- Cover all of your energy requirements and aim for no energy bills
- Create a hybrid system where you can store some energy in batteries and use the energy grid as a backup
- Go off grid completely and not be tied to energy providers

Conservation before creation. Before you do anything in relation to installing a renewable energy system, you should conduct an energy assessment of your home and understand what your energy use is, what is using the energy and when you use it. Then, find areas where you can reduce the energy demand (identify energy reduction strategies) and implement changes to reduce your energy use. Once you have the home working efficiently, then look at sizing a renewable energy solution to suit the energy use that you need. This could save you thousands by enabling a smaller sized system to be installed. A suitably qualified home sustainability assessor will be able to assist by providing a thorough energy audit if you prefer to have some professional guidance.

The primary factors determining what will be right for you will depend very much on your location, the local climate and available budget. Below we provide an overview of each type of renewable energy system available and note the things to look out for when choosing onsite renewable energy for your home.

Types of renewable energy systems

- Off-grid. Usually for homes that do not have access or mains electricity supply, most common in rural areas. Homes that run off-grid generally have renewable energy and/or a diesel generator to provide backup energy generation to the home
- Backup, grid connected. Often seen in areas where there are regular power losses. The backup system can be provided through energy stored in batteries that switch on to take up the energy requirements when the grid fails
- Grid connected. These are most common in urban areas as they provide the opportunity to sell the surplus energy back to the mains electricity grid

To find out more about your area's small scale generation connection process and requirements see the Clean Energy Council's website. www.solaraccreditation.com.au/consumers/small-scale-generation-connection.html

Solar PV

Solar is by far the most popular method of home renewable energy in Australia. In April 2013 there was over 1 million homes with solar PV systems installed, providing a total capacity of over 2,452,000 kW of energy (source: Clean Energy Council, SunWiz analysis)

This significant uptake of solar PV has been due to a number of factors including ever-rising energy bills, increasing environmental awareness, the reduced price of solar panels and until recently, the payments for feeding surplus energy back into the grid. At this point, the key drivers for most households to install solar is to reduce energy bills and to be more environmentally responsible.

Solar power has been around for many years and the technology continues to improve and become more cost effective. Solar PV systems simply convert sunlight into electricity. The main components of a solar PV system are the solar panels (of which there are two main types, crystalline or thin film), and the inverter which converts the energy created from direct current (DC) to alternating current (AC) for use in the home. The solar panels are connected to the inverter unit, which is connected to the home's electrical switchboard.

Energy generated is fed to the switchboard, which is then either sent directly to the grid (or a battery system), or used in the home and surplus is sent to the mains grid or a battery system (depending on the installation). Solar PV panels have no moving parts, are very reliable and require little maintenance. Solar panels can be expected to last for 25 years or longer; inverters generally last 15 years or more.

Panels are usually mounted on a roof but can also be mounted on stand-alone/free standing frames, or strategically placed to collect the sun while providing shade or a feature. The amount of energy they can provide will depend on a variety of factors including how much sun they receive, type of panel, amount of shadows or shade on the panels, orientation and number of panels installed. Some systems may need a frame to optimise solar access. Frames, whether on the roof for stand alone, can be fixed, adjustable or track the sun during the day.

Crystalline silicon photovoltaic panels are the most widely used technology on the residential market. They are built using crystalline silicon solar cells and provide a high efficiency. They generally come in rectangular shaped panels with glass over the top, so they are heavy. There are two main types of crystalline cells, mono-crystalline silicon and multi-crystalline silicon. The difference is in how they are manufactured. Mono-crystalline silicon solar cells provide a higher efficiency than multi-crystalline cells. This type of solar panel tends to perform best in cooler temperatures and needs good ventilation between the modules and the supporting structure to maintain efficiency.

Thin film photovoltaic (PV) cells are more flexible than the crystalline panels, however they have a lower output efficiency. They are made by depositing thin layers of photovoltaic material over a substrate of plastic, glass or similar material, and can be more flexible in sizing and mounting options. Technology and efficiency is steadily improving in thin film PV modules.

What to look for

When choosing a solar PV system there are many variables to consider and you should obtain expert advice prior to making a final decision. The main things to look for are:

- Appropriate north facing space – ensure you have enough good solar access that is not shaded by adjoining buildings, trees or other structures
- If panels are to be installed on a roof check the angle or pitch of the north and west facing areas. If the pitch is not ideal for your location you may need a frame installed
- Get the right size system to cater for your requirements
- Match the capacity of the inverter to the panels, if you want to allow for future expansion (adding on more panels) then choose a larger inverter which enables easy installation for additional solar panels later
- Choose good quality solar panels and check the company has a good reputation and is likely to be around for the duration of the warranty. Ask about service and repair (just in case). Warranties are only as good as the company providing them. Panel warranty should be a 20 year minimum, preferably 25 years
- Look for the newly created Positive Quality (PQ) label on the panels. This is a quality certification from the Solar Council of Australia where they have comprehensively tested the product and ensured that it complies with IEC (International Electrotechnical Commission) and Australian standards. The PQ labels should be found on any module that has been audited by the program. You can check the unique code on the website
- Panel guaranteed output. Look for 90 percent over first 10 years; 80 percent over next 15 years
- Installation and workmanship – minimum five year warranty. If that is not provided, ask why they don't back their product
- Inverter warranty – look for 10 years minimum, preferably 15 years
- Ask for recommendations from neighbours, friends and family. Someone is bound to have solar panels on their roof and it's a good way to find out their views and experiences
- Be sure to get a minimum of two quotes for the same system. Ensure that the quotes are providing the same size/type of panels, inverter and installation
- Be wary of providers that make excessive claims and who don't visit the site to conduct a proper site analysis before quoting
- Ensure the inverter is sited out of direct sunlight, has good ventilation and that it is easy to access
- Check if any government incentives still apply. There may be some local incentives available
- Be sure to use a certified installer – see the Clean Energy Council's list of accredited solar PV installers (**www.solaraccreditation.com.au**)

Further information

- If you intend to connect the solar PV system to the electricity grid, download the free Consumer Guide to Buying Household Solar Panels from the Clean Energy Council at **www.solaraccreditation.com.au/consumers/purchasing-your-solar-pv-system.html**
- The Solar Council website has information on the Positive Quality program and a list of products that comply see **www.solar.org.au**
- The Alternative Technology Association also provides a useful selection of buyers guides for solar, visit **www.ata.org.au**

TIP Check what is going to happen to your electricity meter, billing tariff and bill before you have solar panels installed. That way there will be no surprises.

Operational considerations

Solar PV systems are very self-sufficient, however it's worth knowing how to maximise the benefit of your system.

- If you are on a high feed in tariff (the price per kWh you sell energy back to the grid, is higher than the price you pay for it) then schedule household energy intensive jobs (i.e. dishwasher, ironing, washing) for when there is low, or no solar power generation. This enables you to sell more back to the grid maximising potential feed in benefits
- If you are on a low feed in tariff (the price per kWh you sell energy back to the grid is lower than the price you pay for it), then schedule energy intensive household jobs for when there is high solar power generation. This means you are using the energy at the cheaper rate and only drawing what you really need to at the higher price
- If your feed in tariff is the same as the price you pay for it, schedule your energy intensive tasks for during the day. It won't make much difference to your bill but it will reduce the amount of greenhouse gas your household produces

Maintenance

- Always maintain solar systems in line with the manufacturer's recommendations
- Check the output on occasion to ensure there are no faults (do this by checking the output on a sunny day; the inverter will give you this data)
- Give the panels a clean every 6-12 months to optimise efficiency of the panels. Check the manufacturer's recommendations. You could use a soft broom and clean water to gently brush/wash the dirt from the panels
- Check the inverter has good ventilation as they can become quite hot, and ensure inverter vents are clear of insects or other blockages

Health considerations

There are no known health impacts to humans from generating energy from solar PV systems. However if on a roof to clean panels, take proper safety precautions to minimise the risk of falling.

Wind power

Wind power is the term used for the conversion of wind energy into electrical energy. When we think of wind power we generally think of a big propeller on a stick, or windmills. There is a growing variety of wind turbines and while small scale (domestic) wind power is not as price competitive as solar, or as popular, it is growing as a renewable energy option. Wind is occasionally used in rural areas where it is sometimes connected to a solar system for additional energy generation.

Wind power works by the wind spinning the blades which turns a shaft that is connected to a generator, which then produces electricity. Systems generally consist of a rotor blade, a horizontal or vertical axis, a gearbox, generator, a yaw system, tower and grid or battery connection. Battery connections also have a 'dummy load' for removal of excess energy when batteries are fully charged.

Horizontal axis turbines are the most common. Smaller turbines can provide enough energy to power a home or small business. Wind turbines have a lifespan of around 25 years and produce clean renewable energy. They are reliant on wind to operate.

Wind turbines operate best with smooth 'clean' wind which is generally found along coastal and in rural areas of flat land. Air flow in city and urban areas is generally very turbulent and can often be unsuitable for wind power generation.

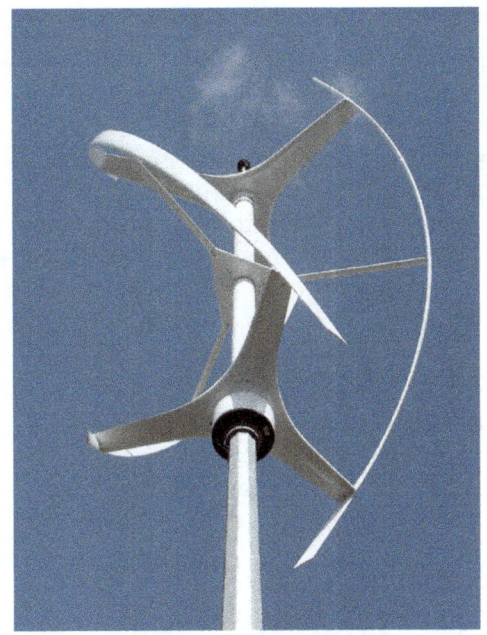

Vertical axis wind turbines.
Image credit: Wind Turbine Zone

Types of wind power

For an urban location, the main difference between vertical axis wind turbines (VAWT) and horizontal axis wind turbines (HAWT) is their response to turbulent winds.

Vertical axis wind turbines (VAWT) are better suited for urban locations, where other buildings and trees cause the wind to be more turbulent (gusty, with severe direction changes).

Horizontal axis wind turbines (HAWT) tend to produce more power with a smaller size, but historically have produced more noise. Technological advances in modern designs have reduced the amount of noise produced.

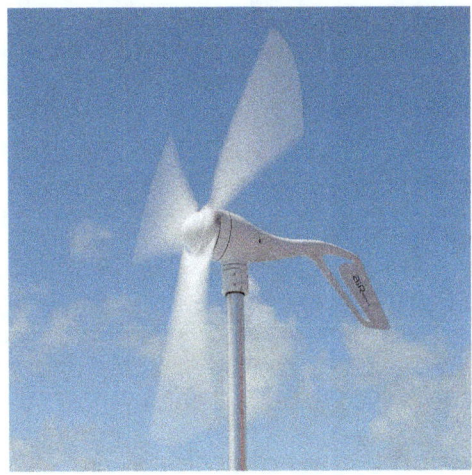

Horizontal axis wind turbines.
Image credit: Wind Turbine Zone

You can normally mount a HAWT higher and get access to faster and smoother air, resulting in more power. Ideally a HAWT should be mounted 10 metres above the height of any obstacle within 500 metres.

Both types of home wind turbine will function better with smooth air, but a VAWT does not need to be rotated to face the wind. Modern wind turbines can produce energy on average between 70 – 85 percent of the time but this is dependent on wind consistency and speed. Turbines can be 'guyed' (supported by guy ropes), attached to a roof or freestanding.

Roof installed systems are available, however they are generally inefficient, have shorter life spans and are unlikely to be financially viable. Be sure to investigate any potential roof system thoroughly before purchasing.

Before you decide to install a wind turbine check the following...

- Check with your local council to find out what local regulations you will need to comply with
- Make sure your site is suitable for wind energy production by having the site properly accessed by a wind assessor and ideally record wind production at the site for at least 12 months
- Determine your home's energy needs (after conducting energy reduction strategies) and look for the right sized system
- Consider if you want to be grid connected or not (if that is an option)
- Consider if the energy generated is to be stored in batteries
- Be sure it is practical and financially viable
- If in an urban area, check with neighbours to see if there are any objections

What to look for

Before you seriously consider a wind generation system you must check the wind maps for your area and ideally monitor the winds for at least 12 months. This will identify if there is enough wind to make the investment viable. See the Bureau of Meteorology's website at **www.bom.gov.au** for wind information.

When considering a wind turbine, look for the following:

- Rated power – the maximum power it is designed to produce. Generally rated in kilowatt hours (kWh)
- Cut in speed – the speed that the turbine blades start to move and produce energy. This can be as low as 4-5 meters per second
- Cut out speed – the speed that the turbine shuts down. Gale force winds, approximately 25 metres per second or higher should trigger a shutdown to protect the turbine from damage. Check the rated speed with the supplier
- Noise – ensure you choose the quietest model you can to minimise disturbance to yourself, neighbours and local animals
- A lightening conductor would be recommended to help protect your wind turbine from lightening damage
- Ask about servicing and maintenance – what parts may need replacing, how often, at what cost (like vehicles, wind turbines have parts that need maintaining)
- Check warranties – industry standard is around five years
- Be sure to use a certified installer endorsed for wind power – see the Clean Energy Council's list of certified small wind installers (**www.solaraccreditation.com.au**)

Operational considerations

As with solar PV, it's worth knowing how to maximise the benefit of your wind power system. Wind energy is a little more complicated because the wind can start and stop during the day and there may not be a straightforward pattern of energy generation. But if you can match appliance use to the generation of energy, you will at the very least reduce the amount of greenhouse gas your home produces.

Things to know if you are grid connected and obtaining a feed-in price:

- If you are on a high feed-in tariff (where the price per kWh you sell energy back to the grid is higher than the price you pay for it) then schedule household energy intensive jobs (i.e. dishwasher, ironing, washing) for when there is little or no wind generating electricity. This enables you to sell more back to the grid, maximising potential feed in benefits.
- If you are on a low feed in tariff (the price per kWh you sell energy back to the grid is lower than the price you pay for it), then schedule energy intensive household jobs for when there is high wind power generation. This means you are using the energy at the cheaper

rate and only drawing what you really need to at the higher price
- If your feed in tariff is the same as the price you pay for it, schedule your energy intensive tasks for when the wind is generating energy. It won't make much difference to your bill but it will reduce the amount of greenhouse gas your household produces

If you have batteries connected, you could consider using any excess energy that may be diverted to a 'dummy load' for heating water or other similar task.

Maintenance

There are several moving parts in a wind turbine that can wear and fail. As a result wind turbine systems will require regular maintenance.

- Ensure you maintain your wind turbine in line with the manufacturer's recommendations. It is likely to be at least an annual service or inspection
- If using 'guy wires' check the wire tension regularly to ensure they are taut
- Position the 'dummy load' where it is out of reach and does not create a risk of fire or explosion
- Check the battery terminals are kept clean, tight and are free of corrosion. Check the electrolyte levels are above the minimum and be sure to use distilled water to top up. Any acid spills should be washed with water and neutralised with sodium bicarbonate
- Batteries may need to be fully charged and drained at specific intervals. Check with the manufacturer and/or installer for proper procedures
- Battery systems may need replacement batteries every 6-10 years (depending on the system and battery). Be sure to dispose of batteries at a battery recycling centre. Your local council or the Detox Your Home website should be able to advise on locations

Health impacts

There have been many concerns relating to the human health impacts of the noise generated by wind turbines ranging from headaches through to cancer. Noise levels from wind turbines have reduced significantly over the years through improved design and sound insulating of mechanical components. However there is still much discussion on potential health implications. There have been several studies conducted, all of which have found that noise level emissions comply with the World Health Organisation (WHO) recommendations for residential areas.

A recent study (March 2014) by the Australian Medical Association found that:

'Domestic and international evidence does not support the theory that infrasound or low frequency sound generated by wind farms causes adverse health effects in people living near them.

'"Individuals residing in the vicinity of wind farms who do experience adverse health or wellbeing, may do so as a consequence of their heightened anxiety or negative perceptions regarding wind farm developments in their area,' said the AMA's position statement."

(Quote from 'The Guardian' **www.theguardian.com/world/2014/mar/17/ama-gives-wind-farms-clean-bill-health**)

There has also been concern about the effect that wind turbines have on birds. To address this, a company in the USA is currently designing a 'bird friendly' wind turbine in an attempt to resolve the issue. It will be interesting to see what they come up with!

TIP Install your wind generator on a tower that is tall enough to ensure you optimise the efficiency of the system by access to good 'clean' wind. Lower towers can significantly reduce the efficiency of a wind turbine due to turbulent wind at lower altitudes.

Further information

- The Alternative Energy Association has a good guide called 'Wind Power, plan your own wind power system' and a 'Small Wind Turbine Buyers Guide' See www.ata.org.au
- Wind Works has some useful guides in wind energy systems – see www.wind-works.org

Geothermal energy

Geothermal energy is a method of using the energy stored in the ground as an energy source for heating, cooling and electricity generation. This section will focus only on electricity generation. Geothermal is slowly gaining in popularity for large scale electricity generation, but currently is cost prohibitive for small scale (residential) generation. The following explains how it works.

Geothermal energy (from Greek roots geo, meaning earth, and thermos, meaning heat) is the energy stored as heat in the earth.

Geothermal power plants use hot water and steam from deep underground, piped up through underground wells. It is used to generate energy through a generator.

Geothermal energy is a good renewable energy source for the following reasons:

- It provides continuous energy
- It is stable and able to provide a long term power base load (not reliant on environmental conditions such as sun, wind and water flow)
- It is very energy efficient
- It's low in greenhouse gas emissions

Geothermal electricity generation on a small scale (for residential market) is very expensive to implement and is currently financially unviable so is yet to be seriously developed in Australia.

Refer to the AGEA for more information - **www.agea.org.au**

Micro hydro

If you have a property that is close to continuous flowing water, typically a river, and ideally a hill, then a micro hydro unit may be suitable. A micro hydro unit works by using the energy of flowing water to create electricity. Properly maintained, micro hydro systems can have a lifespan of up to 50 years.

The process operates by water being collected into a pool, dam or tank which ideally has a high 'head' to assist with creating better water pressure. When released, the water uses gravity to flow downhill through a pipe creating water pressure, depending on the height of the head. At the end of the pipe is a turbine. The force of the water going through the turbine turns a generator that generates electricity.

Why consider a micro hydro system?

There are some micro hydro systems working around Australia but they are not very popular due to the lack of appropriate sites and water. However, if you have a continuous flow of water and an appropriate site there are reasons to consider one.

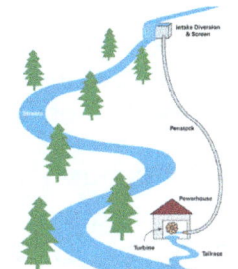

- They can provide continuous power, and can be used to pump water as well as generate electricity
- They are very cost effective and very reliable
- They provide a renewable and low impact energy source

Image credit: www.leparcpronto.com.br

What's the downside?

- Water routing and cabling costs can be difficult to estimate
- Water supply can vary during seasons which can affect generation
- No water flow, no power

If your situation provides this option, be sure to consult a certified installer and micro hydro designer to assess household power needs, flow rates and suitability before making any decisions. You can find a certified installer endorsed for micro-hydro at the Clean Energy Council's list of installers (www.solaraccreditation.com.au)

There are two types of micro hydro turbines that can cater for most needs: reaction turbines, which are submerged into the river; and impulse turbines, which are located away from the main water course. Water is moved through a pipe in to and out of the turbine which can be some distance from the main water course.

What to look for

If you happen to have a suitable supply of running water and the right topography to facilitate a micro hydro system it can be a very affordable source of renewable energy. You will need a good flow rate and high 'head' for the water to fall from.

- **Flow rate** – the rate of flow of the water which is measured in litres per second. Tests should be done to check the flow rate of the water supply to ensure it is adequate for micro hydro. Generally the greater the flow rate the better it will be for producing energy
- **Head** – this is the height that water is stored and gravity fed through the pipes. The higher the head, the more pressure you will have as the water falls and the greater the force on the turbine blades, resulting in more energy generation

If you have a suitable site, flow rate and head availability, then

- Ensure you choose robust pipes and install appropriately
- Protect the pipes from sun, landslides and other physical damage

Operational considerations

- Site the turbine away from the home as the noise from the turbine may cause some disturbance

Maintenance

- Check water intake systems are clear of debris that could reduce water flow

- Check the pipes regularly for damage and leaks and ensure anchors are secure
- Service the generator in line with manufacturers recommendations (bearings will need checking and lubricating)
- Check electrical connections occasionally for signs of corrosion

Health considerations

- Ensure the generator unit is placed far enough away from the home to minimise noise disruption
- The ecosystem health is maintained as the water is returned back to the source

Before making the decision to go micro hydro, ensure you get expert advice and guidance on the suitability of the situation and the energy generation potential.

The final word – remember to

- Check the company's credentials
- Review testimonials and online reviews
- Ask for referral customers to speak with before making your final decision
- Ask friends and family who have similar systems installed, who they used and what their experience has been

Combination and co-generation systems for the home.

Combination and co-generation systems are entering the residential market place and can offer some good alternatives.

Solar systems are now available that are integrated into roof structures and can produce not only solar power, but hot water too. These are very efficient as the water running through the panels reuses the heat generated from the PV cells to warm the water. This helps to cool the panels, making them more efficient. Some are available as integrated roofing systems and expandable as the budget becomes available.

CSIRO is currently testing a solar unit that provides heat, cooling and hot water to a home. There is more on this in the section on Mechanical Cooling.

Personal power plants (co-generation – or Co GEN)

These systems usually use gas as an input fuel to create both heat (re-used for hot water) and electricity simultaneously (cogeneration). It is possible to configure systems to also provide cooling, which are called tri-generation systems. These types of system are becoming very popular in the larger scale commercial world, but are not very common yet for residential use. Although not powered by a renewable fuel, gas produces significantly less greenhouse gas emissions than grid supplied energy, which is generally sourced from coal fired power stations.

These systems are approximately the size of a medium sized washing machine, sit outside the home and are connected to mains gas. Source: www.cfcl.com.au/Assets/Files/BlueGen_Launch_Information_(Web)_May-2009.pdf

> **Further information**
> - Clean Energy Council at www.cleanenergycouncil.org.au/cec.html
> - The Australian Geothermal Energy Association www.agea.org.au
> - The Clean Energy Council at www.solaraccreditation.com.au
> - The Alternative Technology Association at www.ata.org.au
> - CSIRO at www.csiro.org.au
> - Your Home manual from www.yourhome.gov.au

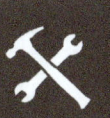

Livable housing

The importance of safety manifests itself in how homes are being designed. Catering for the safety of children and being easily accessed by friends and family regardless of physical ability are now seen as integral to the design progress. This is achieved by simple things implemented at the build stage and which are expensive to change later – for example, the width of doors and corridors.

Such forethought during the build process provides the option for a family to stay in their home longer and creates an environment where safety and mobility are effectively 'built in'. Livable homes are specifically designed to be easily and cost effectively adaptable into a safe and easily accessible house when the need arises.

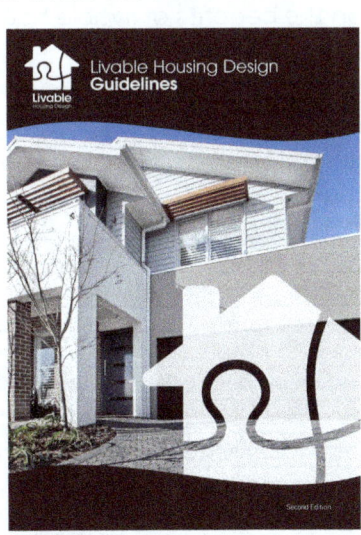

The Livable Housing Design Guidelines compiled by Livable Housing Australia (LHA) is based on universal design principles and is an excellent resource for those building or renovating who might want to 'build in' longevity and accessibility. It provides a room by room guide on what to include and how to do it in order to maximise the livability potential of a home into the future.

Electronic copies of the guide can be freely downloaded from the Livable Housing website at **www.livablehousingaustralia.org.au/**. There is also a free LHA app available.

A livable home is designed and built to meet the changing needs of occupants across their lifetime. It is also easier to enter, easier to navigate in and around and capable of simple and cost-effective adaptation.

Livable homes benefit people from all walks of life including:

- Families with young children
- People with temporary injury
- Ageing baby boomers
- People with disability and their families

The guidelines detail sixteen livable design elements. Each element provides guidance on the performance expected to achieve silver, gold or platinum level accreditation.

These performance levels are voluntary and can be applied to all new homes and dwellings. They range from basic requirements through to best practice in livable home design.

Silver

Contains eight core livable housing design elements and focuses on key structural and spatial elements that are critical to ensure future flexibility and adaptability of the home. Incorporating these features will avoid more costly home modification if required at a later date.

Gold

Enhanced requirements for most of the core livable housing design elements plus additional elements. Gold level provides more generous dimensions for most of the core livable housing design elements and introduces additional elements in areas such as the kitchen and bathroom. There are a total of thirteen design elements in this category.

Platinum

Further enhanced requirements for the core livable housing design elements plus all remaining elements. There are sixteen elements featured in the platinum level. This level describes design elements that would better accommodate aging in place and people with mobility needs. Platinum requires more generous dimensions for most of the core livable design elements and introduces additional elements for features such as the living room and flooring.

A summary of each levels requirements are noted in the table below.

We do not intend to reproduce the Livable Housing Guidelines here, but aim to spread the word on the benefits of livable housing design and promote the benefits that this voluntary certification offers.

For more information see the LHA website at www.livablehousingaustralia.org.au where you will find information on what is involved in getting a home certified, case studies of certified projects and a list of LHA registered assessors.

	Design Element	Silver	Gold	Platinum
1	There is a safe, continuous, level and step-free path of travel from the street entrance and/or parking area to your home's entrance.	✓	✓	✓
2	There is at least one step-free entrance into your home.	✓	✓	✓
3	Where access to your home is through the car park, the parking space has been designed to ensure you can fully open your car doors and move around the vehicle with ease.	✓	✓	✓
4	Internal doors and corridors facilitate comfortable and unimpeded movement between spaces.	✓	✓	✓
5	A toilet on ground or entry level supports easy access for both home occupants and visitors.	✓	✓	✓
6	The bathroom and shower has been designed for easy and independent access for everyone in your home.	✓	✓	✓
7	The bathroom and toilet walls are built to enable grab rails to be installed in the future.	✓	✓	✓
8	Stairways are designed to reduce the likelihood of injury and also enable future adaptation.	✓	✓	✓
9	The kitchen space has been designed to support ease of movement and to support e3asy adaptation.	○	✓	✓
10	The laundry space has been designed to support ease of movement and to support easy adaptation.	○	✓	✓
11	There is a space on the ground or entry level that can be used as a bedroom.	○	✓	✓
12	Light switches and power points are easy for everyone in your home to reach and operate.	○	✓	✓
13	Handles and hardware on doors and tapware have been designed to make them easy for you to open and close.	○	✓	✓
14	The family/living room features clear space to enable you to move in and around the room with ease.	○	○	✓
15	Windows sills are installed at a height that enables you to view the outdoor space from either a seated or standing position.	○	○	✓
16	Floor coverings are slip resistant to reduce the likelihood of slips, trips and falls in the home.	○	○	✓

Source: Livable Housing Design Guidelines.

Adaptable homes

Another area often overlooked is adaptability for future changes, specifically in terms of up sizing and downsizing as family structures change. Imagine a home where the walls can be moved to create more space, or added to separate an area depending on current needs. Imagine that the kitchen can be moved outside for a party and returned in the morning or where a home can be literally split into two homes with a few simple changes. This is true 'adaptability' in structure.

Elements that can be designed in to make a home more adaptable include:

- Easy extension and addition of rooms
- Designing in removable walls (that are non-loadbearing) to facilitate opening up of areas can assist with creating better manoeuvrability
- Inclusion of moveable kitchens (this is very common in Europe)
- If multi-level access is likely to be needed in the future, allow for a vertical shaft so that a lift could be installed between floors. Alternatively, allow enough space for a chair lift to be retrofitted to stairs

Other adaptability ideas include the 'whole home'. We're referring specifically to homes being built that provide for large families, and which also allow the home to be 'split up' (or downsized) once the children have left. With careful original design, a home can be designed so that it can easily be separated into two separate residences. This enables the newly created home to be either rented out or potentially sold in the future (depending on local state and council laws). It also facilitates aging parents to stay in the family home and in a local community where they are comfortable, for longer and without the pressure of a large home to maintain.

We tend to move house because our families and circumstances change. This can be very expensive both financially and to the environment. With a little forethought and careful design, we can create comfortable, efficient homes, which are also highly adaptable; homes that are designed to be flexible from the start and that can provide comfort, efficiency and longevity easily.

Sustainability

Homes that are livable and adaptable provide for sustainability in a variety of ways. They provide for:

- Current needs of the household
- Unexpected and future needs of the household
- Extended use of a family home maximising use of resources used

Health benefits

- Homes that are livable and assessable contribute to a safer, more comfortable living environment, with lower risk of falls
- Contribute to more stable communities
- Relieve the stress of 'having to move'

Further information

Livable Housing Design Guidelines - www.livablehousingaustralia.org.au

Government of South Australia, 2014, Design Guidelines for sustainable housing and livable neighbourhoods, 7/4/14, http://dcsi.sa.gov.au/__data/assets/pdf_file/0005/6386/Design-Guide-2_3.pdf

Australian Network for Universal Housing Design at www.anuhd.org

Wendy A Jordan, 2008, Universal Design for the Home, Massachusetts, Quarry Books

Your Home manual from www.yourhome.gov.au

Tips for building or renovating a sustainable, healthy wet zone

Design for life, not just for now. Where possible, create open spaces that will cater for occupants of all ages and mobility. Create spaces that can easily adjust with occupant needs. We never know what life will throw at us - should a family member need to use mobility aids such as a wheelchair or walking frame or support when showering, good design will have this covered.

Universal design structural considerations easily included in the design phase, will eliminate the need for renovations/additional expenditure should occupants' access needs change.

Basic accessible/universal design considerations:

- Create open plan spaces to allow for movement
- Include minimal door widths of 820mm
- Avoid narrow hallways
- Ensure structural framework is installed within wall cavities that will cater for lifestyle aids if required
- Mount handles and switches at heights suitable for walking adults, children and those in a wheelchair
- Avoid variations in floor heights
- Maximise natural light and ventilation in bathrooms - use windows and operable skylights for light and airflow to minimise stagnant moisture that can contribute to mould and structural impairments
- Choose window frames in wet areas with care – water/moisture and timber frames are not a good mix, unless well sealed and maintained. Opt for frames that cannot absorb moisture (e.g. thermally broken aluminium), minimise maintenance and avoid the health issues and expense of moisture damage
- Ensure an exhaust fan is installed near potential sources of moisture, such as showers in bathrooms and attached to drying appliances in laundries. Vent the fan out to the exterior of the home. Do not vent extraction fans into the ceiling cavity as this may contribute to moisture damage or mould growth in the roof space. Importantly, place the switch for the fan in a convenient location so it will be used
- Wet areas zoned together within the building will reduce use of plumbing materials and minimise heat loss when water is transported

- When designing wet areas such as shower alcoves or surfaces containing taps, consider ways to minimise broken surfaces e.g. joints or grout lines. During the design phase explore large format material options that will work with the dimensions of the space such as glass, stone slabs and large format tiles. If choosing tiles opt for rectified or laser cut tiles which allow for minimal grout lines
- Design the shower recess to be seamless with the floor. This is a beautiful and functional element of a bathroom. It is easier to clean and will facilitate access for family and friends who may require mobility aids
- For surface applications, opt for adhesives, grouts and gap products that are low emission and have environmentally friendly attributes. These will minimise the impact of VOCs on the indoor air, be better for the environment and are a healthier option for your tradespeople to use and for you to live with. Grout products that contain mould resistant additives will help prevent mould growing in the grout over time, which if left untreated can compromise indoor air quality and impact on personal health. When choosing grout products look for colour consistent attributes to avoid the grout discolouring over time as this will impact on appearance and will induce replacement
- Avoid design trends as the space will become dated aesthetically before the materials need replacing. Minimising the reasons for renovating will be a saving into the future and better for the environment
- Design styles that are simple or have classic appeal used with materials in neutral tones will be a long term asset. Use accessories to add a touch of trend, such as light fittings, towels, plants and artwork as these are easily altered without significant cost

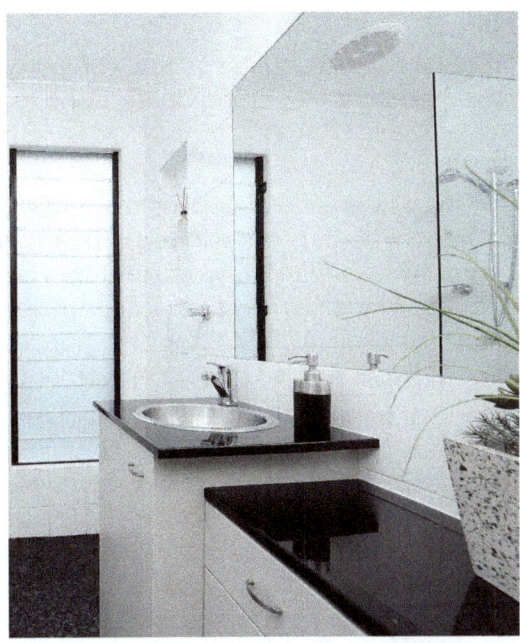

Image supplied by Healthy Interiors

Task lighting

- Placement of lighting in bathrooms is important to prevent shadowing which can make detailed tasks like makeup application and shaving a challenge. Placing lighting at the top of the mirror helps to minimise shadows on your face. Be careful of creating glare; translucent white diffusers are a good option to avoid this problem. Refer to the Lighting section for more detail on bathroom lighting

Insulation

- Select your insulation as required for your thermal needs. Bathrooms and laundries can be noisy spaces. When choosing insulation, opt for a product that insulates while minimising noise transmission, is free from harmful chemicals and potentially harmful fibres

Cabinets
- Opt for E0 board products for new cabinetry. If the reuse of old cabinets is an option these can be updated by replacing doors, handles and/or tops to give them a contemporary look

Tapware
- During the design phase appliances and water ware are usually selected to ensure that structural elements are designed around these items appropriately. Tapware carries the water we use to drink, wash and bathe in so it's important to use products that meet Australian standards. Choose water efficient appliances. If the one you like is not water efficient, install a flow restrictor to enhance efficiency. Use tapware with easy to turn handles to facilitate use if hand movement is restricted
- The world of online sales has opened up many opportunities for bargains. However, cheap imports may use untested metals or plastics, and may leach contaminants into the water. Ineffective tapware can also be costly to replace and if faulty can cause costly moisture damage to surface and structural materials. When choosing tapware, quality fittings are essential. Opt for tapware with metal internal and external components rather than plastic. Metal internal components are more durable. Some water ware products such as adjustable shower rails may contain other plastic parts; often the hoses are made from flexible PVC. Chemical migration from plastics is often induced by heating; hot water and some plastics are not an ideal mix. Many manufacturers do not test for chemical migration from their plastic products into the water. If independent testing or reports are not available, it's best to avoid a potential concern where possible
- When choosing products for your wet areas such as tapware, sanitary ware or whitegoods, look for the Water Efficiency Labelling Scheme (WELS) rating. Water ware that has been rated by WELS will help you select water efficient products saving you future dollars on water usage. Read more about this in the Appliances section

Drainage
- Many architectural waste outlets look great when new, yet can contribute to drainage issues and become a cleaning nightmare. Some of the long shower grate waste outlets become tangled with hair and covered in a slimy film from shower products and are difficult to clean. Waste outlets that are difficult to clean or easily trap particles can build up nasty unhealthy bacteria. Waste outlets that are easily blocked also risk restricting water elimination and flooding. Design with prevention in mind and opt for waste outlets that can fulfil their purpose. People with long hair should have a minimum 100mm waste outlet in the shower to prevent long hair blocking the waste pipe. Opting for an easy to clean waste cover is also preferable
- Consider the use of a grey (used water) water collection system which can redirect grey water to the garden (must be treated for laundry and toilet reuse!)
- For material selection tips read more in the Materials and Finishes section

Tips for building or renovating a sustainable, healthy kitchen

Kitchens are one of the home's most expensive and frequented zones. A lifestyle that embraces sustainability and health needs a supportive kitchen design.

Create a space that avoids trends and fashion, a zone that will appeal throughout the years.

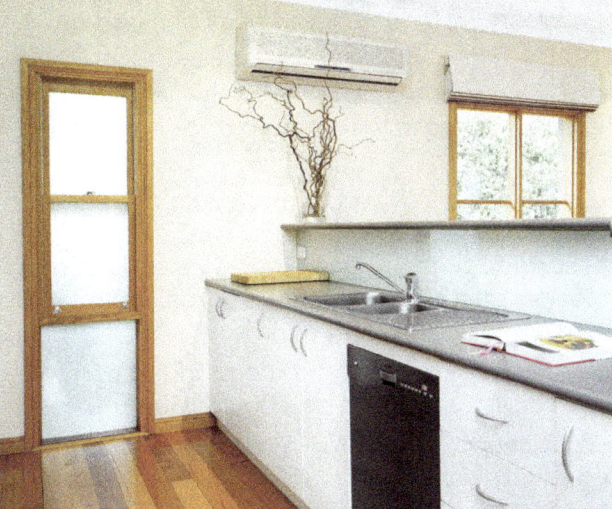

Image supplied by Healthy Interiors

- Use trend accessories that can easily be changed to alter the mood of the kitchen
- When designing a kitchen floorplan, integrate a window for natural light, ventilation and assistance for air extraction if needed, such as when cooking
- Opt for low emission (E0) board for cabinetry carcasses and doors
- Buying a second hand kitchen may be an option for those with creative flair. The reuse of carcass cabinets (internal cabinet framing) is a great way to save money. Used cabinets can be easily upgraded with new doors, handles and benchtop
- Consider future storage requirements for appliances, cookware, utensils, crockery, glassware and food (bulk food buying can save you money)
- Create a space to store your recycling materials, such as rubber bands, plastic cartons, paper rolls, bread clips, glass jars etc.
- Items can be reused for artwork, storage in the shed, craft activities, in the garden or given to the local school or kindergarten art department. Without adequate storage for such items, recycling can be a challenge. A supportive sustainable design makes embracing sustainable practices easy and rewarding
- Design in a waste recycling station and compost bin close to food preparation so organics and recycling waste can be easily separated and utilised
- Opt for quality hardware to minimise replacement. When the day comes that the kitchen is eventually replaced, good hardware should see the product capable of being used somewhere else such as a garage or work area
- Consider the layout style. Straight lines of cabinetry without corners make carcasses easier to reuse at a later date. Corner cabinets are also harder to access and not as user friendly in the kitchen
- Use drawers instead of cupboards where possible as they are easier to access. Pantries or a butler's pantry (small room) are also great options as they can allow for maximum storage with minimal materials and are a good use of space

- When designing cabinet sizes consider appliance sizes and future issues that may arise with an appliance change. There are no 'standard' refrigerator sizes, which can pose a problem if a fridge fails or if a new occupant moves in with a different fridge size. Consider placing a cabinet module next to the fridge that can be easily removed or adjusted without having a major impact on cabinetry
- Ensure appliance specifications are referred to when designing a kitchen so that required space is allowed for around appliances. This is of particular importance with ventilation space around refrigerators as this can have an impact on the unit's efficiency and warranty
- Create lighting zones on separate switches to minimise lights being used when not necessary. Consider task lighting and ambient lighting needs. See the Light section for more information
- Are any materials available that could be reused in the kitchen such as old kitchen carcasses, timbers, bricks or stone? Combining old with new pieces can give a unique style and charm to a new space. Reusing pieces from a home incorporates some history into the design; alternatively salvage yards can provide feature architectural pieces that have shown they stand the test of time
- Second-hand sinks can often be found at commercial second hand kitchen retailers or through online sites such as eBay or Gumtree
- When choosing a benchtop material, consider the size needed and the material supply size. Designing a layout to utilise material sizes reduces wastage. Fix the benchtop with screws and mechanical methods. This makes it easy to remove later for reuse and minimises glues and adhesive used in the area (minimising VOCS)
- When applying a flooring treatment, extend this wall-to-wall under cabinets so that if cabinets are removed or redesigned at a later stage flooring does not need to be altered
- Opt for low emission paints and coatings
- Buy an effective rangehood to remove combustion pollutants. When choosing this item consider the noise factor as they are less likely to be used if noisy. Compare the extraction rate (rate at which air is removed): the higher the better. Compare units that have single or dual fan capacity. Dual fans offer the option to use half of the rangehood when using a small section of a cooktop, which also reduces the operational noise. Choose a unit that has a fan cover that is easy to remove and clean as blocked grills will prevent the unit from operating efficiently
- Choosing quality over quantity for products and finishes in the kitchen will minimise replacement issues and costs; better for your bank balance and community landfill
- There are many additional design considerations to create a universally designed, sustainable home. Refer to the Livable Housing Guidelines and resources list for further information

Further information

Design Ideas for Accessible Homes Publication, Building Commission, Victoria 2002 – www.buildingcommission.com.au

Livable Housing Australia – www.livablehousingaustralia.org.au – Publication: *Livable Housing Design Guidelines*

Water Efficiency Labelling and Standards – www.waterrating.gov.au

WELS product database – www.waterrating.gov.au/consumers

Site health tips

Asbestos

Asbestos is a potentially deadly, naturally occurring substance that is mined and processed into a material that was used to make many products for the construction industry, until it was banned in the late 1980s.

There are two main types of asbestos.

Chrysotile asbestos, also known as white asbestos, and

Amphibole asbestos, of which there are several types, including amosite (known as brown asbestos), crocidolite (known as blue asbestos), tremolite, actinolite and anthophylite.

According to the Australian Government's Asbestos Safety and Eradication Agency, Australia was one of the highest per capita users in the world in the 20th century:

An estimated one third of homes built between 1945 and the late 1980s may contain asbestos in areas such as ceilings, internal walls, roofs, eaves, external cladding, wet areas and vinyl floor tiles. Asbestos was also included in products such as brake pads, gaskets and seals, pipes and pipe lagging.

Asbestos can be found in a range of products in existing houses built before the late 1980s. Asbestos is dangerous when the fibres are disturbed and become airborne which can then be inhaled into the lungs.

Australia has the highest reported per capita incidence of asbestos-related disease in the world, including mesothelioma. There is no known cure, and treatment is about managing the symptoms.

When undertaking a renovation to an older home an asbestos assessment must be done by a professional to identify asbestos risk and have it professionally and safely removed. When selecting an assessor or removalist ensure they are licensed. For details of licensed professionals contact the work health and safety regulators in your state or territory.

Even though there is a ban in Australia for the sale, use and importation of products containing asbestos, there have been cases where such products have been found to have asbestos in them (this is a great reason to buy Australian made products). If you have concerns about a product or material you can have it tested by a National Association of Testing Authorities (NATA) accredited laboratory (visit **www.nata.asn.au**).

TIP — If you are living in an older house and you have not had an asbestos assessment done, please do so. Simply drilling a hole into an asbestos wall to hang a picture could expose you to asbestos.

Radon

The American Cancer Society defines radon as a colourless, odourless, radioactive gas which:

'...forms naturally from decay of radioactive elements, such as uranium, which are found at different levels in soil and rock throughout the world.

Radon gas in the soil and rock can move into the air and into ground water and surface water. Radon breaks down (decays) into solid radioactive elements called radon progeny. Radon progeny can attach to dust and other particles and can be breathed into the lungs. As radon and radon progeny in the air break down, they give off alpha particles, a form of high-energy radiation that can damage the DNA inside the body's cells'.

The Australian Radiation Protection and Nuclear Safety Agency (ARPANSA) reported after a nationwide survey of radon in homes:

'The results show that the average concentration of radon in Australian homes is about 11 Bq m-3. This is less than in many other countries (global average indoor value 40Bq m3) and is not much larger than radon levels in outside air.

'Consequently, there is little cause for concern that the health of the population is at undue risk from radon in homes. However, the survey also found a very wide range of radon levels, from one or two becquerels [Bq] per cubic metre to over four hundred. For those homes having very high concentrations of radon, it may be desirable to take action to reduce the radon levels, in order to reduce the risk of the occupants contracting lung cancer' (ARPANSA, Fact Sheet 2012)

Where homes have elevated levels of radon most of the gases usually get into the interior through the floor. According to the National Health and Medical Research Council (NHMRC) if the annual average radon concentration in a home exceeds 200Bq m3, the homeowner should contact their appropriate radiation health authority.

A radon map of Australia is available from ARPANSA indicating the average indoor radon levels for each postcode – **www.arpansa.gov.au/radiationprotection/Factsheets/is_RadonMap.cfm**

For further information visit **www.arpansa.gov.au**

TIP: For homes with elevated radon levels increasing the ventilation of sub floor spaces can assist to reduce interior levels. Homes built on slabs with elevated levels may need more complex remedies.

Lead

Lead is a heavy metal used in manufacturing batteries, alloys, plastics and protective coatings. Airborne lead from smelting, industrial smokestacks and fumes from burning leaded gases can also contribute lead contamination to air and soil.

There are many industries that have or still do use lead for different purposes, such as plumbing materials (PVC, solder, flashing), mechanical trades, painters, lead lighting, fishing (lead weights),

PVC materials (lead used to make some PVC), fuel, ammunition industries and cosmetics. If the history of your home's property has been subjected to lead, soil testing is advised.

According to the WHO:

'Lead is toxic to the nervous system, the gastrointestinal system, the haematopoietic system (blood making organs), the skeleton, the cardiovascular system, the kidneys and the reproductive system. Signs and symptoms vary with dose and at a given dose by age.'

Lead poisoning has been associated with hyperactivity, behavioural disturbances, learning disabilities, anorexia, anaemia, abdominal pain, seizures, slowed growth and hearing problems. It is considered a neurotoxic pollutant and has been linked to a range of health issues; children and pregnant women are particularly vulnerable. People can get lead into their bodies by breathing or swallowing lead dust.

The NHMRC advises that Australians should have a blood lead level below 10μg/dL.

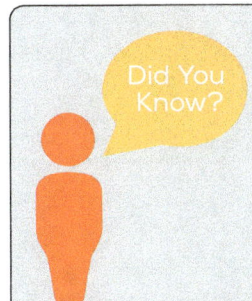

Did You Know? Children six years old and younger are most susceptible to the effects of lead. Lead can accumulate in the body over time. If you have any concerns about lead exposure, talk with your GP and request a blood test.

If you are planning to renovate old painted surfaces of a home such as pre-loved windows and doors, metal trims, walls or painted décor items, ensure you test the surfaces using a lead test kit first. Test kits can be purchased from the local hardware store or you can contact organisations such as The LEAD group - **www.lead.org.au** which offers a comprehensive service for test kits and support.

It is important to know that lead based painted surfaces that are in good condition are not hazardous. Although as the surface deteriorates, lead dust can be generated and is considered a health hazard.

In old homes lead dust can also be found in roof spaces that have collected dust over the years as a result of vehicle emissions.

In the USA, lead contamination is taken so seriously that there are specialised lead removal companies. If you find you need to work on items that are contaminated with lead, ensure you follow safe removal instructions supplied by the relevant authorities or specialised organisations. In Australia, contact:

The Department of Sustainability, Environment, Water, Population and Communities at **www.environment.gov.au**

Australian Dust Removalists Association at **www.adra.com.au**

The LEAD Group - **www.lead.org.au**

Site drainage

Consider the levels of the building site and drainage. Make enquiries with your local council to check if the site is subject to flooding. Examine levels and ensure a drainage assessment has been done and adequate site drainage is implemented as part of any design considerations. Inadequate site drainage and levels that permit moisture accumulation can contribute to structural moisture damage and mould issues.

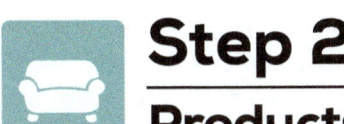

Step 2
Products & furnishings – interior materials

Our home – a big mixing bowl of ingredients

The modern Australian home has evolved and there is an ever-increasing range of products we can choose from, to furnish and decorate with. There are currently two main household issues that Australian families are faced with that have the potential to impact family health.

1. Chemicals used to create the products we are building and filling our homes with
2. Consequences of energy efficiency design changes to Australian housing and indoor air

As we mentioned earlier there are around 38,000 chemicals approved for use in Australia which are used to create products, not forgetting products that are imported using chemicals approved by other countries.

There are many products created and sold that use chemicals that are known to be harmful to health, yet which contain no warning, and in many cases no product labelling. By contacting the consumer hotline number on the back of some cleaning products, insecticides or personal care products and requesting a material safety data sheet you will gain an insight into what you are using and the associated health risks. However, detailed labels for many building materials, household items and furnishings are largely unavailable.

In cooler climates families are being encouraged to seal homes as much as possible to achieve greater energy efficiency. Being an energy efficient consumer is advisable and beneficial, however when restricting passive ventilation we then need to follow through with minimising pollutants (volatile organic compounds, or VOCs) that are trapped inside our houses.

Indoor air quality is a health concern that is well documented but not publicised by national and global organisations. Construction materials, paints, stains, fabrics, carpets, furniture, foams, heating, and household products all contribute VOCs into our household air. Toxicity varies with the product and unfortunately we do not have sufficient labelling laws in Australia to inform consumers about the chemicals used in the manufacturing process, or emissions testing (air quality) data on labels.

Toxicity and VOCs are not necessarily related. Low VOC does not necessarily mean lower toxicity than a high VOC coating or vice versa. Toxicity depends on the type of solvent or ingredients used and the proportion of these ingredients in a product.

This chapter is focused on highlighting health considerations of material selections. Here you will find questions to ask before you buy and issues to consider when shopping so that you can make informed decision about the materials and products you do and don't want to live with.

This section will help guide you in your decision making. **It is really important to remember that we inhale, ingest and absorb things that we come into contact with.** Although this sounds simple it is often forgotten and should be remembered whenever we are shopping.

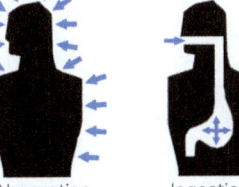
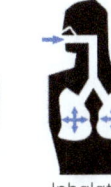

Absorption   Ingestion   Inhalation

From the ground up there are decisions to be made about materials used in a home. One product at a time we make decisions about products we use to build, decorate, furnish and live with. Many products we buy today are made with chemicals that have not been tested in relation to human health.

Our home is a place where we spend a significant amount of time and contains thousands of products, each potentially containing chemicals/pollutants to which we are being exposed. The attitude of 'a little won't do any harm' may not necessarily be true when we consider the culmination of pollutants in the home – a big mixing bowl of ingredients!

A great place to start when examining a home's health is with the foundations and structural elements of the building.

Structural framing – timber vs steel

The environmental impacts and benefits of timber verses steel is a contentious issue.

Steel is the world's most recycled material yet timber is one of the world's most renewable resources.

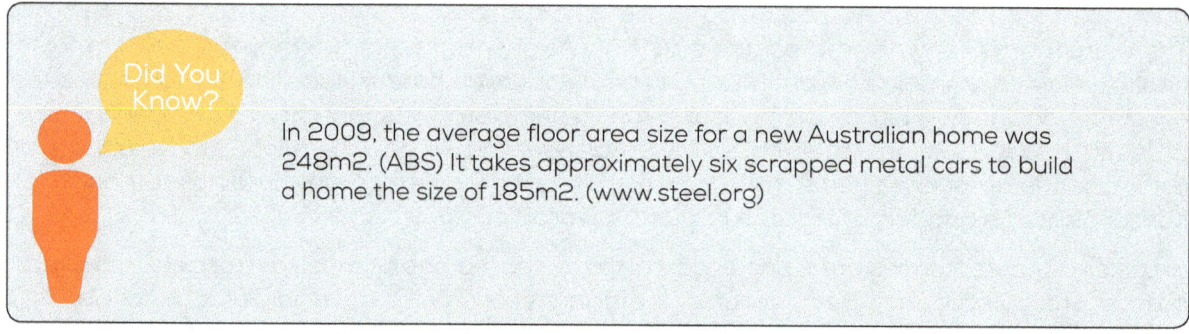

Did You Know?

In 2009, the average floor area size for a new Australian home was 248m2. (ABS) It takes approximately six scrapped metal cars to build a home the size of 185m2. (www.steel.org)

From a very basic resource perspective we can consider the energy used to create steel products (embodied energy). This includes collection of raw materials, processing of these materials and the manufacturing required to create the product. Steel has a very high embodied energy. In comparison, timber framing uses significantly less embodied energy than steel.

Building biologists have expressed concerns regarding the connection between metals and magnetic fields in the home and the impacts on human health. This is a subject worthy of further exploration for anyone considering a steel framed home.

From a health and environmental perspective timber is a great choice, having many attributes that we often take for granted such as strength, light weight, ease of use, it can be recycled or upcycled and it's a material that breathes. Timber also contributes to the fight against climate change by absorbing carbon dioxide.

Sustainable timber

When selecting timber for your project whether it's for structural purposes, furniture or decorative purposes, there are some important considerations beyond aesthetics to be addressed.

The initial question is, will you buy a local timber species or imported timber product?

Buying local products has many benefits over imported species. Apart from supporting local business and jobs, local products use far less energy. Think about the extra manufacturing time, resources and costs needed to prepare timber for large scale and distance transportation. From a health perspective some imported timbers require fumigation before entering the country, exposing the product to pesticides, whereas local species do not undergo fumigation when used locally as the kiln drying process is sufficient.

Buying sustainable timber will help preserve the health and functions of global forests, which inevitably has a positive impact on our health. Trees are the lungs of the earth, they clean our air and provide us with oxygen to breathe. Many communities and people rely on responsible forestry and fair trade for their livelihood and quality of life.

Responsible forest management schemes provide independent verification that timber is sourced from responsibly managed forests. These schemes provide resources for tracing products from the forest origin through the supply chain to the end customer to ensure independent assessment of good forestry practice. Certification of this process is called 'chain of custody'.

There are two significant international schemes to look for when purchasing timber products:

The Forest Stewardship Council® (FSC®) www.au.fsc.org

FSC® is an international, non-profit organisation founded in 1993 by environmentalists, social interest groups, responsible retailers and leading forest companies to develop standards for responsible forest management. FSC® makes sure that environmental, social and economic needs are balanced, and that long-term and healthy forest management plans are put into practice.

To find products or suppliers that are FSC® Certified you can check **the www.info.fsc.org** international database or the FSC® Australia website **www.au.fsc.org** and click on the 'Buy FSC® Certified' section. Products should also be labelled with the FSC® logo.

PEFC

The Program for the Endorsement of Forest Certification (PEFC) is a not-for-profit global certification system, the 'world's largest forest certification system with standards that seek to transform the way forests are managed globally and locally.' To find products or suppliers that are PEFC certified you can check the **www.pefc.org** international information register and look for the logo on the product.

The Australian Forestry Standard (AFS) is an Australian registered certifying body and is also the PEFC national governing body for Australia. According to the Australian Forestry Standard the world is losing millions of hectares of forest each year. For more information about the certification standards visit **www.forestrystandard.org.au** and watch the video called 'Going bush explains forest certification' in the online resources section.

For a list of Australian businesses that have achieved 'chain of custody' certification by the Australian Forestry Standard or PEFC, visit the Australian Forestry Standard website at **www.forestrystandard.org.au**

In addition to sustainable sourcing, consider your functional needs along with the durability of the timber, colouring and natural characteristics (knots, veins, checking and pockets). For insights into the timber grading system visit the hardwood flooring grades fact sheet at the Australian Timber Flooring Association website, **www.atfa.com.au**

The Forest & Wood Products Association provides online resources, such as a species comparison database and technical guides at **www.woodsolutions.com.au**

Simply put, trees are essential to the environment and essential to our health. Look for one of the certifications outlined above when buying your timber to ensure this precious resource is harvested and managed in an ethical, responsible way.

Solid vs engineered

Solid timber is a rich material with unique colouring and characteristics, significant strength and durability. From a health perspective a benefit of solid timber over engineered products is that it is a material free from resins and glues (excluding joinery requirements).

If you need to use products such as MDF (medium density fibreboard), particle board or plywood which all use resins/adhesives in their manufacturing process, opt for E0 classified product (very low emission). The term E0 refers to a formaldehyde emission rating that a composite wood product has been given.

The various composite boards have differing standards in relation to emission requirements.

The following table is from the Australian and New Zealand Standard for Exterior Plywood- AS/NZS 2271. It lists the formaldehyde classes and the requirements exterior plywood manufacturers must meet (in mg/L) in order to claim that class.

Formaldehyde emissions from marine plywood	
Emission class mark	Maximum formaldehyde emission
E_0	0.5 mg/L
E_1	1.0 mg/L
E_2	2.0 mg/L
E_3	Above 2.5 mg/L

Table supplied by Engineered Wood Products Association of Australasia

The other Australian standards for structural, interior and marine plywood, particleboard and fibreboard also contain an E0 classification. Note that the E2 and E3 classifications above are hardly (if at all) used in product made by Australasian manufacturers. A Super E0 classification is also emerging in some sectors.

When choosing product that claims it has a low emission rating, look for independent certification on the label to indicate that the claims have been verified.

When using timber products (especially for flooring) it is best to allow timber products to acclimatise to the installation environment for a few days before installing. This allows for the product's moisture content to equalise with the environment; providing for a more stable material. It also allows emissions to reduce from composite board products as these are at their highest immediately after manufacture.

There are many opportunities that present themselves throughout an interior where timber products are used – wall and ceiling linings, floors, doors, windows, architraves, skirting boards, cabinetry, benchtops and furniture.

Architraves and skirting finishes are selections that contribute to every room in a home. Hardwood architraves and skirting boards are more expensive compared to composite products such as MDF, however hardwood is considerably more durable when knocked, does not contain adhesive emissions and can be reused if removed. If budget permits, hardwood trims are a great option.

If you are building a new house or room you may opt to avoid skirting boards by adding a shadow line finish on the wall above the flooring (where plaster trim is used at the base of plasterboard sheeting). This can be used with an aluminium door jamb system (no architraves) for a minimalistic look.

If using MDF products ask trades to cut the product outdoors to avoid fine dust particles (containing toxic adhesives) indoors. Contain dust to an area where it can be easily removed.

Flooring and wall linings are other large surface areas where timber is often used. With the development of engineered timber floor boards there is a debate over which is a more sustainable or healthier option. Engineered timber flooring has a thin layer of timber on the top with an engineered substrate (board) adhered to the back of the timber. These products consist of layers which require adhesives. If opting for engineered board request information as to whether the adhesives are low emission.

Many people feel that engineered boards e.g. floorboards are more sustainable than solid timber given that engineered boards often only use a thin layer of timber as opposed to a solid piece. However on the flip side we have the manufacturing processes of the substrate board and adhesives to consider. In some instances engineered boards will be sold pre-coated.

Our first question from a health perspective is, what is the coating made from?

The second question: is the coating low emission?

Boards that are prefinished remove the need for onsite finishing, therefore having the benefit of reducing off-gassing in your home.

Engineered floor boards across brands are made in different ways, some will have a thicker top layer of solid timber than others. This may be an issue if you ever need to resurface your boards. The installation systems for engineered boards can also vary.

Consider:

Solid timber boards	Pros	Cons
	• Natural material • Thicker sandable surface (if repairs or resurfacing required) • No glues used to make the product • Can be reused/recycled	• Can expand and contract (bend, warp) with environmental changes • Adhesives may be used to install (depending on method used) • Requires onsite finishing treatment

Engineered timber boards	Pros	Cons
	• Ideal for floating or direct stick (e.g. onto slab/existing flooring) • Prefinished - no chemical applications required onsite • Engineered for stability • May use recycled waste wood	• Adhesives used to manufacture the board • Adhesives used to lay the product • Limited sandable surface – once reached product needs replacing

Industry innovation is needed to establish new ways to manufacture composite board products without the toxic additives.

Researchers from the University of Leicester in the UK have developed a biodegradable composite panel that uses resin made from the starch of potatoes and other natural sources. It is exciting to hear that we may have more environmentally friendly and less toxic product options available in the marketplace in the future. To find these new innovative products and encourage demand, we need to continue to ask questions of suppliers.

Further Information

Queensland Government, Department of Agriculture & Forestry – www.daff.qld.gov.au/forestry/using-wood-and-its-benefits/wood-properties-of-timber-trees Online database providing descriptive information about timber species and technical data to help you choose the best timber for your required application.

Engineered Wood Products Association of Australasia (EWPAA) – www.ewp.asn.au – Provides technical information about engineered wood products, i.e. plywood, mdf, particle board, laminated veneer lumber, along with useful factsheets on relevant topics.

Australian Timber Flooring Association – www.atfa.com.au – Guide to products available, industry information and technical notes.

Forest & Wood Products Australia – Wood Solutions – www.woodsolutions.com.au – Species fact sheets, comparison database and technical guidance

Forest Stewardship Council® (FSC®) – www.au.fsc.org – Database of FSC® Certified timber suppliers

Australian Forestry Standard – www.forestrystandard.org.au – AFS Sustainable Forest Management Certification Register

PEFC – www.pefcregs.info – PEFC Council Information Register to find PEFC Certified products

Timber coatings

In many applications timber requires a protective coating to protect it from deterioration, either from the elements or wear and tear while in use.

It is important to understand that there are hundreds of products on the market that can be used to coat timber - too many to compare here.

However the following are features you may like to look for in a timber coating to assist in selecting a product that minimises the pollutants in your home.

- Full declaration of ingredients
- Low allergenic product – preventative action is wise
- Biodegradable – ideal for the environment
- Natural ingredients over petro chemically derived
- Product tested and independently certified to high standards e.g. European standards
- Water based products are usually preferable over solvent based products (remember to wash up responsibly to prevent contamination of water ways and environment).
- Products that allow timber to breathe can prevent issues with coating displacement due to the natural movement of timber to different environments.
- Low emission

In previous years two-pack polyurethane coatings on timber flooring have been popular. You are likely to know someone who has had their floor resurfaced and had to leave their home for days, only to return to odours/fumes that linger for weeks. Today polyurethane coatings are available in either a water based acrylic or solvent based form. The polyurethane coats the timber with a solid film – a plastic bag effect to the timber. These products can vary significantly in emissions (fumes). Water based products tend to have lower emission levels, however all products are unique so check the labels.

In recent years oils and waxes are becoming more popular and are offering a timber finish that allows timber to breathe while avoiding many of the chemicals associated with polyurethane finishes.

Beyond the initial finishing of a floor we also need to consider the maintenance regime. With polyurethane products flooring usually requires sanding back before a coating can be repaired. However, many of the oils and waxes available claim that sanding is not required, possibly a buff only and in some cases just a mop with product to rejuvenate.

The Australian Timber Flooring Association states on its website:

To meet Green Building Council of Australia (GBCA) criteria, coatings must contain less than 140 grams per litre of VOC, while adhesives must contain less than 100 grams per litre.

When comparing VOCs levels, remember to take into account the number of coats to be used.

The following is a coating selection chart from the 'Coating Choices' fact sheet by the Australian Timber Flooring Association that refers to emissions at application. This can be downloaded at www.atfa.com.au/wp-content/uploads/2012/10/is-coating-choices.pdf

COATING SELECTION CHART

Timber Floor Coatings

Property	Penetrating oil / wax & hard wax	Oil based finishes	Oil Modified Urethane	Polyurethane Solventborne 1 pack	Polyurethane Solventborne 2 pack	Polyurethane Waterborne 1 pack	Polyurethane Waterborne 2 pack
Durability (Ability to resist wear)	Low-Med	Low-Med	Medium	Very High	Very High	Med-High	Med-VH
Ability to accept careful foot traffic 3 days after coating. (Ave. temperature 20°C)	Low	Low	Medium	Medium	High	Medium	High
Timber colour 'richness'	Low-High	High	High	High	High	Low-Med	Low-Med
Darkening with age	High	High	High	Low-High	Low-High	Low-Med	Low-Med
Ability to cure in cold & dry weather	Low	Low	Medium	Medium	High	Medium	High
Ability to cure in cold and damp weather	Low	Low	Low	Medium	High	Low	Low
Edge bonding resistance	High	High	Med-High	Low-Med	Low	High	Med-High
Rejection resistance	High	Medium	Medium	Low-Med	Low-Med	Medium	Medium
VOC emission at application	Low-High	High	Med-High	High	High	Low	Low-Med
Inhalation hazard when coating is applied	Low	Medium	Medium	High	Very High	Low	Medium
Odour on application	Low-Med	Medium	Medium	High	Very High	Low	Low-Med
General product cost	Med-High	Low-Med	Medium	Medium	Medium	High	Very High

Source: The Australian Timber Flooring Association, 2008.

Each product has its own unique combination of ingredients and characteristics. Remember to assess a product on its own merits.

It is important to remember toxicity and VOCs are not necessarily related. Low VOC does not necessarily mean lower toxicity than a high VOC coating or vice versa. Toxicity depends on type of solvent or ingredients used and the proportion of these ingredients in a product. This is important because ideally a healthy home uses a floor coating that doesn't compromise the indoor air quality over time within the home, and does not leach fine particles into household dust. Therefore the toxicity of coatings is just as important as the VOC emissions.

Further information

Australian Timber Flooring Association – www.atfa.com.au
Ecospecifier Global – www.ecospecifier.com.au
Healthy Interiors – www.healthyinteriors.com.au

Plastics and your health

Plastics can be found in products that affect nearly every aspect of our lives. Consumers eat food prepared with plastics, sit and eat on plastics, wear plastics and use plastics in their jobs.

Plastics are found throughout the home in many materials and finishes which is why it's important to understand the following to be able to choose wisely.

Plastics are made using a group of chemicals known as phthalates. The Center for Disease Control and Prevention (CDC) defines them as follows:

'Phthalates are a group of chemicals used to make plastics more flexible and harder to break. They are often called plasticisers. Some phthalates are used as solvents (dissolving agents) for other materials.'

Phthalates are used in many products found throughout the home such as vinyl flooring or joinery wrap, adhesives, wallpapers, wall decals, window coverings, detergents, plastic clothing, personal care products (shampoo, conditioner, nail polish, hair spray), cookware, food storage containers, food packaging, window films, toys, and don't forget inside the car.

What has largely gone unnoticed, yet has been widely documented, is that some phthalates have been associated with the ability to disrupt normal hormonal function, otherwise known as endocrine disrupting chemicals (EDC). Some studies have found that phthalate chemicals can migrate from products into household dust.

The CDC states that 'exposure can occur by eating and drinking foods that have been in contact with containers and products containing phthalates and...from breathing in air that contains phthalate vapours or dust contaminated with phthalate particles.'

A study published by Environmental Health Perspectives (Bornehag et al, 2004) found that children with the highest levels of phthalates in their bedroom dust were between two and three times more likely to be diagnosed with asthma, rhinitis or eczema compared with children with the lowest levels.

'In humans, a study in the USA that investigated levels of phthalate metabolites (breakdown products) in urine concluded that human exposure to phthalates was greater than previously assumed.' (Blount et al, 2000).

A study by Oie et al in 1997 hypothesised that exposure to the phthalate DEHP in the home, especially from inhalation of particulate matter containing DEHP, may increase the risk of inflammation of the lung airways and as a consequence, increase the risk of asthma. (Allsopp et al, 2001)

It's worth noting that in the United States, the National Toxicology Program (NTP) and The International Agency for Research on Cancer (IARC) have classified PVC (polyvinyl chloride) as a carcinogen. PVC is a widely used plastic and can be found in many products in the home – such as furniture, joinery, window coverings, wallpapers, clothing and toys.

Given international concerns, a precautionary approach is wise. Minimising the use of plastics where possible throughout the home is a precautionary approach to health while also making a positive contribution to the long term health of the environment. Plastic production has a considerable impact on the health of the environment, through pollution and waste management.

Refer to the navigating plastics tip sheet in the Shop Wise Resources section for an overview of the different types of plastics.

Flooring

Flooring is one of the most important interior selections in a home as it makes a significant impact on the aesthetics, receives considerable wear and is one of the largest surface areas.

What is sustainable flooring?

The phrase 'sustainable flooring' often refers to the materials a floor is made from, and the production process. A floor that is made from renewable, responsible materials and processed using minimal energy and resources (low embodied energy) that provides for end of life recyclability would be considered sustainable.

To achieve a healthy, sustainable floor we need to add further elements to our consideration.

What chemicals are used to create the floor?

and

Is there any risk of interior contamination from these chemicals in the form of ingestion (via dust), inhalation (via air) or absorption (via topical treatments)?

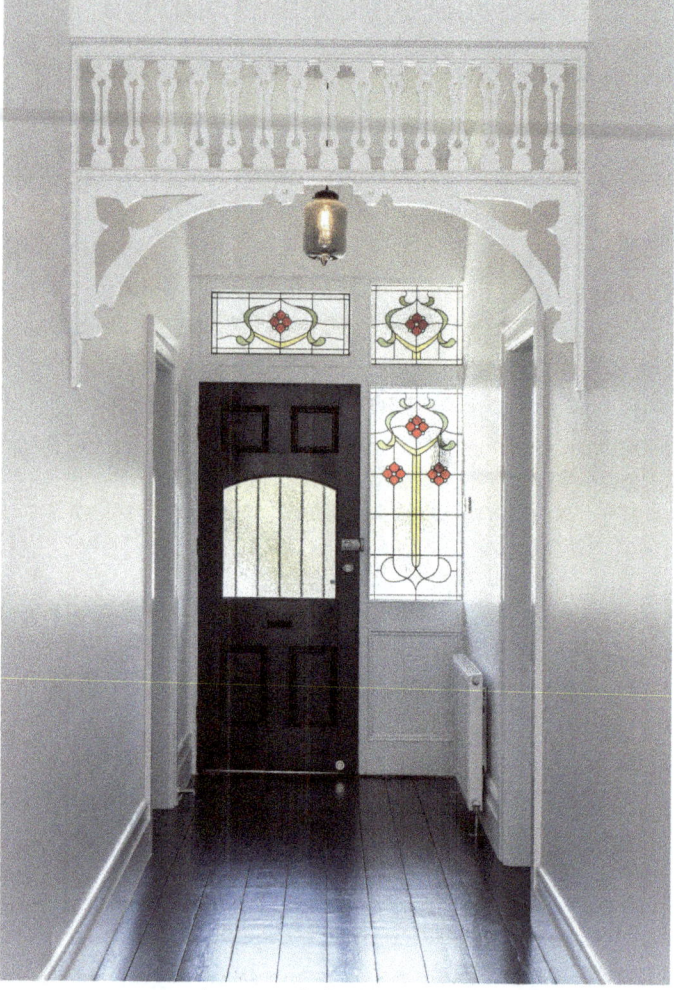

Image credit: Healthy Interiors

If you are building a new home or renovating, you have an opportunity to reduce the potential pollutants in your home by making informed product decisions about your flooring material.

For people with allergies, sensitivities and respiratory health concerns, minimising the potential exposure to dust and associated pollutants with flooring is a significant consideration, especially for babies and children as they spend a significant amount of time close to the floor. Taking a precautionary approach to material selection will assist to minimise pollutants throughout the home and is a great healthy home strategy.

When choosing a flooring material, the space, occupant and material needs to be considered to achieve a healthy sustainable outcome.

The following are some flooring considerations:
- Site conditions
- How will the floor be used?

- Who will be using the floor?
- Do occupants have any allergies, sensitivities or respiratory complaints?
- Consider material attributes linked to occupant: inhalation, ingestion, absorption:
- What is the material made from?
- How durable is the material and what is the likelihood of replacement?
- Does the surface emit VOCs?
- What is the installation process?
- What maintenance is required?
- Does the flooring mass have any thermal properties to assist with heating or cooling?
- Is the product biodegradable? (Not just the material, the finished product)
- Can the product be recycled?

There is no one flooring material available that provides a 100 percent natural, efficient, sustainable solution to flooring, so a list of priorities needs to be identified. Flooring can be categorised into hard floors e.g. timber, tile, stone; and soft floor coverings e.g. carpets and vinyls.

Hard flooring

As discussed in the sustainable timber section, hardwood floors (new or recycled) are a great natural choice and a reasonably healthy option provided that the finishing product applied to the timber is chosen wisely. Wood is a natural resource that requires minimal production energy compared to many other flooring types and is biodegradable and long lasting.

Hard flooring alternatives to timber floors are:

- Polished concrete
- Tiles – ensure tiles are pre sealed to avoid onsite chemical use
- Stone/slate – with sand and cement mix bonding – avoid toxic adhesives
- Linoleum
- Bamboo
- Cork
- Laminate
- Vinyl

With the list above remember to consider the finishes on these products and the installation method to achieve a healthy option product.

Polished concrete

Compared to other flooring choices which require regular replacement, concrete floors offer many years of durability.

The sustainability of concrete floors begins with the main component of the floor: limestone, an abundant mineral in our environment. Recycled product such as fly ash (a by-product of coal burning plants) is now also being used (in part) as a concrete substitute, contributing to the environmental appeal of this product. Be sure to ask for recycled content in your concrete floor.

Concrete flooring can be finished in a variety of different ways. The concrete surface is sanded (grinding process) and may be finished with topical products that alter the colour, texture or surface finish such as matt or gloss.

VOC emissions for sealant products can range from 100 g/L to 400 g/L (very high), therefore understanding what a product is made from is important when choosing product that minimises pollutants.

Polished concrete floors are a popular choice for modern homes and offices. When creating a concrete floor there are many finishes to choose from including terrazzo style, oxide coloured or natural colour sealed.

A variety of finishing products (for decoration and protection) are available. Two variants of concrete sealants are solvent based sealers and water based sealants (solvent based are usually higher in VOCs).

A terrazzo effect is achieved by mixing stone or crushed product such as glass into the concrete mix before the concrete is poured. Colour effects can be manipulated by using different coloured crushed material or varying types of stones.

For decorative topical treatments epoxy and polymer (plasticised) coatings are often used, these are usually much higher in VOCs and may contain phthalate chemicals.

To achieve a low emission concrete floor, opt for mechanical polishing and carefully selected (low emission) water base sealer or natural oil.

If opting for a concrete floor in a new build, details of the desired finish should be communicated on drawings and to trades at the beginning of the project. Extra care is required at the pour stage for mix colour preparation and to ensure levels and finish are suitable for an exposed floor.

Some concrete floors (depending on finish and type of use) can last many years without having to be resealed. Cleaning maintenance of concrete flooring is easy and can be maintained without the use of toxic cleaners.

From a design perspective, concrete flooring has thermal mass qualities that can be maximised with energy efficient housing design. Concrete flooring also provides the option for in slab heating which offers radiant heat (without air movement) to minimise dust circulation. Note that concrete slab heating is expensive to install, is generally not very efficient (a good proportion is lost into the ground) and can be very expensive to run.

A concrete floor surface offers options; providing a floor surface of its own or it can be used as a foundation for other surface materials to be laid on top. Concrete is a recyclable product and can be reused in other products at its end of life.

Choosing manufacturers that have environmentally friendly practices, use recycled materials and safe additives is good for the environment and human health.

For further considerations when choosing a coating, refer to the Coatings section.

Tiles

Tiles are a great hard floor sustainable option as they are durable, recyclable and inert (they don't off-gas) and usually no topical treatment is required onsite. Most tiles are made from clay or a mixture of clay and other materials that are then kiln fired. Although tiles require significant energy consumption to create the product, given their durability they can generally outlast many other surface finishes. Some manufacturers reuse waste products from the tiling process or incorporate recycled materials such as glass into tile designs. Tiles can also be recycled for other uses such as road base material.

A significant consideration when choosing tiles is to opt for tile styles, colour and textures that will remain appealing over the years to eliminate the need to remove tiles due to aesthetics. Look for locally manufactured products (although not always possible) to minimise embodied energy.

Characteristics of tiles

- Durable
- Hygienic
- Resistant to stains, scratches and moisture
- UV resistant
- Available in glazed or unglazed options
- Easily maintained with non-toxic cleaners
- Long lasting material
- Moisture/damp resistant
- Allergy friendly: can be maintained dust and chemically free

There are many options when it comes to choosing tiles.

With regards to colour density, full body porcelain tiles carry the colour and pattern throughout the tile which prevents contrasting colour being revealed if scratched or chipped.

There are also many types of tiles – wall, floor, extruded or pressed, glazed or unglazed. Water absorption is a common characteristic for all types of tiles. Generally the lower the water absorption, the greater the tiles' resistance to mechanical and environmental stresses.

Porcelain is the name given to low absorption ceramic tiles. The lower the absorption rate of a tile the more places you can generally use them e.g. floors, walls, interior, exterior.

Porcelain tiles are a popular flooring choice given their durability. Ceramic tiles with a higher than 3 percent water absorption level should be carefully considered before laying on floors as they may not be hard wearing enough.

Large format tiles are becoming more popular as they reduce grout and maintenance required over the life of the product.

To prevent onsite finishing chemicals, ensure that tiles purchased do not require sealing or topical anti slip treatments. If on-site treatments are required be sure to have the property well ventilated during and after the process so that fumes can be removed from the indoor environment.

Opt for low emission water proofing membrane products, adhesives, grout and silicone products where possible. The links in the resources section can assist with finding low emission options.

With limited labelling in this sector it can be challenging to differentiate between tiles to find product that is made with 'green' characteristics. Look for independently certified products e.g. Ecospecifier GreenTag, where responsible manufacturing and toxicity has been assessed.

When questioning the tile supplier about certifications, it is important to identify if they have been locally accredited. If international certifications apply, do they extend to local issues such as shipping, warehousing and local merchant behaviour such as minimising waste, freight miles and product stewardship program?

Stone

Natural stone has many attractive environmentally friendly attributes such as durability, recyclability, easy maintenance and long-term appeal.

The Natural Stone Council (NSC) in America has identified the following durability performance for flooring made from the following stones (with proper maintenance):

Slate: 100 years
Granite: 100 years
Limestone: Lifetime
Marble: 100 years
Sandstone: Lifetime

All the above stones do not emit volatile organic compounds which makes them a healthier base material than some other flooring options. However, stone flooring usually requires adhesives and sealants which can introduce chemicals into the home and bring with it VOCs that impact on indoor air quality.

Consider the functional properties of the stone you choose. Different stones have varying properties that can impact on functionality and longevity. For example, marble is porous and acid sensitive, therefore not ideal for kitchen benches or floors.

What to consider

Compressive strength required for the application e.g. structural use

Hardness – durability required and workability of the stone

Appearance - select your stone from large slab samples as each piece of natural stone has unique colouring and characteristics

Size – consider the sizing required and that joining or matching pieces for some applications may cause pattern or colouring issues

Supply source:
- Where is the product coming from?
- How much is available?
- Is there a local alternative?
- Is it from a responsible manufacturer?

Porous stones will require sealant to avoid staining. Opt for sealants that are low emission where possible and query if the sealant will change the colour of the raw stone after application.

Structural considerations must be considered when using stone as the weight may require additional reinforcing.

When using stone for flooring, slip resistance must be considered when selecting the finish. Some stones can be sandblasted or exfoliated to achieve a grit finish that assists with preventing slippery surfaces.

Maintenance – understand the maintenance required for your stone selection and assess if any ongoing maintenance requirements will impact on indoor air quality.

> **Further information**
>
>
> Natural Stone Council (America) – www.naturalstonecouncil.org
> Australian Stone Advisory Association (ASAA) – www.asaa.com.au

Linoleum

Linoleum is a sheet or tile floor covering made from linseed oil derived from the flax plant. Renewable and recyclable materials are used. The product is commonly made with a mix of resins, limestone, cork, wood powder, coloured pigments and linseed oil. The ingredients are combined to create a mixture that is rolled out onto a backing to create a material. It is then cured and surface treatments applied.

Linoleum was one of the most popular floor coverings in the 1900 -1950s. This material has natural anti-bacterial properties and is often biodegradable (subject to manufacturer additives).

Each supplier will have differences in their product and installation requirements. Installation may involve adhesives or heat welding.

What to consider
- Colour and design that will not date quickly
- If installation glues are required, are they low emission?
- What are the topical finishing treatments made from?
- Are particular cleaners required to keep the product in warranty?
- Tile or sheet product?
- How will the edges be finished e.g. skirting board or cove finish?
- Does the company have an end of life recycling scheme?

Bamboo

Bamboo flooring is made from bamboo grass. It is easy and quick to grow with minimal water, which is one of the reasons this material is considered a sustainable option. However, given this material is a fibre it requires processing to bond the fibres together to create a durable flooring material. Bamboo flooring can be constructed in different ways, either solid lamination of fibres into a board or as an engineered bamboo board consisting of a top layer of bamboo adhered to a board substrate.

Bamboo flooring is available in a range of different sizes and colours and can be described as either 'horizontal' or 'vertical' referring to the way the individual strips of bamboo are laminated. Horizontal bamboo planks have strips of bamboo laid flat to show the natural growth rings of the plant. Vertical bamboo has strips of bamboo turned to their sides and laminated together to show long slender rows.

As a material, bamboo offers strength and durability, however is subject to colour fading. Ultra violet coatings are added by some manufacturers to slow this process.

The durable adhesives used to bond bamboo together have the potential to release VOC emissions; many of the binders used contain formaldehyde. The type and toxicity of the finishing coat used to seal the product also needs to be considered.

If choosing a bamboo floor opt for product manufactured using responsibly harvested bamboo. Query the composition of chemicals used to bond the fibres together and what has been used on the finishing top coat. When all the elements of the bamboo processing come together they combine to create a flooring product that will have its own emissions profile, opt for a product that is transparent and can provide answers to the issues raised above.

We have access to local and global products that use different chemicals and have different standards. Being informed is essential to selecting a product that will minimise pollutants in your home.

Cork

Cork flooring is made from cork harvested from the exterior of a cork oak tree. This material is a renewable, sustainable, natural material which provides durability, sound absorbency, inherent fire resistance, thermal benefits and softer under foot than other hard floors. However, floor use of cork requires a protective coating that is often applied using polyurethane products or PVC. Both of these products have been associated with releasing VOC emissions into indoor air and with possible migration of toxins into household dust. When investigating cork flooring products consider the following:

- Type of sealer – is a low-VOC water-based option available?
- Are glues required for installation? Are they low emission?
- How often does the floor need maintenance coats?
- Is the maintenance coating low emission?
- If the product is made with a board core, is this a low emission product?
- Has the finished product had emission testing done?
- What non-toxic cleaners are accepted for use to remain within product warranty?
- Sheet flooring or tiles? (Tiles provide for easy replacement)
- If bonding of edges is required, what product is being used?
- If a silicone edge is required, is this a low emission colour matched product?
- Is the product made from cork oak forests certified as maintained responsibly?

Laminate flooring

Laminate flooring can be more economical than solid timber or timber veneer flooring, however there are some long term disadvantages. Laminate flooring is less durable than timber flooring and difficult to repair. This type of flooring also requires more energy in the manufacturing process compared to traditional timber flooring options.

Laminated flooring involves a mechanical process of lamination or bonding of the film or image (with the colour, texture or print) onto a board product. Glues that are considered toxic (often containing formaldehyde) are generally used in the process. A top coating is required to protect the print image and in many cases is coated in a polyurethane finish. There are many different finishing products used in the marketplace, so consumers should request emissions and toxicity information for individual brands that are being considered.

Vinyl flooring

Compared to many flooring options, vinyl is often one of the cheapest and can be found in sheet or tile format. Vinyl flooring is made from polyvinyl chloride (PVC), it is combined with plasticisers, pigments, stabilisers, fillers and can contain fungicides. There are significant concerns with PVC as a material including toxic manufacturing pollution, accumulative waste issues, and the material has been linked to a range of health concerns such as hormonal disruption and respiratory illness such as asthma. PVC also releases VOCs which can contribute to a reduced quality of indoor air within a home.

The Healthy Building Network in the USA highlights that:

'Dioxin (the most potent carcinogen known), ethylene dichloride and vinyl chloride are unavoidably created in the production of PVC and can cause severe health problems, including:

Cancer
Endocrine disruption
Endometriosis
Neurological damage

Birth defects & impaired child development
Reproductive and immune system damage'

Given PVC flooring cannot be composted at its end of life, it contributes to landfill or is burnt, releasing carcinogenic dioxins into the environment.

Using products that are not biodegradable or that can't be reused or recycled makes no sense for the health of the collective air we breathe or the water we drink. The use of materials and products that accumulate as waste is a nasty legacy of years of unhealthy practices and the pollution of spaces that future generations will be unable to enjoy.

Overview

The following is a Sustainability Assessment of different floors by www.choice.com.au. Reproduced with permission (table published June 2010).

SUSTAINABILITY ASSESSMENT OF DIFFERENT FLOORS		
FLOOR TYPE	ADVANTAGE	DISADVANTAGES
Carpet	• Provides warmth (by insulating the floor) and acoustic benefits • Carpet can sometimes be recycled; some brands of carpet contain recycled materials such as PET plastic • Natural-fibre carpets such as coir, sisal and seagrass are non-toxic and can be from a sustainable resource	• Low thermal mass benefits • Is one of the least durable floor systems • High energy requirement for cleaning • Some synthetic carpets and dyes can be toxic • Can be high waste in installation • Is sometimes difficult to recycle
Timber	• Can be recycled - and it's often possible to buy recycled timber • Relatively hard-wearing and durable • Easy to clean • Low embodied energy	• May be sourced from unsustainable forestry, unless it carries proper certification labels • Low thermal mass benefits • Some finishes or composite products can be petroleum-based and toxic
Bamboo	• Comes from a fast-growing, more sustainable resource than timber or plastic flooring • Hard-wearing and durable • Easy to clean • Low embodied energy	• Some bamboo floorboards may have been finished with toxic glues
Linoleum, rubber or cork ("resilient floors")	• Made from renewable materials such as linseed oil, rubber, cork and wood fibre • Low toxicity • Fairly durable • Easy to clean • Low embodied energy	• Not recyclable • All these products are imported to Australia • Some rubber, cork and wood fibre floors contain petroleum-based materials
Ceramic tiles	• Good thermal mass • Low toxicity • Easy to clean • Highly durable	• Higher embodied energy • Local environmental impacts of quarries
Polished stone (granite, sandstone etc)	• Good thermal mass • Low toxicity • Easy to clean • Highly durable	• Higher embodied energy (especially if imported from overseas) • Local environmental impacts of quarries
Polished concrete	• Good thermal mass • Easy to clean • Highly durable	• High embodied energy of concrete, as well as the polishing process • May be finished with a toxic polyurethane sealant
Vinyl	• Low maintenance, easy to clean	• Can contain toxic plasticisers and lead-based stabilisers

Summary flooring considerations

- What is the material made from?
- What is the topical finish treatment made from?
- Can the finished coating break down and release particles into household dust?
- Has the product been independently tested as low emission?
- Ask for a copy of the product emissions test certificate.
- Can the product be cleaned without toxic cleaners?
- What maintenance is required on the surface over time? Can it be locally sourced?

Further information

Good Environmental Choice Australia – www.geca.org.au
Ecospecifier Global – www.ecospecififer.com.au
Choice – www.choice.com.au

Adhesives, caulks and grouts

Adhesives used throughout the home can impact on the health of indoor air for many months after construction. Choose low VOC products and be wary of a group of chemicals often used in adhesives referred to as phthalates, such as dibutyl phthalate (DBP) and butyl benzyl phthalate (BBP).

Formaldehyde (a known carcinogen) is also often used in adhesives and resins. Phenol-formaldehyde glues generally release less formaldehyde then urea-formaldehyde glues.

Certification bodies are a great resource to establish what they know about the environmental and health aspects of a product. Ecospecifier Global is an example of an Australian based certification body that provides a database on a range of products, including adhesives.

Further information

EcoSpecifier Global Product search database – www.ecospecifier.com.au
Australian Tile Council – www.australiantilecouncil.com.au
Natural Stone Council (USA) fact sheets – www.naturalstonecouncil.org
Australian Timber Flooring Association – www.atfa.com.au
Forest & Wood Products Australia – Wood Solutions - www.woodsolutions.com.au

Carpet

Australians have a range of carpet products to choose from, manufactured both locally and abroad. When shopping for carpet it's important to remember that manufacturers around the world have different product and quality standards and this includes different standards for acceptable emissions.

Some countries have implemented guidelines for indoor air quality; other countries have voluntary guidelines. It's a good idea to query where a carpet has been made. As a general rule, there are no specific import standards. Under Australian consumer law, products must be durable, safe and fit for their intended purpose. If consumers identify a product concern they can report the matter to the Australian Competitor & Consumer Commission (ACCC).

The importance of asking where a carpet has been made and what has been used to make the carpet is due to differing international chemical standards and lack of detailed labelling.

The 2001 Hazardous Chemicals in Carpets report by Allsopp, Santillo and Johnston published by Greenpeace Research Laboratories in the UK, revealed that carpet samples they tested were found to contain organotins, permethrin, brominated flame retardants and formaldehyde.

Permethrin (pyrethoids) are used on some carpets as a mothproofing treatment. Carpets are frequently sold with pest proof guarantees for many years, therefore the pesticide applied at the manufacturing stage remains active for long periods. The Environmental Protection Agency (EPA) in the US has found that one member of the pyrethroid class, permethrin, is 'likely to be carcinogenic to humans.' (USA EPA, 2012)

Carpets may be sold with chemical treatments for:

- Dust mites
- Odour elimination
- Mould or mildew growth prevention
- Insecticide (moth proofing)
- Stain resistance

There is debate over whether chemicals used and found in carpets are significant enough to cause any health issues. We do know that some people are more susceptible or sensitive to chemicals within the home environment than others.

Understanding what a carpet is made from provides consumers with information to make informed decisions suitable for individual circumstances.

There are two different categories of carpets:

- Natural materials such as wools, linen, cotton, jute, sea grasses
- Synthetic fibres such as nylon and polyester

Natural fibres have some alluring characteristics. Natural fibres such as sisal, sea grasses or wool carpet, with natural fibre backing such as jute, are great sustainable options.

Nylons and polyesters are made from petro chemically derived raw materials, often requiring bonding agents to hold them together. These carpets tend to be more durable and stain resistant than natural fibres, yet contain plasticised materials.

The Hazardous Chemicals in Carpet report (Allsopp et al, 2001) highlighted the following:

'...a ... report by the British Society for Allergies noted that it is likely that increase in exposure to synthetic and pollutant chemicals makes a substantial contribution to increases in allergic disease (Eaton et al, 1999). The presence of the above chemicals in carpets (refer to the report for the extensive list) highlights an important product sector which will need attention to prevent human exposure to hazardous chemicals and possible health consequences.'

To minimise pollutants when selecting carpet, consider product that is from a natural source, free from chemical treatments and PVC.

Look for low VOC emission credentials – check the carpet meets the Australian Carpet Classification Scheme (ACCS) Environmental Classification criteria as low emission. Don't forget that the underlay also contributes to the overall air quality after installation. Use a low emission (preferably biodegradable) carpet underlay.

VOC minimisation tips from the Carpet Institute of Australia:

- Carpet installed with maximum ventilation
- Vacuum after installation
- Operate ventilation system (if available) at room temperature for 72 hours after installation
- If carpet adhesives are used, ask for low VOC emitting water based adhesive
- If you are sensitive to VOC emissions, leave the premises during and immediately after carpet installation

People living with asthma and allergies have varying degrees of sensitivities to pollutants in the home therefore there is no one golden rule to suitable flooring. However, reducing exposures to pollutants seems common sense.

The debate over hard floors verses carpet for allergies is a contentious issue. Some argue dust is more visible on hard floors prompting removal, whereas others say that dust is mobilised on floorboards whereas carpet holds dust within the pile until vacuumed, preventing it from becoming airborne and aggravating allergies.

If opting for carpet choose a low pile variety that is easily cleaned compared with long pile styles. Natural fibres reduce the potential of exposure to phthalate and VOCs from synthetic products. Also consider the environmental impact of the carpet, does the supplier have a 'take back' recycling scheme? What happens to the product when it is no longer needed? These environmental considerations are elements of what is often referred to as cradle to cradle attributes. Refer to the certifications section to learn about the cradle to cradle product certification label.

For all carpets, query what has been used to make it, opt for a product with the least treatments as outlined above. For imported carpets query if the carpet has been treated with fumigation chemicals when it was bought into the country.

Maintenance tips:

- Ensure your vacuum cleaner is maintained in good working order
- Use the appropriate vacuum cleaning head for the type of carpet
- Use a HEPA filter vacuum unit
- Regularly replace the HEPA filter on the vacuum as per manufacturer's instructions
- Have carpets professionally cleaned; the Carpet Institute of Australia recommends every 18 months
- Professionally clean carpets (with non-toxic chemicals) in warm weather to assist with drying and prevent mould growth
- Don't wear shoes on carpeted areas, to minimise dust pollutants
- Regular vacuuming along skirtings, under furniture to minimise dust and allow early identification of minor infestation of insects

Underlay

Natural underlays made from recycled textiles, hessian or jute are a more sustainable and often healthier option than synthetic underlays which all have differing levels of VOCs. Foams such as polyurethane foam or latex foam can emit a strong 'new carpet smell' for some time after installation. Some natural fibre underlays such as jute are also biodegrable when they are no longer needed rather than contributing to landfill.

Underlay materials can be vastly different in the materials and chemicals used. Products commonly used are made from rubbers, foams, textiles or jute.

- Place babies on a blanket on top of the carpet surface to prevent their face coming into direct contact with carpet materials (supervision of babies required)
- If removing carpet or underlay from the home, respiratory protection should be worn such as a P2 mask available at the hardware store

Further information

Carpet Institute of Australia Limited – www.carpetinstitute.com.au

Hazardous Chemicals in Carpets, 2001 – Report compiled for the Healthy Flooring Network by Greenpeace Laboratories – www.greenpeace.to/publications/carpet.pdf

Cabinetry – furniture

There are so many materials used today to create furniture for our homes - timbers, glass, metals, resins, plastics, synthetic fibres, leather, grass fibres, paper/cardboard, wools and many others. An exciting opportunity exists to be selective and combine materials for function, beauty and health.

For large structural furniture such as cabinets and functional items like shelving and beds, timber or wood derived products are commonly used. Manufactured board products tend to be cheaper than hardwood timbers and are therefore popular.

Types of composite boards and what to look for:

MDF – Medium density fibreboard

MDF is made by adding wood fibres with resins and pressing it into various sheet sizes.

Plywood

Plywood is made by bonding together multiple thin veneer layers of softwood, hardwood, or a combination of both. The type of veneers and adhesives used determine the types of suitable applications e.g. interior or exterior use. Ply can be purchased in various sizes and thicknesses.

Melamine board

Melamine board has a top surface that is made from decorative sheet paper that has been covered with a transparent layer of melamine resin. The outer decorative layer is adhered to a particle board or MDF board. Edges of the board are usually finished with a melamine tape strip glued to the edge or a PVC edge tape.

Laminate board

Laminate board is constructed using a process of high pressure bonding of resin impregnated paper to a board finish; usually MDF is used. The paper carries the colour or design of the laminate and usually has a plasticised hardwearing transparent top coat. Edges of the board are usually finished with a melamine tape strip glued to the edge or a PVC edge tape, often referred to in Australia as an ABS (acrylonitrile butadiene styrene) edging.

Timber veneer board

Very thin slices of timber are glued to a board substrate such as MDF to achieve a solid timber look without using a solid product. Timber veneers are also available in designer ranges where the veneer has been treated with dyes and designs for an engineered appearance which at times has a very different to the look of natural timber veneer.

Furniture made from pressed wood products (such as particle board, MDF or ply) contain adhesives or resins to bind the particles. These products have the capacity to release emissions from the adhesives when they are not sealed (query individual product specifications).

Formaldehyde is often a component of the adhesive to create pressed board product. Formaldehyde is classified by the International Agency for Research on Cancer (IARC) as carcinogenic to humans. Look for formaldehyde free options or E0 classified board as outlined in the timber section of this book. Product Safety Australia (Australian Competition & Consumer Commission) states on its website that to gain categorisation as a 'low formaldehyde emission' product, finished pressed wood products must meet test criteria levels of less than 1ppm formaldehyde.

Pressed board products can be finished with a range of surfaces such as laminate, vinyl wrap or painted/stain finish.

What to consider when choosing the finish for your furniture:

If choosing products that are laminated, query the emissions rating of the laminate as this is the surface area exposed to your indoor environment. Does the supplier use low emission glues and resins?

Vinyl wrap finishes, sometimes referred to as thermo wrap (applied using heat) is a material of great debate. This is a type of plasticised sheeting applied to board products to achieve a seamless wrapped look. To achieve this the product contains various plastic softeners (phthalate chemicals) that are heated to mould around the substrate. Some of these finishes also contain PVC. The USA EPA has classified the vinyl chloride mostly used to make PVC as a Group A human carcinogen.

Ask - Does the wrap product contain PVC?

If the answer is yes, does the PVC also contain lead?

One of the social concerns about PVC is that during the manufacturing process and the eventual

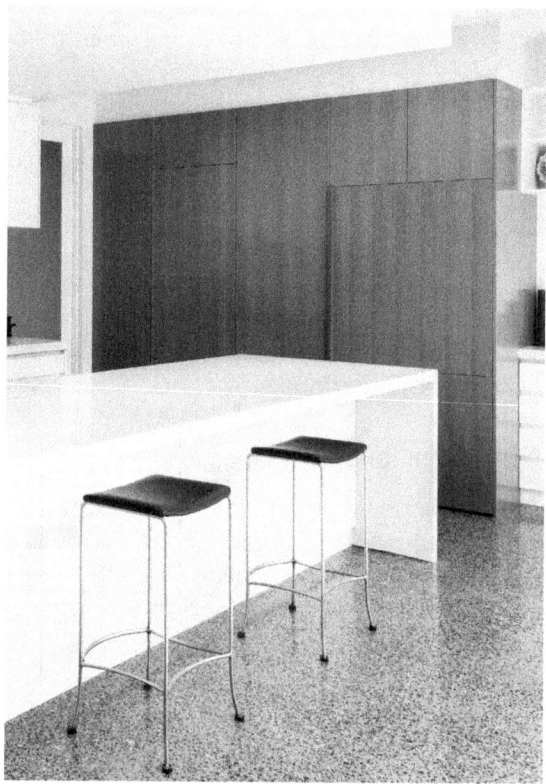

Image supplied by Healthy Interiors

disposal at the end of a product's life, PVC releases cancer causing (persistent environmental pollutant) dioxins into the atmosphere when it is disposed of (burnt). There has been a considerable amount of documentation produced globally identifying concerns over PVC manufacturing, factory worker illness, factory community illnesses and persistent dioxin compounds in the water and air. The World Health Organisation states that 'Dioxins are highly toxic and can cause reproductive and developmental problems, damage the immune system, interfere with hormones and also cause cancer'. For further information on dioxins refer to the World Health Organisations fact sheet no.225 - **www.who.int/mediacentre/factsheets/fs225/en/**

PVC contains phthalates (plastic softeners). There have been some studies that have found phthalate chemicals within indoor dust, highlighting that some phthalates can migrate from plasticised products. Some phthalates are considered endocrine disruptors and have also been linked to respiratory health concerns. The notion that some plastic products within the home are releasing these chemicals is of international concern.

We know reducing our use of plastics is good for environmental health, yet understanding the manufacturing process, community impact and potential personal health impacts of plastics makes choosing alternatives a sensible and easier choice.

If you are opting for laminated products, laminated furniture is usually on a particle board or MDF substrate. Query if the substrate is E0 or formaldehyde free. Ask if the board is Australian made or imported. Imported board may not have been made to Australian standards and may contain higher levels of toxic additives.

An interesting experiment you can try is to smell furniture as you shop, this will soon highlight the differences between furniture emissions and illustrate how these items can impact on the indoor air in a home. Just keep in mind that not all VOCs have an odour, although avoiding items that do is a great start.

Furniture manufactured in Australia is made to relevant standards (some only voluntary). Keep in mind that furniture made in other countries may contain chemicals that are not necessarily approved for use in Australia nor meet Australian chemical standards. There are no mandatory furniture labelling laws in Australia that require all materials and chemicals used on a product to be disclosed. Asking questions of the retailer or supplier is essential to understand what you are buying.

At a recent design expo an importer displayed a range of children's beds made in amazing shapes that would excite most children. The beds were made from pressed board and a combination of plasticised coatings and gloss paints. Although they were visually exciting to look at the beds had been made with a cocktail of pollutants – formaldehyde, phthalate chemicals (plastic softeners) and solvents…hardly an ideal environment for a child to play near let alone sleep on every night. The 'new' smell was evident, which as you know now are VOCs – a hazard to health.

When selecting furniture, opt for pieces of quality that will be durable and minimise replacement. Natural hardwood timber products that are stained or finished with naturally derived oils or waxes are a great option. Hardwood is generally a more expensive option than pressed board products, although reclaimed timber is a great way to minimise waste and costs.

Beyond timber products other materials such as glass, metal and stone used for cabinetry are also great options to minimise indoor pollutants.

When specifying, designing or buying cabinetry, built in cabinets minimise the potential for dust, debris and pests to accumulate.

Summary:
- When choosing pressed board products, opt for E0 classified product (or better)
- When choosing laminates, opt for E0 substrate and low emission laminate
- If choosing timber veneer on board products opt for low emission stain/finish on E0 board
- Minimise the use of plastics
- Ask for product credentials – has the product been tested as low emission?
- Opt for reclaimed/recycled hardwood timbers where possible
- Opt for low emission, naturally derived paints/stains where possible
- Use your nose when you shop!

Benchtops

There is a wide variety of materials used for benchtops and many things to consider when weighing up the pros and cons of each. Questions that can assist you to assess both the environmental impacts of the product and potential health characteristics are:

- What are the raw materials?
- Where are the materials from?
- What is the manufacturing process? Energy consumed, waste and ethics, etc
- Where is the product made?
- Is there a local alternative?
- What is involved in the installation process? Will this create additional pollutants?
- Are there any use implications and impacts on indoor air quality?
- Does the installed product release VOCs?
- What maintenance is required?
- Can the benchtop be easily repaired?
- What happens to the benchtop when not required? Is it recyclable?

If you are new to the world of benchtop options the following is a guide to get you started.

The story behind a product provides clarity as to what you are choosing to live with from a health perspective along with a greater appreciation for the history, impact or innovation of a particular material.

Types of benchtop materials

- Acrylic resin
- Bamboo
- Ceramic tile
- Concrete
- Engineered stone
- Laminate
- Natural stone – granite, marble
- Recycled glass and stone
- Recycled paper and resin
- Solid timber
- Stainless steel

Acrylic resins

Often referred to solid surface material, acrylic benchtops can provide seamless customised moulded applications in a large range of colours. Plasticised products can offer appealing characteristics such as stain resistance, antimicrobial properties and seamless large spans. These products can often be repaired in place but usually cannot be recycled.

Plastic materials require high energy processing. While some plasticised products can be repaired, altered and reused they can usually not be recycled, which puts a substantial burden on the environment at the end of the product's life. Plastics are also made primarily from petrochemicals sources, a resource that is limited and contributes substantially to pollution while being mined, manufactured and transported.

Pollutants from some plastics have been linked to a range of health concerns, including endocrine disrupting (hormonal disruption) health issues. If opting for an acrylic resin product, request independent testing information on VOC emissions and the acrylic end use toxicity.

Questions to ask:

- Is this product safe for direct food preparation?

- Can the product leach pollutants?
- Can the product leach pollutants as it ages?
- Has any testing been done to check this?

Pro – colour consistency and seamless sections
Con – plasticised product that is not biodegradable, VOC enquiry required.

Bamboo

Bamboo is a grass fibre that is easily and quickly grown with minimal water which is why it is often referred to as a sustainable material option. Bamboo has a range of appealing characteristics such as aesthetic warmth, durability, heat and water resistance properties. Bamboo also has natural anti-bacterial and anti-fungal attributes. Scratches or dents can also be repaired as required.

To achieve a benchtop material from bamboo fibre, adhesives and compression are used to create the material. The solvents, glues and finishes used to manufacture bamboo benchtops vary, therefore to identify if additives used are low emission and/or nontoxic, questions need to be asked about the manufacturing process and products used.

Bamboo benchtops can be custom made to specific sizes, minimising wastage.

Pro – fast growing fibre and natural material
Con – often toxic adhesives are used to create the material from the fibre

Ceramic tile

Tiles consist of natural clays and sands and in some cases recycled glass or aggregate. The manufacturing process of creating tiles is energy intensive due to firings required and the transportation of heavy product. Tiled bench tops require a sealed tile to avoid staining from use. When selecting tiles, consider that larger tiles will result in less grout required. The type of grout used should also be considered. Opt for a low emission option that is durable and suitable for food surfaces. If buying an imported tile product ask for confirmation that lead has not been used in the glaze as different countries have varying regulations.

Pro - does not release VOCs (topical sealer exempt)
Con - grout is porous and can harbour bacteria, requiring maintenance

Concrete

Concrete can be moulded into custom shapes and coloured to a variety of shades, although the toxicity of the pigments should be explored. The toxicity of the finishing sealer also needs to be questioned to ensure that it is suitable for food grade surfaces and is low emission. Installation techniques can vary and onsite grinding may be required. Opt for installation procedures that minimise onsite dust. While concrete is very durable and can be crushed into aggregate for reuse at end of life, it is an energy intensive material. If opting for concrete, incorporating a percentage of post-industrial fly ash (left over material from coal fired power plants) makes it a more sustainable product.

Pro - seamless appearance is possible and very durable
Con – heavy and requires sealer maintenance

Engineered stone

Engineered stone benchtops are often also referred to composite benchtops. These products are usually a combination of stone powder, crushed stone and binding agent, such as resins. They are usually less porous than natural stone. Composite materials are generally cheaper than natural stone and are made to offer a broad range of colours and textures. This range of benchtops has also seen the introduction of blending recycled glass and semi-precious stones with crushed stone to achieve unique effects. The type of resins used can also vary from petrochemical-derived resins to bio resins made using vegetable derived ingredients e.g. from corn.

Slab sizes vary and some suppliers will offer salvaged pieces that can be available at a reduced cost. These pieces are often offcuts from large jobs.

Pro - no resealing required, engineered stone is more stable and uniform than natural stone
Con - the presence of resin binders requires questions about toxicity and emissions

Laminate

Laminates are resin impregnated paper adhered to a board backing. Laminates are a popular choice for benchtops due to affordability, durability, stain resistance and colour/texture options available. However, once laminate is damaged it is difficult to repair. The substrate (board) used under the laminate is often a particle board product, in most instances water resistant particle board. This type of product usually contains formaldehyde in the adhesive. Look for laminate products that offer an E0 classified substrate (or Super E0 if available). This means it has minimal formaldehyde content.

There are laminate products made from recycled sources which lessen the environmental impact. Question the glues used in the lamination process, opting for products that use low VOC glues during the manufacture and/or installation process.

Avoid the use of glues for installation where possible, opting for mechanical fastening applications. Look for laminate benchtops that have been certified as low emission, preferably from a company that takes pride in environmentally responsible manufacturing. When exploring the substrate materials that laminates are adhered to, seek out responsible forestry certified board products.

Laminates are generally not heat resistant and different manufacturers will give varying assurances as to laminate chemical resistance. Scratches and indentations cannot be repaired therefore the lifespan is shorter than other more durable options. However, for many the affordability of laminate is appealing. From a design perspective, laminate is supplied in specific sheet sizes so minimisation of seams/joins in the surface is a consideration.

Pro - wide choice of colours, pattern and textures
Con - difficult to repair and may release emissions – enquiry required

Natural stone

Natural stones such as granite and marble are removed from the earth and considerable energy is used to transform them into construction-ready product. Stone used for benchtops is not a renewable material and at this stage is not widely being recycled. At end of life, slabs can however be cut down and used for other applications. Granite is a popular choice used for benchtops and is often selected for its unique colour and pattern variations, prestigious appearance and natural qualities. The surface does require sealing to protect it from staining; therefore ensuring the sealer is suitable for food grade use and is a low emission product is recommended. Opt for low dust installation measures.

Stone does not off-gas however there have been international concerns raised over radon emissions from granite. The US EPA has noted that:

'It is possible for any granite sample to contain varying concentrations of uranium and other naturally occurring radioactive elements. These elements can emit radiation and produce radon gas, a source of alpha and beta particles and gamma rays. Some granite used for countertops may contribute variably to indoor radon levels.'

Radon has been linked to health concerns, though there is suggestion that small amounts of granite within a home have negligible risk. Testing of radon levels from a granite slab can be done and requires specialty equipment. If this is something of interest contact a local building biologist and ask if they have the appropriate equipment and knowledge for this testing.

Slab sizes for natural stone vary and some suppliers will offer salvaged pieces that can be available at a reduced cost.

Pro - unique colours and patterns
Con - porous, needs sealer maintenance, unknown quantity of radon in granite

Recycled glass and stone

Recycled glass and stone is used across various industries offering materials for benchtop use.

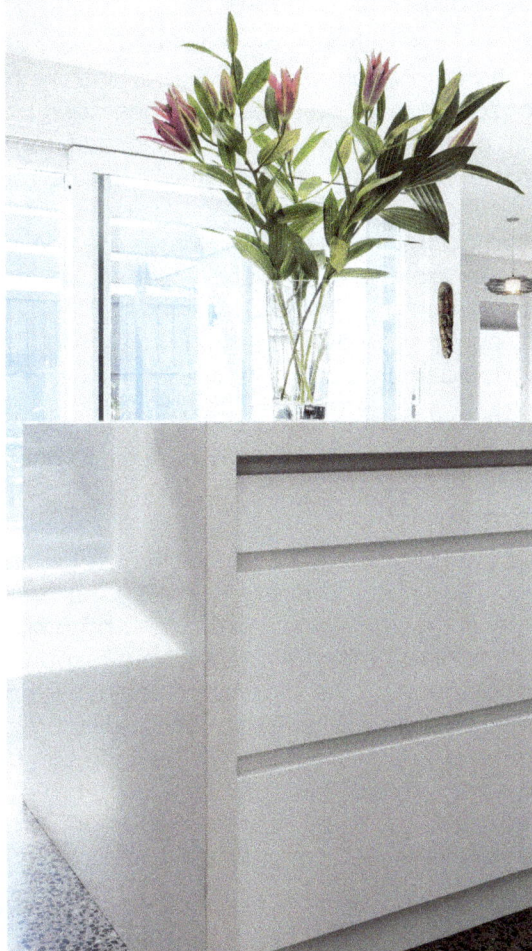

Image supplied by Healthy Interiors

Colourful glass mixed with cement or resin based products create a terrazzo effect. This effect can be found in engineered stone products, custom cement products or ceramic tiling. Terrazzo inspired products are often a good 'eco' choice as they can contain quite high levels of recycled content, especially if the product is made locally with locally recycled materials and minimal transportation. When exploring these types of products consider the type of binding agent used and query the toxicity. Can the manufacturer supply documentation that shows they have considered the toxicity of the materials for food surface area use? What is the product sealed with (to prevent staining)? Is it a low emission finished product? Is the product factory sealed or is onsite sealing required? Onsite sealing can generate pollutants within the home that can be avoided by factory sealed products.

Pro – recycled material
Con – resin intense, enquire about resin toxicity

Recycled paper and resin

We are entering exciting times where innovative manufacturers are finding ways to create construction materials from previously unused materials. Benchtops are now available using post-consumer recycled paper that has been bonded with resin to create durable, stain resistant, heat resistant surfaces. A class of commercial synthetic resins used to create many laminates and wood bonded boards are referred to as phenolic resins. These resins contain phenol and formaldehyde, both associated with a range of health concerns. We are starting to see composite resins emerging that are using naturally derived products in an effort to find more environmentally friendly ways to manufacture – e.g. biopolymers and resins made with cashew nut shell liquid and corn oil. These innovations will help us to reduce our reliance on petroleum based products and drive product advancement to reveal products that are safer and healthier for human use.

Pro – recycled material use
Con – limited colours, resin intense, need to ask about resin toxicity

Solid timber

Timber, new or recycled, is a valuable asset in a healthy home. If opting for a timber benchtop untreated hardwood that is from a responsible, sustainable source (such as FSC® certified) is ideal. A range of oils and waxes using naturally derived ingredients are also available in the marketplace. Timber is a renewable resource, however a limited resource, and as the global population grows, plantation zones will have high demand. The characteristics of being lightweight with natural strength and individual beauty are appealing. Timber should be protected from continual wet areas, which can be addressed by appropriate sink selection. Compared to some of the other benchtop options, customised timber benchtops can be more expensive, although a great opportunity to recycle hardwood from a construction site or salvage timber with a story from a local salvage yard.

If using salvaged timber for benchtops ensure the timber has not been previously exposed to chemicals. Opt for mechanical installation fixing rather than adhesives. At the benchtop's end of life it can be cut up and used for other uses (upcycled) or if kept free from toxic surface treatments can be made into woodchips, left to biodegrade naturally or transformed into outdoor art. The range of options make this a sustainable material choice.

Pro – strong, natural renewable material
Con – not heat resistant or scratch resistant, needs sealer maintenance

Stainless steel

To create stainless steel, raw materials are mined and transformed in a manufacturing process to create the material. This process has environmental impacts and high energy use. However, due to the recyclability and recycling uptake of stainless steel, the material has a lower environmental impact than if production was based purely on primary virgin materials. Stainless steel is 100 percent recyclable. A study undertaken by the Stainless Steel Forum (ISSF) found that the recycled content of stainless steel globally is 60 percent or more for certain countries.

Stainless steel benchtops do not off-gas emissions, are durable, hygienic and give an industrial, professional ambience with low maintenance. Stainless steel does develop scratches from use over time and gives the benchtop a less reflective surface which is loved by many.

Pro – low maintenance, does not release VOCs and is recyclable
Con - shows scratches and fingerprint marks; needs to be kept clean

Products that utilise recycled product are fantastic, yet don't forget that just because a product is marketed as a 'green' or 'eco' product that it is not necessarily a healthy home option. We need to remember we ingest, inhale and absorb pollutants in our surroundings. The ideal scenario is to find product that has 'health' credentials and 'green' credentials.

Paint

There is plenty of choice in the marketplace for interior paints, including plant/mineral based products and petro chemically derived paints, all offering different attributes. The choices are varied with attributes such as colour availability, differing application methods, durability, washability, breathability, finish, price and emission levels.

Low VOC paints are available in naturally derived or petrochemical options. Factors for consideration include health sensitivities (ingredients), coverage, cost, colour and durability.

Lead

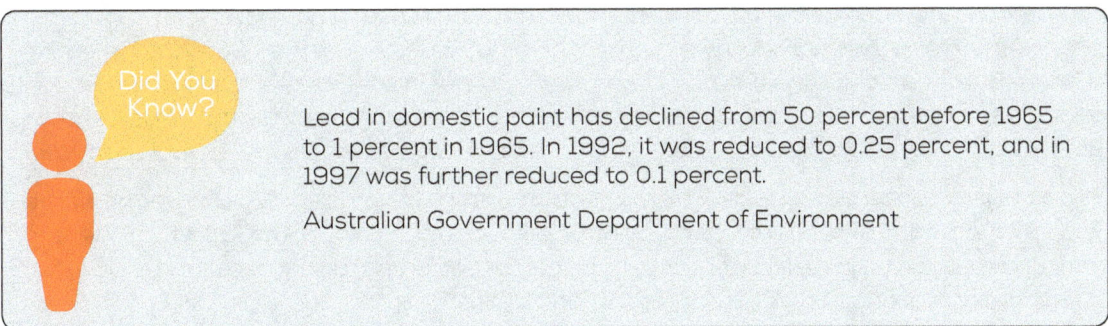

Did You Know?

Lead in domestic paint has declined from 50 percent before 1965 to 1 percent in 1965. In 1992, it was reduced to 0.25 percent, and in 1997 was further reduced to 0.1 percent.

Australian Government Department of Environment

If renovating a home that was built prior to 1970 it is wise to conduct a lead test on previously painted surfaces to establish if lead is present. Paints manufactured prior to 1965 could contain up to 50 percent lead. Lead is considered a neurotoxic pollutant and has been linked to a range of health issues; children and pregnant women are particularly vulnerable.

Before renovating old painted surfaces, a lead test should always be done. Refer to the earlier section, Site Health Tips – Lead. If lead is present in old paintwork, safety precautions must be taken to minimise personal lead exposure, lead dust and spreading the pollutant around the home.

The Australian government has a booklet available for download, called The Six Step Guide to Painting Your Home. This is available at www.environment.gov.au/resource/lead-alert-facts-lead-house-paint

Things **not to do** to surfaces containing lead.:

- Dry sand or scrap
- Sand blast
- Work outside on a wet or windy day
- Use a high temperature heat removal system (or open flame)
- Allow children, pregnant women or nursing women near disturbed surfaces

TIP The LEAD Group provides resources for lead testing, information, lead-safe removal resources and support www.lead.org.au

For many years we have been encouraged to read our food labels and get to know the ingredients and additives that we are consuming. Reading the labels on paints and coatings used throughout a home is just as important because potential pollutants from these products can make their way into our bodies through inhalation of fumes/VOCs or inhalation/ingestion of dusts. As we have seen with lead pollutant concerns, we know that when paint starts to break down (it can be seen to be cracked or have a powdered residue), the paint ingredients are migrating into dust that can be inadvertently inhaled or ingested.

What to consider when purchasing

Supporting documents such as the MSDS (material safety data sheets) are legally only required to list hazardous chemicals that individually make up more than 1 percent of the volume of the entire formula (unlike European guidelines). A paint company may put in several chemical masking agents and biocides, and not have to list any of them because individually they are less than 1 percent of the volume. As a combination, though, these can make up a large volume of the actual product.

VOCs in paints is a contentious issue – from a health perspective not all VOCs are the same. There is a large amount of research and scientific evidence to support the idea that there is a significant distinction, in terms of health impacts, between naturally occurring VOCs, for example comparing orange oil VOCs, and synthetic VOCs.

In terms of implications for health, further to choosing product that minimises VOCs, the argument for choosing naturally derived products makes common sense when striving to minimise potential harmful pollutants that may migrate into household dust.

Reasons for selecting lowest toxicity and low VOC paint selection:

- Supports the manufacturing of cleaner, less toxic raw materials within industry
- Better for workers' health – manufacturing workers and paint applicators
- Less risk to occupants health from exposures – VOCs and dusts
- Offers improved indoor air quality compared with other products
- Product is less toxic than others when it is no longer used – product lifecycle

What is a low VOC paint/coating?

From the Environment Protection & Heritage Council, 2008:

'VOC emissions from coatings result from the presence of solvents (and other organic compounds) in solvent-based and water-based coatings. Solvents are used in coatings as a vehicle to transfer the coating to a substrate and are released to the atmosphere by evaporation following application.'

There are no legislatively based or mandated standards that prescribe a maximum VOC content of coatings in Australia. There are only voluntary VOC limits for a range of coating products established by the Australian Paint Approval Scheme (APAS). APAS certifies paints and coatings made in Australia to ensure the product meets its voluntary performance specifications, administered by the CSIRO. The APAS document D181 details the limits of maximum VOCs for APAS approved products.

Green Painters has outlined a range of the variations of VOCs across different products. In petrochemical solvent based paints, VOCs can be as high as 35-550 grams per litre. Water based paints generally have VOC levels of 30-80 grams per litre.

The certification body Good Environmental Choice Australia's paints and coatings certification criteria requires that the total volatile organic compounds in a product must not exceed those stated in the following table (these amounts do not include tints or colourants).

Coating Type	VOC limits g/L	
	Interior Coatings	Exterior Coatings
Ceiling	5	N/A
Wall – flat and low sheen	5	10
Wall – gloss, semi-gloss and satin	5	15
Trim	75	75
Fillers and primers	30	30
Sealers and undercoats	30	30
Stains and varnishes	75	75
Durable external topcoats* – flat and low sheen	–	45
Durable external topcoats* – gloss, semi-gloss and satin	–	60
Powder coatings	10	10

* Durable coatings are those with a warranty of at least 10 years. Table supplied by Good Environmental Choice Australia.

Tints and colourants are not included in the calculations above, however for certification, GECA approved products must have tints or colourants with a VOC limit below 5 g/L.

To know if a product has been approved by GECA, look for the certification logo.

Further information about GECA standards for paints and coatings can be found at **www.geca.org.au**

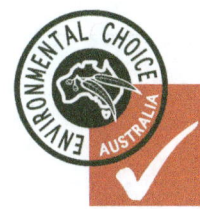

There is a significant difference between the maximum voluntary guidelines for VOCs in coatings and the voluntary low emission levels that can be found certified by organisations such as GECA and Ecospecifier.

Solvent based paints/coatings may contain ingredients such as benzene, toluene, xylene, glycol ether, phenol, formaldehyde and methylene chloride, all of which are carcinogens. Water based paints may still contain harmful ingredients, however given reduced VOC levels they are a good place to start when navigating your choices.

When choosing products, consider that a product with half the VOC content of another product may not be a wise choice if you have to apply two or three coats against one coat for the higher VOC product.

Consider the VOC grams per litre on the label along with what the paint is made from and the coverage rate. If this information is not provided on the label of a product you want to use, contact the company directly to request this information so you are informed, and companies will start to realise consumers want transparent labelling. Often paint ingredients will not be listed on the label and some investigation is needed. Also be aware that material safety data sheets for paints and coatings can be general in nature e.g. stating aromatic hydrocarbons rather than specific benzene. Be sure to check that the colour (tint) added to the base tin does not significantly increase the VOC levels of the product.

Eco labels are fast becoming a way that consumers can identify attributes of paints and coatings. It is interesting to note that the European Eco certifications are generally progressive and products largely must meet high environmental and performance standards, often with stricter compliance requirements than here in Australia. Some paint and coating companies supply global markets yet do not necessarily offer their healthier products for sale in Australia. Australia may receive products that are not accepted by countries with higher standards – raising 'dumping ground' concerns.

Further to chemicals highlighted above, there are two ingredients you may like to note are being reviewed internationally:

Triclosan antimicrobials – this chemical is sold under trade names claiming to stop the growth of bacteria, fungi and mildew and to deodorise. The WHO and United Nations Environment program included triclosan as an endocrine disruptor in its State of the Science of Endocrine Disrupting Chemicals report, published in 2013.

Nanoparticles are being used in some paints offering crack-resistance, anti-graffiti properties, strength and light weight attributes. Titanium dioxide (TiO_2) nanoparticles are widely reported to be used in Australia in cosmetics, sunscreen, household products and surface coatings. According to the 2013 Nano Titanium Dioxide fact sheet by the Australian, National Industrial Chemicals Notification and Assessment Scheme:

'TiO_2 nanoparticles may be inhaled during normal spray application of surface coatings, but this is not expected to pose concern due to the film-forming nature of paints when applied on surfaces...Based on reports in some rodent studies of increased lung tumours after inhalation, the International Agency for Research on Cancer (IARC) has classified TiO_2 as possibly carcinogenic to humans (Group 2B).'

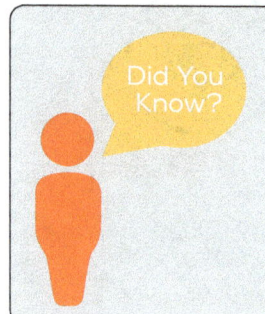

Did You Know?

Close to 800 chemicals are known or suspected to be capable of interfering with hormone receptors, hormone synthesis or hormone conversion.

United Nations Environment Programme and World Health Organisation – State of the Science: Endocrine Disrupting Chemicals – 2012 report.

What to consider when painting

- If paint stripping is required, do a lead test first (buy kit from hardware store)
- If paint stripping is required, opt for a removal system that minimises dust such as a wet topical removal product, and wear protective clothing
- Opt for zero VOC or low VOC paint product (the lower the better). Decide if you want a product made from natural or petro chemically derived ingredients
- Look for independent product certifications such as Good Environmental Choice Australia (GECA) or GreenTag
- Do you want the surface underneath your paint to be able to breathe? Some paints allow surfaces underneath to breathe while others seal the surface (there is contentious debate about the health impacts on a building with breathable vs non-breathable coatings)
- No matter what product you choose, air the room regularly for as long as possible before use
- Whichever paint you choose, follow the full proprietary paint system. Deviating from the product paint system (all associated products, method and process recommended for the application) is likely to void product warranties and may cause issues that result in rework
- Calculate your paint purchase to minimisation wastage – better for the budget and the environment
- Keep some touch-up paint for any repairs to scratches or dents
- Choose environmentally friendly paint accessories like brushes, trays and drop sheets. Roller trays and plastic drop sheets are available made from recycled materials

Further Information

Good Environmental Choice Australia – GECA is an Australian certifier of environmentally preferable goods and services measured according to their product criteria. The online site provides a 'Find Products' resource for items they have certified – www.geca.org.au

EcoSpecifer Global – Sustainable products database for consumers and industry, highlighting products with sustainable and low emission attributes based on various criteria. GreenTag product certification data – www.ecospecifier.com.au

Green Painters – Green Painters is an organisation offering a range of online resources related to sustainable painting products, trade skills and consumer information and resources – www.greenpainters.org.au

Healthy Interiors – Interior design health focused website containing a 'Featured Products' section of the website showcasing healthy option products – www.healthyinteriors.com.au

Australian Paint Approval Scheme (APAS) – APAS is administered by the CSIRO and certifies paint coatings to ensure they meet stringent performance specifications – www.apas.gov.au

Window coverings

Many window covering products use plasticised materials or plasticised coatings to achieve a block-out capability for fabrics. The concern with these applications is that window coverings hang in windows and receive considerable direct heat. Heat causes plastic to off-gas, therefore releasing VOCs into indoor air. Plastics also contain phthalate chemicals, otherwise known as plastic softeners. In recent years, studies and organisations have highlighted health concerns of phthalate chemicals in relation to products migrating phthalates into household dust which has been linked to respiratory illness and endocrine (hormonal) disruption.

Curtains or drapes tend to collect more dust than blinds and curtains. For people living with asthma or allergies, opting for blinds on the windows can reduce dust levels and the circulation of dust.

When selecting window coverings it makes common sense to look for materials that have minimal VOC emissions and do not contain plasticisers that may potentially migrate phthalates into household dust.

Like so many other products in the building industry now, the window coverings sector does not currently provide labels that outline the full list of materials used to create their products. Consumers need to make their own assessments about product suitability for their home on the basis of material and industry knowledge.

Window coverings generally fall into two supply categories: pre-made and custom made.

When buying custom made, assess the labelling and look for any independent product certifications about the product's sustainability or health attributes. You may need to ask the supplier for additional information if full disclosure about the type of material, coatings or treatments is not included on the label.

For custom made blinds and curtains, consumers have the choice to combine various materials and finishes to create their own window covering solution.

Textile manufacturing involves the use of many chemicals throughout the process of pre-treatments, dyeing, finishing and printing. The steps of textile production can also take place in different countries, all with differing standards and legal requirements regarding harmful substances. Given these circumstances, problems can arise with the safety of chemicals used in manufacturing textiles. These issues impact on the environment, however given we get up close and personal with our fabrics through the use of clothing, bedding and soft furnishings in the home, any residue of harmful substances has the potential to impact on our health.

Oeko-Tex is a global certification body that tests textiles for harmful substances. Products tested by this agency carry a 'Confidence in Textiles® Standard 100' logo.

This certification is not mandatory, therefore consumers need to be aware that where product does not have this certification, additional questions as to the origin or the fabric, standards met and chemicals used may need to be asked of the supplier.

Verification of Oeko-Tex certified product claims can be checked at **www.oeko-tex.com**

Window covering selection considerations:
- If using fabrics opt for material that has been Oeko-Tex certified
- For wooden blinds opt for product with finishing coatings that are nontoxic and low emission
- Avoid PVC and plasticised products where possible
- Avoid flame retardant chemicals, especially those topically applied as they can migrate into household dust
- Avoid stain resistant treatments
  Consider the cleaning requirements of your window covering – can they be cleaned with nontoxic cleaning methods?
- Consider the insulating properties where used to maintain internal comfort levels

To reduce the direct heat that interior window coverings receive in the summer months, consider the installation of exterior window shades to protect your soft furnishings. Exterior window shading in the summer months can also reduce your cooling needs and reduce your cooling bills. This is discussed further in the passive cooling section.

Further information

Oeko-Tex - www.oeko-tex.com

Furniture

Furniture for the home is usually acquired through ready made purchases or custom made items.

The questions raised and considerations highlighted in the previous material sections apply to buying furniture for the home. When choosing materials for the home you are in a position to query what a material is made from and how it has been made. When buying ready made furniture for the home you are also in a position to query the same elements:

- What the product has been made from?
- How has it been made?
- Where was it made?

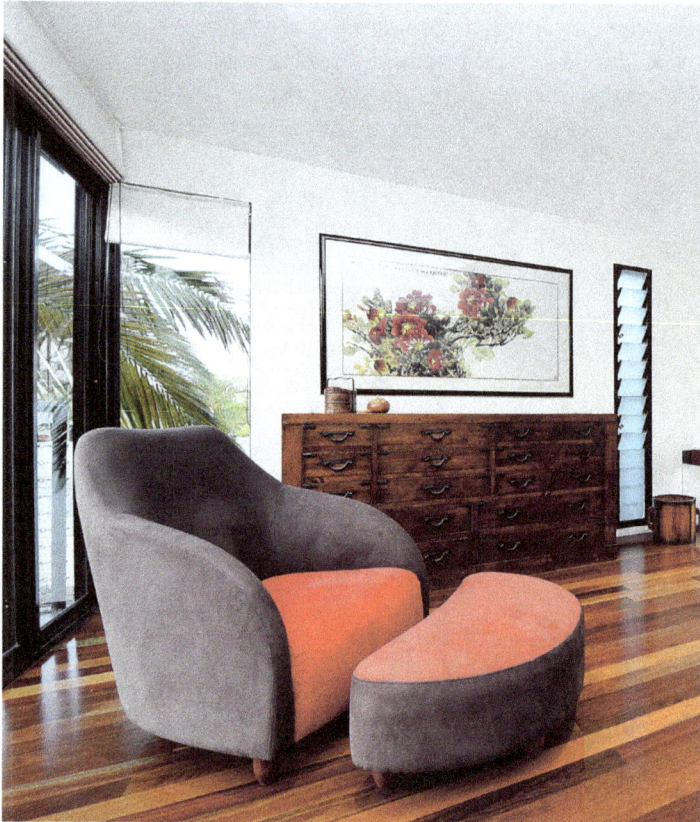

The answers to these questions allow you to make informed decisions as to the health and sustainability attributes of a piece of furniture.

The table, right, is an example of a health focused furniture acquisition:

Image supplied by Healthy Interiors

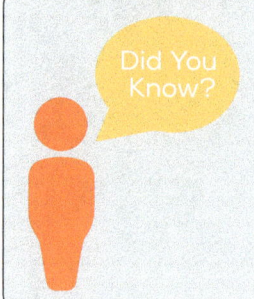

Did You Know?

Reused pre-loved sofas may contain lurking pollutants such as lead and toxic banned flame retardants. New sofas may contain indoor pollutants in the foam, textiles, stains and adhesives. Furniture imported from overseas such as sofas are fumigated with toxic chemicals to kill any insects that may have made the trip on or in the article. Many Australian brands import furniture. Some Australian companies that make their furniture may also import some as well. If looking for an Australian-made sofa ensure you clarify it was made in Australia.

Tips for a healthy, sustainable sofa

1. Needs analysis – reusing or reviving preloved furniture is the most sustainable option.
2. If opting to reuse or revive preloved items do a pollutant check to remove toxins that could be lurking; such as lead in old paints/coatings and flame retardants lurking in old foams.
3. Space analysis – assess the size of the space the sofa will be placed in, consider any moves you may need to make and if the item is likely to be relocated at any stage in the future.
4. Consider the size and shape of the piece or pieces that will provide the flexibility you require given the room size and type of use e.g. lounging, sleeping or sitting only.
5. Opt for a classic shape that is timeless - quality furniture will last many years and replacement for aesthetic purposes only is costly and contributes to landfill.
6. Opt for a fabric design that is timeless. Patterns tend to be linked to fashion and will date quickly. Replacing or recovering a sofa due to fashion changes is costly and an inefficient use of materials.
7. Opt for a fabric that is Oeko-Tex certified – free from harmful textile additives.
8. Avoid textiles with chemical treatments such as crease resistance, UV resistant, antibacterial or stain resistant treatments. Many of these have been linked to a range of health concerns.
9. Opt for a fabric that is easy to spot clean, consider textured fabrics to help hide any marks that may arise over time
10. Opt for natural fibre materials where possible, avoid plasticised materials as they may leach phthalate chemicals or contribute to VOCs within indoor air. Natural fibres will also break down easier at the end of a products life when the item is discarded.
11. Opt for a solid timber frame that is made from certified timber – such as FSC® (Forest Stewardship Council) or PEFC certified product. This ensures supply is from a responsibly sourced and managed resource. Some frames may be made using MDF board, pressed board or ply which contain adhesives and likely to contain formaldehyde.
12. Opt for environmentally friendly seat/cushion filler. Foams to be CFC-free, preferably without flame retardants – opt for independently certified and verified product. Alternatives to foam are feather and down, wool or kapok. Query the cleaning process and chemicals potentially used to prepare fibres.
13. Opt for a sofa made from water-based adhesives that are low VOC.
14. Consider the 'small stuff' - are components used such as glides and feet made from recyclable materials?
15. Avoid fumigation chemicals used on imported items – buy local!

    Carbon miles matter – the energy used to pack and ship sofas, along with the fuel and pollution generated is considerable. Buying local is healthier for the environment, less burden on energy resources, healthier for people and supports local jobs/families.
16. If buying a new sofa ask your supplier if the manufacturer has a product stewardship program, where the product is taken back and recycled for reuse.
17. Opt for products that have product claims verified and certified by an independent organisation.

Water ware and plumbing

Water is a valued resource so opting for plumbing devices and accessories that help minimise waste is ideal. Products that we choose to use with water have the potential to impact water quantity, quality, water costs and indirectly impact our heath.

Considerations for healthy water:

- Is the water journey free from lead contamination?
- Has any chemical treatment been added that may impact on health?
- Is the water in contact with plastic that can migrate pollutants when heated?

Lead is a naturally occurring metal that can be found deep within the ground. Lead has been mined and used in a wide range of consumer products for many years. Science has since realised that lead is unsafe and contributes to a wide range of health conditions including impaired child development, muscular conditions, nerve disorders, neurological conditions, fertility and decreased kidney function. Lead has been used over the years in a range of products utilised by the building industry, such as lead flashing, ceramic tiles, lead roofing, sheet metal, PVC, lead solder used on pipes, leaded brass or bronze components.

In order to avoid lead contamination of water, the journey to the outlet needs to be examined and potential sources of lead removed.

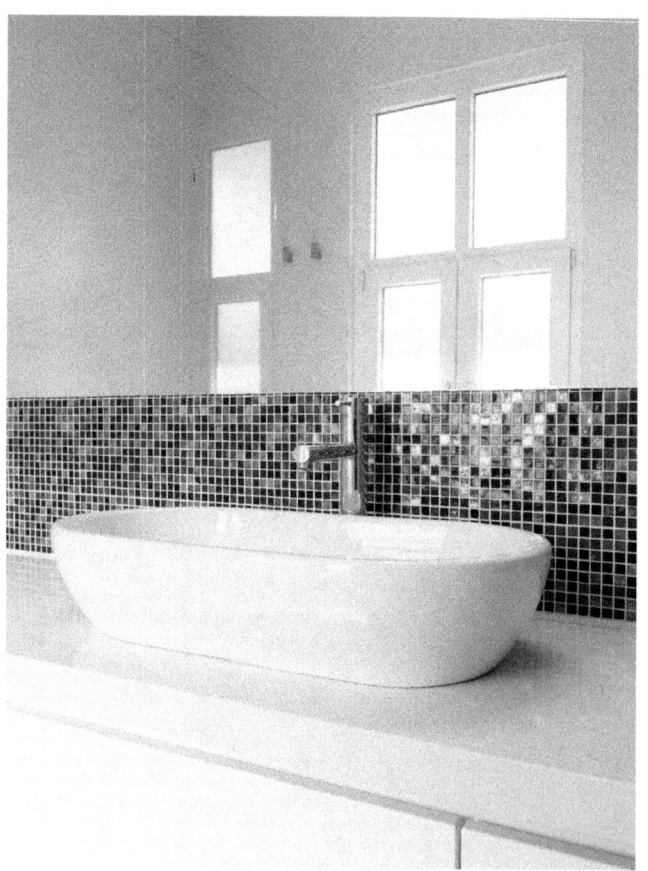

Image supplied by Healthy Interiors

If your home was built prior to the 1930s, when copper pipes replaced lead pipes, check to ensure that all lead has been removed. Lead based solder on brass fittings and copper pipes was continued in use until 1989. As a result of corrosion there is potential for any lead to leach into the water after prolonged contact. In older homes it is advisable to avoid consuming water from first use after water has sat in pipes overnight or for prolonged periods.

Droughts, water scarcity and increasing water bills have motivated many to install rainwater tanks. For those living in rural communities, rainwater tanks often collect drinking water. It is particularly important for those harvesting their own drinking water to investigate and eliminate potential contaminates that the water may collect, from moving over roof and gutter surfaces and from storage in tanks.

Many old homes contain lead flashing on the roof. This is often forgotten when rain water is collected. Rainwater is also often used for home gardens. Ensuring rainwater collected is free from lead is also important for those using the water on edible plants or for feeding animals.

'The National Health and Medical Research Council (NHMRC) guideline level for lead in drinking water is that it should be a maximum of 10 micrograms per litre (which is also written as 0.01 milligrams per litre or 0.01 mg/L)' Lead Advisory Service Australia, 2002

If you would like to have your water tested for lead you will need to contact a testing laboratory and provide them with a sample. Testing costs can vary depending on what you are testing and how many investigations are needed.

The following are examples of laboratories that provide heavy metal testing:

Spectrometer - **www.spectrometer.com.au**
Sydney Analytical Laboratories – **www.sal.com.au**
National Measurement Institute – **www.measurement.gov.au**

The LEAD Group Incorporated is a great resource and can also provide lead testing information **www.lead.org.au**

Further to considering heavy metal contamination of water, it is also important to be aware of plastics. Some plastics can leach phthalate chemicals. Phthalates have been linked to a range of serious health concerns and many are considered endocrine altering chemicals (ability to alter hormones). There are many types of plastics used to create a wide variety of products. These all vary in their stability and their capacity to leach toxins in different conditions.

When plastics are heated they are more likely to leach toxins. There are many products that contain plastics within the plumbing accessories sector such as pipes, tapware, shower heads and adjustable hoses. The lack of labelling and product transparency makes it difficult to ascertain if these products are made from plastics that do not leach phthalates or other contaminants when heated with hot water. In circumstances where information is limited, all we can do is minimise use of products that may be an issue.

Avoid PVC piping (especially for pipes carrying drinking water). Better alternatives include polyethylene and copper.

When buying tapware in Australia check for the product's Water Efficiency Labelling and Standards (WELS) rating. WELS products must carry a WELS label showing the water efficiency star rating and the water consumption or flow rate of the product. The WELS Act obliges suppliers to test and register products and to ensure that they are correctly labelled in advertisements and at the point of sale. A prerequisite of WELS registration of tapware is that products have WaterMark Certification.

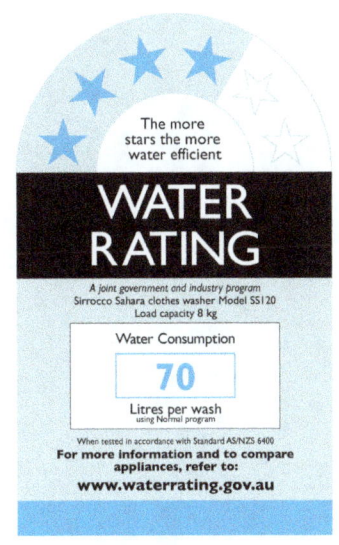

WaterMark Certification provides proof that a manufacturer's tapware design, material and construction meets the requirements of the Australian Standard AS/NZS 3718 Water Supply – Tapware.

When choosing tapware, check that the item complies with the Standard by looking for a WaterMark licence number, WaterMark logo, and the product Standard engraved on the product, usually in a position that will not be visible when the tapware is installed.

Online availability of products and rogue importers may offer bargains, but buying tapware that has not had the relevant safety and quality tests could inevitably cost you more dollars and impact on health. Testing required under the WaterMark certification scheme ensures that materials used to make the product are safe. The types and combination of metals used to make tapware vary globally, not all of them are suitable for drinking water, and some may leach heavy metals.

Buying a product that does not have WaterMark approval can also result in a financial loss as while retailers are allowed to sell non-WaterMark products, licenced plumbers are not authorised to install these products. WaterMark certification provides confidence that you are purchasing a product that meets relevant Standards and which can be installed by a licenced plumber.

Some additional tips:

- Specify and use 100 percent lead-free solder to connect plumbing pipe if soldering is required
- Specify and use lead-free roofing and flashing
- For copper pipe applications, reduce or eliminate joint-related sources of copper corrosion and/or use mechanically crimped copper joint systems
- Avoid PVC pipes

Water filtration

In Australia there is a range of chemicals used in the treatment of our public water supply. The list is extensive and can be viewed in the Australian Drinking Water Guidelines Report available on the National Health and Medical Research Council (NHMRC) website at www.nhmrc.gov.au.

Two of the chemicals commonly associated with water and health concerns in Australia are fluoride and chlorine.

Fluoride added to the public water supply is a contentious issue. Fluoride is banned in many countries and others have held off as a precautionary approach. Despite fluoride once being disposed of as toxic waste, Australia is now one of the most heavily fluoridated countries in the world. The introduction of fluoride into the water supply was largely due to dental industry claims it would improve dental health. There are mounting health concerns associated with fluoride. Fluoride has been linked to a range of health issues such as fluorosis of the teeth (white patches), bone cancer, thyroid complaints, and cardiovascular and endocrine system impairments. In the USA mothers who intend to bottle feed are routinely advised to avoid fluorinated water when preparing bottles.

There is considerable data available online about both sides of this issue. The Fluoride Action Network has collated some interesting research associated with health concerns, at **www.fluoridealert.org**. There is also an Australian information group, **www.australianfluorideaction.com**.

Removing fluoride from water is difficult and can be expensive. When exploring filter options, question:

- the process of the filter
- the journey the water takes
- what the water is exposed to as it passes through the filter

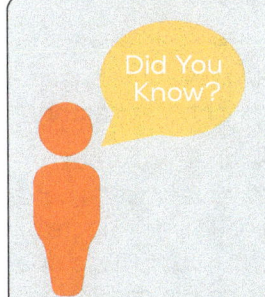

Did You Know?

A recently-published Harvard University meta-analysis funded by the National Institutes of Health (NIH) has concluded that children who live in areas with highly fluoridated water have 'significantly lower' IQ scores than those who live in low fluoride areas.

(Choi et al, 2012)

Chlorine is also another chemical added to our public water supply. It is added to perform a disinfectant function to prevent the spread of disease-causing bacteria.

Chlorine added to the water supply reacts with other naturally-occurring elements to form toxins called trihalomethanes (THMs), which eventually make their way into our bodies. THMs are a suspected carcinogen and have been linked to a wide range of human health concerns such as asthma, eczema, bladder cancer and heart disease.

THMs can be absorbed by the body through:

Inhalation – when showering or bathing (VOCs)
Absorbed – when high levels are in contact with the skin
Ingested – consumed in food prepared with water

How can you reduce your exposure to THMs?

- Tapware selection - aeration of the water at the tap
- Boiling drinking water for a minute and allowing it to cool
- Water filtration system – activated carbon filters for drinking and bathing water

The American College of Allergy, Asthma and Immunology indicates that some people can be sensitive to chlorine and that skin sensitivity to chlorine can present the following symptoms:

- Skin redness, tenderness, inflammation, and/or itchiness at the site of contact
- Skin lesions or rash
- Scales or crust on the skin

People with asthma, EIB (exercise-induced bronchoconstriction) and allergic rhinitis, who already have sensitive airways, might also have the following symptoms:

- Coughing, especially at night, with exercise, or when laughing
- Trouble breathing
- A tight feeling in the chest
- Wheezing, or a squeaky or whistling sound during breathing
- Runny nose
- Itching
- Sneezing
- Stuffy nose due to blockage or congestion

Eczema, dermatitis and asthma are common aliments many families struggle with. Given chlorine-treated water is documented as a potential irritant, sufferers may find it beneficial to minimise exposure through the use of shower, bath and drinking water filters.

Consumers can independently test their water supply if concerned about chemical levels. To have your water tested contact a National Analytical Testing Authority (NATA) authorised chemical laboratory. Chemical laboratories are listed under 'analysts' in the phone directory.

There is a range of benefits to using water filters; they can not only remove chemicals but also have the ability to remove heavy metals, pesticides and bacteria from your water. There are many different types that perform different functions. There are several filter products on the market using differing filtration mediums, all having different removal capability, so be sure to read the label to understand what your filter is made from and what it can filter out of the water.

When choosing a water filter consider:

What is the filter made from?

Are independent testing results available for the removal of contaminants? (to avoid unsubstantiated claims)

Has any independent migration testing has been done to ascertain if any of the filter materials leach into the water as part of the filtering process?

Has the filter been independently certified, for example by NSF International **www.nsf.org/about-nsf/what-is-third-party-certification/**

Swimmers who frequent indoor chlorinated pools may be interested to know that chloramines (what chlorine turns into when combined with organics) and chlorine by products in the air above indoor swimming pools have been linked to respiratory symptoms. The Centres for Disease Control and Prevention (CDC) in the USA highlight that:

'The symptoms of irritant exposure in the air can range from mild symptoms, such as coughing, to severe symptoms, such as wheezing or aggravating asthma.'

Look for indoor swimming pools with alternative disinfectant systems, e.g. ultraviolet light and ozone chemical free (natural) pools.

Lighting

Lighting is an important functional design element in a home, used for a variety of functional and decorative purposes. It is important to have some understanding of how lighting can work for you and the different functions and moods it can create.

Types of lighting

Ambient lighting (also referred to as general lighting) is used to create a particular atmosphere and generally illuminates the overall space. It should provide enough light brightness to support the room's basic activities. Lamp types used to provide ambient lighting include LED, CFL, fluorescent strips, and halogen. Incandescent globes are still used despite their inefficiencies.

Task lighting is used to provide high levels of light illuminating a specific function, for example meal preparation. Common areas within a home that require task lighting are the kitchen, bathrooms, reading zones and home office. Lamp types that are suitable for task lighting include LED strip lighting and lamps, some fluorescent types, halogen and spot lights.

Accent lighting is used to highlight spaces or items such as artwork, architectural features or plants. Lamp types used to provide accent lighting are usually track lighting, spot lights in the floor or ceiling, or occasionally table or floor lamps. These usually have a narrow beam spread and have a higher lighting lumen output.

Decorative lighting effects

Wall washing – this is used to illuminate large surfaces such as a wall or several objects on the wall that provide a focal point. The lighting source lights the wall at wide angles and provides an even level of brightness to the area. Spacing will depend on the wall and height of the ceiling. This is mostly used in public buildings, however it can be used in a home to make a room seem brighter or more spacious.

Wall grazing – where concealed lighting is used to highlight various areas by skimming light across the surface. For example, where a lighting source lights a wall at a narrow angle and accentuates details through use of shadows. This technique is often used for accentuating textured surfaces such as brick and stone. The angle of lighting is adjusted to make the shadowing more or less pronounced.

The type of lighting and desired effect required for each space in the home varies according to the uses of each room. Identifying how different spaces within the home are to be used, and the décor style you would like to achieve, will help you to establish the types of lighting you need for functional purposes and the types of lighting you need for general and decorative lighting.

A wide choice of light fittings and globes is available which makes it very easy to get frustrated and confused with lighting selections. The following are a few basic terms to understand when shopping for lighting.

Lighting terminology

Lumens – the amount of light that is emitted from a bulb. A high number of lumens means it has a brighter light; lower lumens is a dimmer light. For example:

- A 100 watt incandescent bulb would provide around 1600 lumens
- A 40 watt incandescent bulb would provide around 450 lumens

The diagram below provides an example of the amount of lumens per light type.

Lux: the measurement of the amount of light over a given area. Generally measured in lux per m2, so 1 lux = 1 lumens per m2

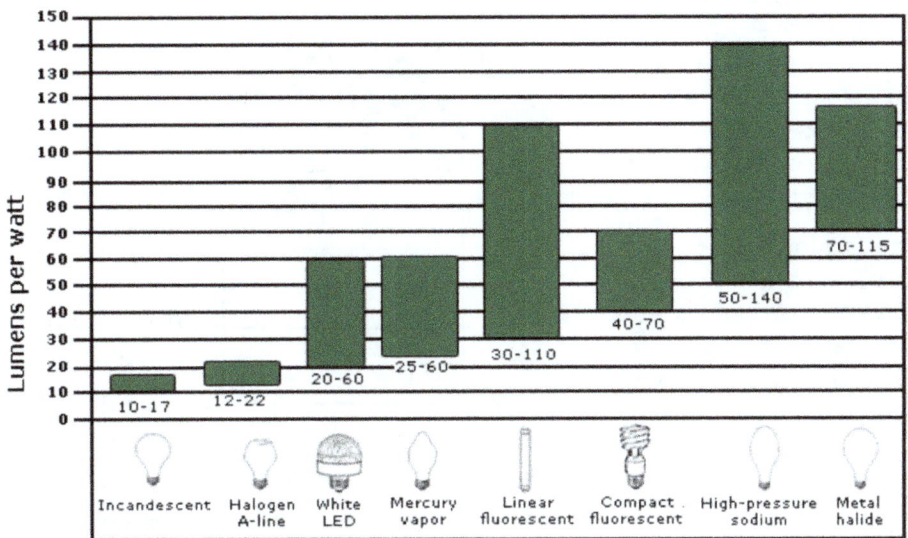

Image source: WA5MLF

Efficacy: the ratio of light output to power input measured in lumens per watt. For example:

- The efficacy of a 50 watt halogen downlight emitting 900 lux would be 900/50 = 18 lumens per watt
- The efficacy of a 10 watt LED bulb emitting 900 lux would be 90. 900/10 = 90 lumens per watt, which is significantly more energy efficient than other bulb types

Efficiency

This is the percentage of power that is converted to light. For example:

- The old incandescent light bulbs had an efficiency of around 5 percent and it converts the other 95 percent to heat
- A 50 watt halogen downlight has about 3.5 percent efficiency, and the remaining 96.5 percent is wasted heat
- A LED is now around 80 percent efficient with just 20 percent being wasted as heat

The **beam angle** is the outer angle of the light emitted from the light source when it is at 50 percent of its centre beam intensity. For example:

- A halogen downlight typically has a 60 degree beam angle
- LED downlight globes have a beam angle ranging from 20 degrees to 180 degrees depending on the globe

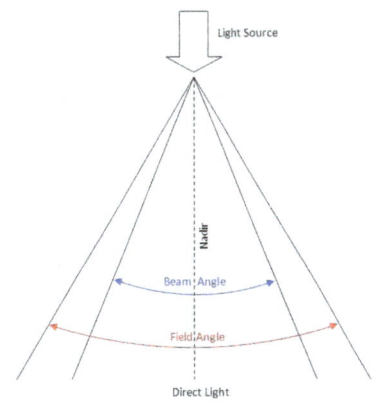

Image source: High Technology Lighting

Colour temperature

This is measured in 'degrees Kelvin'. Kelvin temperature is a numerical measurement that describes the colour and appearance of the light produced by the lamp and the colour appearance of the lamp itself, expressed on the Kelvin (K) scale. This indicates the hue or colour of a light source. The warmer the colour the closer to the red end of the spectrum it gets. Colour temperature range for a household is best between 2800 and 4000 degrees Kelvin, which provides for a 'warm white' colour.

The Colour Rendering Index (CRI) is a measure of how well a light source can accurately display colours compared to natural light. It is expressed as percentage. The higher the CRI, the better the visual perception of colours. For example:

- CRI between 85 and 100 is excellent
- CRI between 60 and 85 is considered good
- CRI between 0 and 59 is considered poor

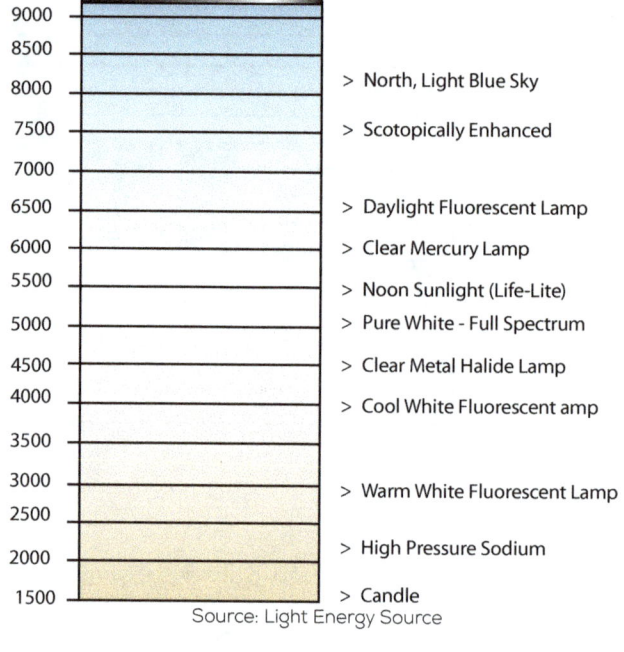
Source: Light Energy Source

Natural light

We use the term 'natural light' to mean sunlight entering the home through windows, glazed doors, skylights or solar tube type lighting. This is the nicest and most valued form of lighting achieved in a home. Where possible ensure your primary living spaces (family room and kitchen) have access to substantial natural sunlight.

When designing spaces with natural lighting sources, be mindful of furniture placement and effects of UV on furniture, such as fading or surface deterioration. For spaces that receive considerable direct light this is something to consider when choosing the type of glass for your windows as products are available that assist with minimising UV transmission.

Types of electric lighting

There are many different types of electric lighting available on the market. This section reviews those that would be suitable for households.

The following information is reproduced with permission from the Australian Government Department of Industry Energy Efficiency website:

> The Australian Government, Department of Industry is targeting any light bulbs that have an efficiency level of less than 15 lumens per watt (lm/w). Lumens (lm) are a measure of light output and watts (W) are a measure of energy input.
>
> The traditional pear-shaped incandescent bulbs (General Lighting Service lamps) are the least efficient - these bulbs waste 90 per cent of the energy they use, mainly as heat. They were phased out first, with an import restriction that applied from 1 February 2009, followed by a sales restriction from November 2009.
>
> More efficient types of incandescent bulbs known as halogens will continue to be available, but the least efficient of this group will be phased out over time. Mains voltage (240 Volt), and low voltage bulbs (12 Volt - typically used in downlighting), are the common types of halogens. NOTE: low voltage does not mean low energy use.
>
> To find out more, go to www.ee.ret.gov.au/energy-efficiency/lighting

Light emitting diodes (LED)

LEDs are the latest in energy efficient lighting. In its most basic form it's a semiconductor device that converts electricity into light. LEDs use approximately 85 percent less energy than a halogen or older incandescent types. LEDs also have a significantly longer lifespan

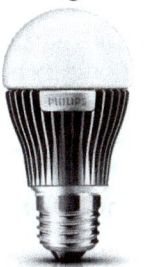

of between 30,000 and 50,000 hours. A halogen has a lifespan of between 1,000 – 2,000 hours, and the older incandescent types just 1,000 hours.

LEDs are often used to replace halogen downlights and come in a range of colours, wattage, brightness and quality. LEDs need a 'driver' as opposed to a 'transformer' to moderate the power. The 'driver' is an electrical device that regulates power to the LED ensuring a constant amount of power as the electrical properties change with temperature. It is a kind of 'cruise control' for an LED lamp.

Image credit: Philips LED globe

Some LEDs will work with standard transformers, however the lifespan of the LED bulb is usually greatly reduced. Best practice is always to replace any halogen fitting and transformer with an LED fitting and driver. However you can sometimes get away with just replacing the lamp and the transformer, and reusing the fitting (dependent on the lamp type).

Fluorescent strip lighting

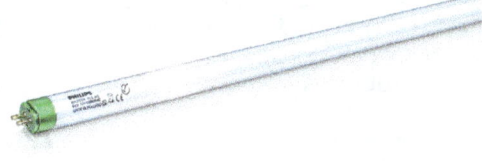

Often called fluorescent tubes, these are low pressure mercury vapour lamps that use fluorescence to produce light by converting electrical energy. These require a 'ballast' which is generally in the centre of the fitting to regulate the current through the lamp. Fluorescent tubes provide a very efficient light source.

Image credit: Philips lighting

Unfortunately fluorescent lamps contain mercury, and because of this they are considered hazardous waste and should be disposed of through the appropriate recycling waste stream. They should not be put into landfill or standard recycling bins. There is further information about disposal later in this section.

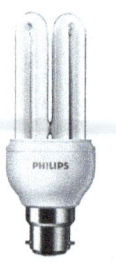

Image credit: Philips Lighting

Compact fluorescent lamps (CFL)

These low energy lights (also known as low energy lighting) consist of fluorescent strips (as above) curled into a compact shape to fit into standard light fitting sockets.

CFLs are approximately 80 percent more energy efficient than old incandescent bulbs and last between 8,000-15,000 hours. The CFL is a good option for an area that has lighting on for periods of time to provide ambient light. As with fluorescent strip lighting, these contain mercury and should be disposed of carefully at end of life.

CFLs and fluorescent strips are not suitable for short bursts of lighting in areas such as toilets or security lamps on sensors that tend to go on and off a lot. If they are used in these situations they will fail and need regular replacement.

Disposal of mercury-containing products

Fluorescent lighting contains a small amount of mercury. If a fluorescent light breaks in your home, safe clean up and disposal procedures are required to prevent toxic mercury exposure.

The Australian Government's Department of Industry has detailed safe disposal instructions on their webpage for cleaning up broken fluorescent light bulbs along with national product disposal information. The following is reproduced with permission from their webpage.

Safety steps for cleaning up broken CFL bulbs containing mercury

- First, open nearby windows and doors to allow the room to ventilate for 15 minutes before cleaning up the broken light bulb. Turn off air conditioning or heating equipment which could recirculate mercury vapours back into the room.
- Use disposable rubber gloves rather than bare hands.
- Do not use a vacuum cleaner or broom on hard surfaces because this can spread the contents of the light bulb and contaminate the cleaner. Instead, scoop up broken material (e.g. using stiff paper or cardboard) if possible into a glass container which can be sealed with a metal lid.
- Use a disposable brush to carefully sweep up the pieces.
- Wipe up any remaining glass fragments or powders using sticky tape, a damp cloth or damp paper.
- On carpets or fabrics, carefully remove as much glass or powdered material as possible using a scoop and sticky tape. If vacuuming is needed to remove residual material you will need to discard the vacuum bag or thoroughly wipe clean the vacuum cleaner canister afterwards.
- Finally, dispose of any clean-up equipment such as gloves, brush, damp paper and sealed containers containing pieces of broken light bulb in your outside rubbish bin—never in your recycling bin.

While not all of the recommended clean-up and disposal equipment described above may be available (particularly a suitably sealed glass container) it is important to remember to remove broken CFL and clean-up materials to an outside rubbish bin (preferably sealed) as soon as possible. This will reduce the potential contamination indoors.

For more information visit the Australian Government, Department of Industry - Energy Efficiency website http://ee.ret.gov.au/energy-efficiency/lighting/energy-efficient-alternatives/disposing-used-and-broken-compact-fluorescent-lamps-cfl

CFL and fluorescent globes should always be recycled to recover the mercury, phosphor powder and other materials contained. Be sure to recycle mercury-containing lamps and bulbs. Most councils have a recycling facility available, contact your local council to find out where and how to dispose of these products properly. Alternatively call Planet Ark's Recycling Near You Hotline on 1300 733 712 or visit **www.recyclingnearyou.com.au**. It is very important they do not go to landfill as the mercury can contaminate the soil.

Halogen globes

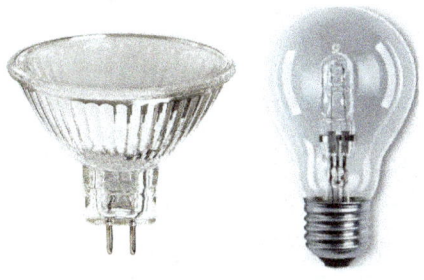

Image credit: Crompton

Many halogen globes (also referred to as tungsten halogen or quartz halogens) look like the older incandescent variety and they are often used for downlights. The low voltage halogen downlight is the most commonly used light bulb in Australia, but low voltage is not low energy and they are not energy efficient. With the exception of incandescent bulbs, they are the most inefficient form of lighting.

Low voltage halogen downlights run through transformers so they cannot be retrofitted with CFL bulbs. Some LED types can replace them but they generally don't last as long as they should because the transformers work differently to the LED drivers as noted above.

When considering the replacement of a halogen downlight with an LED it is better to replace the whole unit. Remove the halogen globe, fitting and transformer and replace it with an LED globe, fitting and driver. Some LEDs can reuse the fitting, but the globe and transformer should always be replaced.

The standard 50 watt halogen that graces so many homes in Australia is now banned from import due to the energy inefficiency, and the fire risk to homes. The following is an indication of the heat halogens can generate:

- A 50W globe can reach up to 300°C in the ceiling
- A 35W globe can reach up to 85°C in the ceiling
- A 20W globe can reach up to 65°C in the ceiling

TIP If you still have 50W halogen globes in your home, but don't want the expense of changing over to LED, change the 50W globes in the main living areas, and other spaces you need well lit, to 35W globes. You will hardly notice the difference in light levels. Then change the hallways and areas that don't need to be so well lit to the 20 watt globes (you will notice a degradation of light level). This removes the heat and fire risk, and saves some energy.

Incandescent

These are the old 'Edison' type of light bulb with a filament wire strung between two metal bars in the centre of the globe which produces light when heated by electric current. Until recently these bulbs were widely used in households and businesses.

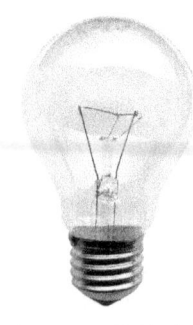

Image credit: Neolux

They generally have a low efficacy of around 16 lumens per watt. The average lifetime of an incandescent bulb is around 1,000 hours, which is significantly less than CFL (around 10,000 hours) or LED (up to 80,000 hours).

Due to government regulations in Australia, as of November 2009 you are no longer able to purchase standard incandescent globes. These globes are extremely inefficient because they only convert approximately five percent of the energy they produced into light, while the remainder is converted to heat, resulting in an extreme waste of electricity. Incandescent bulbs can no longer be purchased in Australia.

Solar lighting

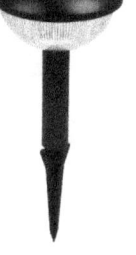

Image credit: Winlights

Solar lamps or lights are generally portable lights that use an LED bulb, a solar photovoltaic (PV) panel and a rechargeable battery. These may be integrated into a single fitting or all completely separate units, depending on the type.

These lamps recharge during sunlight hours and store the energy in the battery, ready for use when the sun goes down. They will usually operate from dusk until the stored energy is depleted which can be several hours.

Solar lights tend to be used for decoration around the garden area, or occasionally for shed or garage lighting if power is not readily available. Solar lighting is very popular because it costs nothing to run (after initial purchase price) and they are easy to install. It's a very energy efficient method of providing light to an area, whether or not there is a power supply, and the range of solar lights available for a variety of uses is growing.

Lighting health considerations:

- Avoid lighting with plastic shades as heat encourages plastic to off-gas
- Avoid adjustable downlights as these often leave gaps around the light into the ceiling space where roof cavity dust and pollutants can fall into the house
- Always choose a 'warm white' colour for inside the home to avoid headaches and nausea from the extremely 'blue' white lights

Lighting plans

Do you need a lighting plan?

A lighting plan is a scaled drawing that details the location and type of each fixed lamp in a building, including switching and dimming. When undertaking a new building project or major renovation, a lighting plan allows you to communicate the type of light fittings you have chosen for your home, where these are to be installed and where the switches are to be located. Lighting plans can at times be incorporated on an electrical plan, which would include other electrical requirements and locations for smoke alarms, exhaust fans, power points, ceiling fans etc. When a lighting plan is created by a professional the level of lighting in each room is carefully considered to ensure the selections are suitable i.e. not too much, not too little.

The image right is a sample lighting plan, courtesy of Eco Decisions.

Object   :
Installation   :
Project number   : Demo Lounge room
Date   : 06.02.2014

Room 1

Summary, Room 1

Result overview, Evaluation area 1

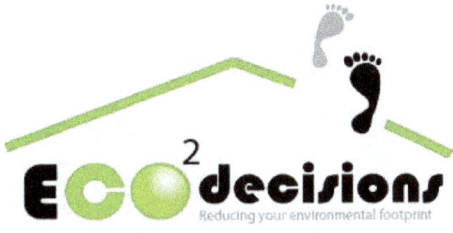

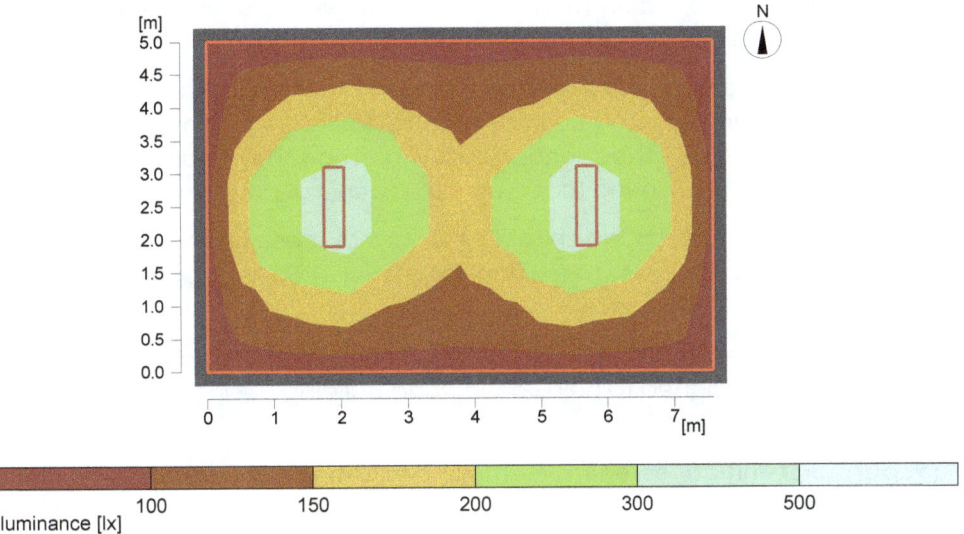

General
Calculation algorithm used
Height of luminaire plane
Maintenance factor

Total luminous flux of all lamps
Total power
Total power per area (37.90 m²)

Average indirect fraction with light colours
2.40 m
0.80

7884 lm
84.0 W
2.22 W/m² (1.26 W/m²/100lx)

Evaluation area 1   **Reference plane 1.1**
                                Horizontal
Em   176 lx
Emin   95 lx
Emin/Eav (Uo)   0.54
Emin/Emax (Ud)   0.27
UGR (4.2H 6.3H)   <=21.8
Position   0.75 m

Major surfaces   Em   Uo
m 1.5 (Ceiling)   59 lx   0.89
m 1.1 (Wall)   93 lx   0.62
m 1.2 (Wall)   100 lx   0.58
m 1.3 (Wall)   93 lx   0.63
m 1.4 (Wall)   100 lx   0.57

Ph 03 9770 5686, mob.0404 538822, ecodecisions@aapt.net.au
EcoDecisions, 27 Hoadley Ave, Frankston Sth. Victoria.

lounge.rdf

As of May 2011, changes to the National Construction Code (NCC), in the Energy Efficiency section, Volume 2 Part 3.12 came into effect, limiting the amount of energy used for lighting per square meter of ceiling space. The limits are:

- 5 watts per m2 for indoor lighting
- 4 watts per m2 for outdoor areas
- 3 watts per m2 for garage lighting

The amendment to the NCC is a very deliberate move to reduce the amount of energy used in new homes for lighting. These requirements are easily achievable when you take the time to consider the adequate lighting requirements of a space and have a lighting plan done.

Some concessions to the rule are available, referred to in the trade as 'adjustment factors', if you choose to include lighting controls such as motion detectors or dimmers. Note that the limitations to the NCC only include fixed lighting that is permanently or directly wired in. It does not include lamps or other lighting that plug into a general power outlet (GPO).

Any good lighting designer or electrician should be aware of these changes. Homes that do not meet these requirements are likely to fail final inspections. Some local councils require a lighting plan to demonstrate compliance.

The Australian Building Codes Board (ABCB) has also created and released a useful lighting calculator which has been designed to help lighting and building designers to meet the code. It is available to download for free from this link:

www.abcb.gov.au/major-initiatives/energy-efficiency/lighting-calculator

Room by room lighting considerations

General lighting

If your budget allows, choose good quality LED products as your preferred primary light source. LEDs are significantly more energy efficient than other lighting types and offer a wide variety of lighting styles to choose from, including standard lamp type globes, downlights, strip lighting, security lamps and even chandelier styles. There really is something for just about every situation. Choose one with a high CRI (between 85 and 100 for the best light) and a warm white colour temperature.

Another good option is the fluorescent lamp (either strip or CFL). After LED, these are the most energy efficient light sources available. However, remember to dispose of them safely and properly when they need replacing.

Living/family rooms

The living space is used for many purposes – a place to relax after work, or a play area for children; the uses are endless. But whatever the purpose, the lighting should be flexible. Opt for a combination approach to lighting and include a mix of ceiling lighting and task lamps.

Choose fittings that work with your devised décor scheme to add interest to the room. Dimmers can be used to control brightness and alter the mood of the lighting.

Floor or task lamps are flexible lighting options that provide task lighting for activities such as reading. Spot lights are functional and decorative additions for the purpose of highlighting artwork or features within the room.

Dining room

The dining room, like the living room, is also used for a variety of purposes. Be it a romantic dinner for two, a celebration with friends and family, or just somewhere to sit and relax with a coffee, it's important that the lighting in this space is also flexible and comfortable.

Depending on the room and dining furniture, pendants may be suitable. When choosing lighting consider where people will be sitting and ensure any exposed light bulbs are not going to cause glare issues to those using the space.

Dimmer switches in a dining space provide for maximum functional flexibility and lighting mood control.

Kitchen

Otherwise known as the heart of the home, the kitchen is one of the most used, most expensive spaces in a home. It's a zone that requires effective task and general lighting. Kitchen spaces are often designed to flow into living spaces therefore the integration of feature lighting in the kitchen 'for wow factor' has gained appeal.

Start by considering the task lighting required over benchtops, sinks and cooking zones.

If opting for decorative feature lighting in the kitchen space consider the décor style you aim to achieve and the overall design of the space. Feature fittings in the kitchen space can provide light for general lighting or task lighting. Opt for lighting styles that take into account the following:

- Décor style
- Ceiling height
- Cabinetry design
- Cabinetry colors and color contrast if required
- Placement
- Lamp styles available – types of lamps the fitting can use and beam spread
- Location and style of task lighting

Architectural highlight lighting

This is the use of continuous LED strip lighting to highlight lines or features within a space, e.g. under the base of the kitchen cabinets to create a floating effect at night.

Overhead cupboard downlighting

Concealed continuous LED strip lighting or LED downlights concealed into the base of the overhead cabinets eliminates shadowing that can occur with general ceiling lighting where overhead cabinets are present. These options provide concealed direct task lighting over benches.

Pendant lighting can be used to provide task of general lighting in a kitchen and are often used to provide a visual divide between areas.

Any spot lights used should be placed where the light is needed, considering glare to occupants and be adjustable for flexibility. Consider shadowing issues when placing spot lights in the kitchen and ensure they are separately switched.

Bathrooms

Bathrooms are another space that need careful consideration. This space is where we bathe and prepare ourselves for the day ahead so it's important to be able to see properly. There are two types of lighting in a bathroom, ambient and task. The ambient light is used for general illumination while bathing or showering. Task lights are important when doing jobs such as shaving or applying makeup.

The bathroom is an excellent place for skylights or solar tube lighting located near the mirror as natural lighting is the best type of light to do personal hygiene tasks by. However, this may not be an option and active lighting is required for times when it is dark.

Ambient lighting in the bathroom is generally best placed in the centre of the space and should be separately switched to the task lights. Task lighting is usually located around the mirror. There is a variety of placement options with bathroom lighting. We cover the main ones below.

Task lighting for a bathroom mirror can be achieved through a variety of methods.

- Sconce type lights placed to both sides of the mirror at face height provides good lighting and minimal shadows on the face as long as the mirror itself isn't too wide
- Putting task lighting at the top of the mirror helps to minimise shadows on your face. Be careful of creating glare. Translucent white diffusers are a good option to avoid this problem. If lighting is projecting from a mirror cabinet, this may not be the best solution
- If you place lighting on the mirror itself, ensure it is kept simple, is of good quality and well finished. This is because the whole of the light, including the back of it, will be reflected in the mirror. Keep in mind that the globe may need replacing at some point, so ensure it is easy and safe to do this. Otherwise use LED as they will last a very long time
- If using recessed lighting put it as close to the mirror as you can to avoid shadowing and to help create a brighter space

If the above methods are not suitable for your situation, other options include using an adjustable wide angle light over the vanity basin with a frost or wide lens (to minimise shadows), or if the ceiling is low use wide angle LED downlights directly behind where you stand at the mirror to get the reflection back onto your face.

Have the bathroom exhaust fan separately switched from the lights.

Hallways

Entrance halls and internal halls are another great place to bring natural light into the home through skylights, solar tube lighting or well-placed clerestory windows.

To provide evening lighting there are several options. Standard ambient type lighting through the use of ceiling mounted fittings, pendant fixtures or wall sconces can provide good lighting for these spaces. LED panel lighting is also a good option as it gives an even light and when using neutral white LED can look like a skylight.

Alternatively, low level recessed LED lighting or recessed LED strip lighting can provide a soft glow for general lighting. Movement sensors can be installed for spaces intermittently used to assist with night time visibility and provide a sense of security for the home.

Stairs

Areas where steps and stairs are located should always be well lit to reduce the risk of tripping and falls. Efficient options include LED strips along the tread of the step or recessed along the wall. Installing sensor lights (that sense movement and daylight) will activate stair lighting as necessary when someone approaches the stairs.

Decorative pendant type lighting also works well placed above stairs at the centre point or at the landing depending on the style of the staircase. Wall mounted lighting in combination with tread lighting is an additional option. The type of lighting used should suit the intended use of the occupants and provide a safe stairwell.

Bedrooms

Using energy efficient ceiling or wall ambient lighting to provide general illumination, including a dimmer provides additional flexibility to suit moods.

Tasks lamps are ideal for those who like reading in bed. These can either be freestanding on bedside tables, fixed to the wall above the bed or wall mounted beside the bed. Bedside lamps are available in many styles including pendant, adjustable or fixed. Bedroom furniture heights and locations should be considered at the electrical rough in stage to ensure fittings function properly with selected furniture.

Home office

The home office needs to provide quality lighting for productivity, especially in the workspace. Bad lighting here can cause eye strain, headaches and reduce productivity. Australian standards for an office specify between 240 and 320 lux at the desktop. There are free smart phone apps available that can provide reasonably accurate lux readings using a phone. Search for lux meter and download the one that appeals to you.

Use ambient lighting to light the space generally (when natural light is not available).

Task lighting should be used when working, especially in zones with computers, filing cabinets and other intensive tasks. When choosing task lighting for the office consider the tasks undertaken and positioning to avoid glare, reflections and shadowing. If light is coming from behind you it's likely to cause reflection and glare on your computer screen.

Lamps that are adjustable and can be moved provide flexible light for a variety of tasks.

Natural light is always best to work by if it's available. Sometimes it can get too bright so ensure you can diffuse the light with a blind or other window treatment if it provides too much glare.

Garage

The garage is usually used for storage - and of course the car.

Simple lighting is more than suitable for garage lights. Aim for energy efficient types of lighting such as LED or fluorescent lamps. If you have a workbench in the garage you may like to consider adjustable task lamps for the workspace.

Sensors or timers are useful for garage lights to provide light when accessing the garage at night, these usually switch off automatically after a few minutes and are ideal for security and energy efficiency.

External security

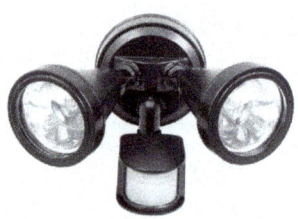

Image credit: Mance Electrical

Security lights are generally used as a form of outdoor lighting to provide security for a home as a preventative measure against intrusions. When we think of security lights we think very bright light, mounted high on a wall or roof and, when triggered through motion sensors, will throw lots of light onto a specific area.

Ensure that externally mounted security lights are weatherproof/resistant to survive outdoor conditions. These lights need to be bright and are often fitted with 150W halogen globes which are highly inefficient, although usually only on for short periods of time. These globes can be replaced with more efficient LED bulbs (minimum 20W) or the whole fitting could be replaced with solar powered security lights.

There is a weatherproof rating for outdoor appliances called an IP rating. Weatherproof fittings are rated IP65 or 66; be sure to check the weatherproof ratings before purchasing exterior lamps.

The main things to remember with outdoor security lighting are:

- Use timing switches or motion/daylight sensors to ensure they only come on at night
- Adjust the settings so that they don't go off when cats or possums go past
- Ensure steps and any other hazards are well light to prevent injury
- Always use weather proof fittings (do not use internal lighting outdoors)
- Ensure all wiring is secured and well hidden
- Marine grade stainless steel increases the life of outdoor lighting if corrosion due to salt in the air is an issue

Do not use CFL type globes in a security light that is connected to trigger sensors. They will not work well (there is generally a 'warm up' period), and they will fail quickly as they are not designed for frequent on/off use.

Garden lighting

There is a wide variety of landscape lighting that includes up lighting, downlighting, moonlighting, accent lighting, shadowing, silhouetting, cross lighting and path lighting. A landscaper will be able to advise you on what would suit your needs.

The most commonly used garden lights are solar garden lights. These, as noted earlier, are very easy to install, use renewable energy and cost nothing to run.

The main things to remember for garden lighting (similar to external security lighting), are:

- Only use them when you need them (e.g. if entertaining or for security)
- Ensure steps and any other hazards are well light to prevent injury
- Highlighting garden features around the home creates the sense of an outdoor room, an inviting backdrop for outdoor entertaining areas

Some general advice about outdoor lighting (compliments of Beacon Lighting):

- Never use indoor lights for outdoor applications
- Clean exposed outdoor bulbs every three months to remove any dirt and pollen. If bulbs are dirty the light efficiency decreases dramatically
- Check cords and electrical outlets when you clean your bulbs to ensure everything is working efficiently
- If you have children or pets ensure any loose cords are tucked out of sight to avoid tripping hazards and safeguard pets against the temptation to chew electrical cords
- If you have fittings that are 304 or 316 marine grade stainless steel, ensure all fittings are treated before installation with a neutral oil such as WD40. Once your fittings are installed, remove any blotches or stains with a soft cloth soaked in neutral oil. Repeat this process up to four times a year to maintain superior quality and finish
- Install simple switches in easily accessible locations near door or windows. Mounted indoors, you can easily switch them on and off without stepping outside
- Use motion detectors to automatically turn on when someone approaches your front door or garden path. Most modern sensors have the ability to be adjusted so that they don't turn on when pets or branches move past the sensor. You can also set the light level so that they only activate after sunset, which saves you money
- Timers are perfect for automatically turning your lights on at a specified time

Further information

Australian Government, Department of Industry, Energy Efficiency – www.ee.ret.gov.au/energy-efficiency/lighting

Beacon Lighting – www.beaconlighting.com.au

National Electrical Contractors Association (NECA) – www.neca.asn.au

Appliances

Our homes contain many appliances. They range from those that keep us warm to those that clean and are the significant contributor to energy use in the home.

Research has shown that appliance use in a typical home is around 30 percent of total energy use (not including hot water, lighting or heating/cooling). (Source: Energy Use in the Australian Residential Sector 1986 – 2020 – Department of Environment, Water, Heritage and the Arts (DEWHA) 2008).

This section will provide information on what to look for and tips on usage to get the best from your appliances. Note that hot water, lighting, heating and cooling is covered separately.

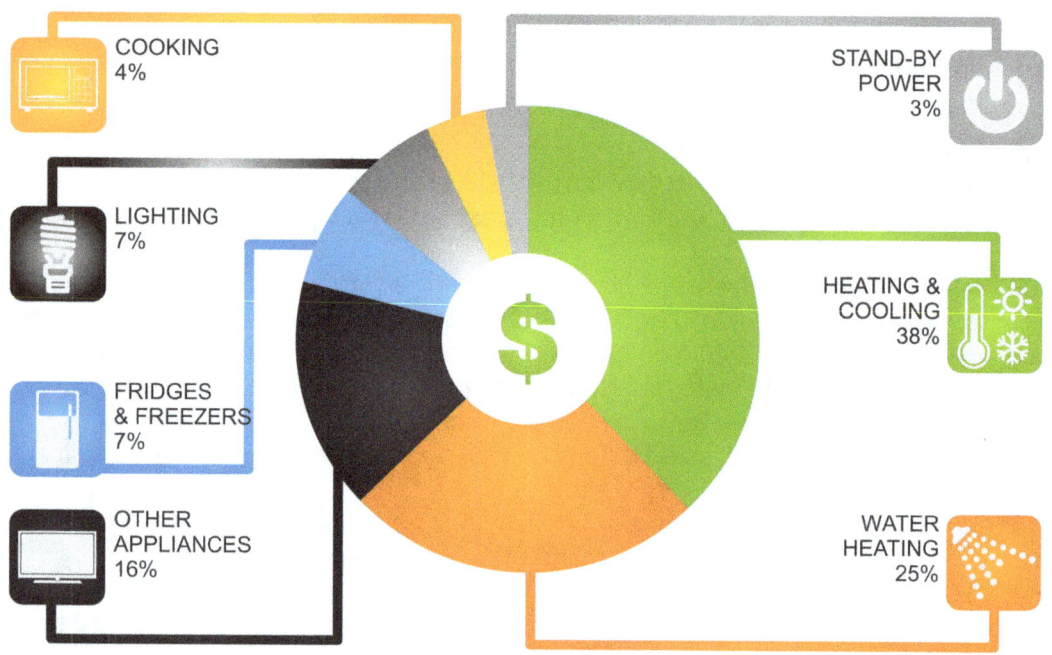

Data source: www.switchon.vic.gov.au

There are many opportunities to minimise energy use in the home, primarily through the products we choose to purchase, and how we use them.

There is a variety of rating labels and independent certification schemes available that highlight product attributes. It's worth understanding what these mean and keep them in mind when purchasing products. The value of certification schemes is summarised in the Our Behaviour – Consumer Choice section of this book. For appliances, a significant source of information is provided on the energy and water rating labels. A summary of Australia's current energy rating labelling scheme, sourced from the Australian government's Energy Efficiency website is below.

Energy rating labels and minimum energy performance standards

In Australia, the Greenhouse and Energy Minimum Standards (GEMS) legislation sets out specific product requirements for energy performance.

One of the key tools relating to appliances that is readily available for consumers is the energy rating label. Not all appliances will have these labels, but those that do provide very useful information and can assist consumers to make informed choices.

Simply installing appliances with energy (and water) saving features can significantly reduce a home's operating cost. When shopping for appliances, look at the energy rating label on the appliance or look up the brand and model on the Federal Government's website at: **www.energyrating.gov.au**

Be aware that a large appliance with the same star rating as a smaller model uses more energy and generates more greenhouse gas. This makes it easier for large appliances to get a higher star rating. For example, when comparing different sized refrigerators, all with a 4 Star energy rating, operating costs would be:

A 300 litre model uses 420 kWh/pa costing $126 pa or $ 1,260 over 10 years*

A 400 litre model uses 500 kWh/pa costing $150 pa or $ 1,500 over 10 years*

A 500 litre model uses 600 kWh/pa costing $180 pa or $ 1,800 over 10 years*

* Note: calculations based on 0.30 cents per kWh with straight multiplier, not taking account of compounding costs or rate increases.

The following text on the Energy Rating Labeling Scheme is from the Commonwealth of Australia (Department of Industry):

The Energy Rating Labelling Scheme is a mandatory scheme for a range of appliances, which currently includes:

- Refrigerators
- Freezers
- Clothes Washers
- Clothes Dryers
- Dishwashers
- Air Conditioners
- Televisions

When offered for sale, these appliances must display a label that shows the star rating and other useful information about energy consumption. The label gives the appliances a star rating between one and ten stars. The greater the number of stars the higher the efficiency. It enables consumers to compare the energy efficiency of domestic appliances on a fair and equitable basis. It also provides incentive for manufacturers to improve the energy performance of appliances.

The energy rating label was first introduced in 1986 in NSW and Victoria. It is now mandatory in all Australian states and territories and New Zealand for refrigerators, freezer, clothes washers, clothes dryers, dishwashers, air-conditioners (single phase only) to carry the label when they are offered for sale. Australia also applies a mandatory label to televisions.

Three phase air conditioners and swimming pool pumps may carry an energy rating label if the supplier chooses to apply for one. This is currently a voluntary program.

The energy rating label has two main features that provide consumers with the following information:

- The star rating gives a comparative assessment of the model's energy efficiency
- The comparative energy consumption (usually kilowatt hours per year) provides an estimate of the annual energy consumption of the appliance based on the tested energy consumption and information about the typical use of the appliance in the home. Air conditioners show the power consumption of the appliance in straight kilowatts (not over a time period)

The star rating of an appliance is determined from the energy consumption and size of the product. These values are measured under Australian Standards which define test procedures for measuring energy consumption and minimum energy performance criteria. Appliances must meet these criteria before they can be granted an energy rating label.

Note: energy consumption figures assume certain conditions. For example, with refrigeration they assume good ventilation, and that the motor and seals are in good condition. To find the true usage the appliance would need to be monitored while in operation with an appropriate energy usage meter.

About Minimum Energy Performance Standards (MEPS)

MEPS specify the minimum level of energy performance that appliances, lighting and electrical equipment must meet or exceed before they can be offered for sale or used for commercial purposes. MEPS are mandatory for a range of products in Australia and New Zealand. These products must be registered through an online database and meet a number of legal requirements before they can be sold in either of these countries. To find out the MEPS requirements for a particular product check the relevant Australian GEMS determination or the New Zealand regulations.

Why are MEPS important?

MEPS are an effective way to increase the energy efficiency of products. By specifying a minimum energy performance level they prevent inefficient products from entering the marketplace and help to increase average product efficiency over time. For consumers, this means that products available in the market use less energy and have lower running costs over the life of the product.

Using energy efficient products also reduces greenhouse gas emissions and our impact on the environment. With the introduction of MEPS consumers now have information to hand and can make better informed decisions, whilst manufacturers are encouraged to make their appliances more energy efficient.

The first MEPS standards were introduced in 2001 when appliances were required to comply with Tier 1 MEPS and energy rating labelling requirements. From April 2013 the updated Tier 2 MEPS requirements came into force, introducing a more stringent rating level. Hence, an appliance rated and labelled before 9th April 2013 might have earned a 4 star rating, where under Tier 2, that same appliance would only achieve a 1 star energy rating. So ask if the label is related to the old (Tier 1) or new (Tier 2) star rating.

For more information on MEPS see www.energyrating.gov.au/programs/about

For more information on Energy Rating see www.energyrating.gov.au

Source text: Commonwealth of Australia (Department of Industry)

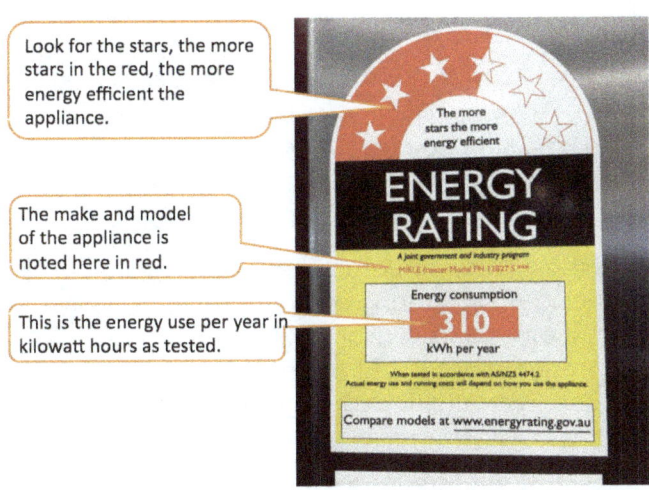

Image: © Green Moves Australia 2014.

Reading the labels

The more stars, the more efficient the appliance when compared to other competitive models of the same size.

Kilowatt hours (kWh) per year – this is the estimated total electricity use over a 12 month period. The lower the number the more energy efficient the appliance is when compared to other competitive models of the same size.

Occasionally you will see some fine print on a label below the kWh per year figure (usually in red text). This notes the testing cycles, for example a washing machine usage is based on one wash cycle per day.

Operating cost – an approximate cost can be calculated by multiplying the annual energy consumption figure (in the red rectangle on the label) by your actual electricity price (obtained from your energy bill). Alternatively, for comparison purposes you could use an approximate rate of say 0.30 cents per kWh.

Here's an example: using the label above (which is for a freezer).

Energy consumption is 310 kWh, and we'll use the cost rate of .30 cents kWh.

The calculation would be 310 kWh x .30 cents = $93.00 pa to run this freezer.

Note, for appliances that are not 'always on', the actual operating cost will vary depending on the number of hours the appliance is in active use.

Greenhouse gas (GHG) emissions – the GHG rate varies depending on which state you are in and the electricity supply source you are using. If you are using grid connected electricity, as a rough estimate assume that each kWh equates to one kilogram of GHG emissions. If you are using 100 percent renewable energy, GHG emissions will be zero.

Further information

Australian Government Energy Rating website – www.energyrating.gov.au
Australian Department of Industry website – www.ee.ret.gov.au/energy-efficiency

Water Efficiency Labelling Scheme (WELS)

WELS is Australia's water efficiency labelling scheme (similar to the energy efficiency scheme) requires the water efficiency of certain products to be registered and labelled, highlighting a product's water efficiency on the product label. The National Water Efficiency Labelling and Standards Act 2005 sets the standards for the WELS system and can be found at the Australian Government's ComLaw site. www.comlaw.gov.au/Details/C2005A00004

The WELS system is managed and enforced by the WELS regulator. The WELS regulator has a range of powers and resources and the role includes monitoring compliance, investigating breaches of the WELS Act, imposing fines and penalties for breaches, withdrawal of a product from the market, deregistration of the product on the WELS scheme and publicising convictions. The regulator can choose to utilise administration or educational options as an alternative to legal action.

Minimum water efficiency applies to some appliances (specifically toilets and washing machines). The water-using WELS products are listed below:

Plumbing products
- showers
- tap equipment for use over a basin, sink or tub (excluding over a bath)
- flow controllers

Sanitary ware
- toilet (lavatory) equipment
- urinal equipment

White goods
- clothes washing machines
- dishwashers

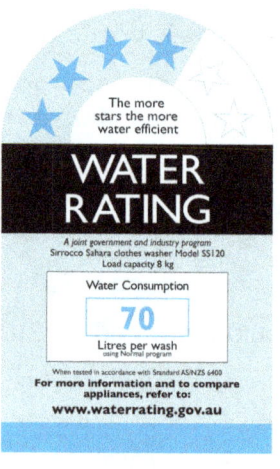

Sample label

Products that are WELS rated allow consumers to compare the water efficiency of different products. WELS labels should be visible and available on the appliance at the point of sale or where advertised. Where an appliance has both energy and water rating labels, both should be shown.

For more information on the WELS system, see www.waterrating.gov.au

Some states and territories offer rebates for water efficient appliances. Contact your local water companies or local governments to see what is currently available.

Information on the WELS scheme has been obtained from the Water Rating website and is attributed to the Commonwealth of Australia 2013.

Best practice for appliances

Regardless of the appliance, there are some general considerations you should think about when looking to purchase new equipment. These are:

- Fit for purpose/appropriated sized. Is the appliance the right size for your needs? For example, a retired couple may not need a large dishwasher, but a young family is likely to need a large capacity dishwasher. Choose the right size appliance for the job it needs to do
- Opt for the most efficient model you can afford, especially if it is used a lot. Read the energy rating label, and consider how often the appliance is on for. For example, a refrigerator is always on so it is ideal to have the most energy efficient model you can afford. Refrigerators can cost anywhere from $80 a year to over $1,200 a year to operate, so choose carefully
- Quality is also important as it relates to the longevity of the appliance. This minimises having to replace the appliance regularly, saving money and reducing waste in the longer term. There are several mainstream brands available that offer lengthy warranties and include 'eco' cycles. Manufacturers are now very mindful of creating products that have a lighter environmental footprint during the manufacturing process, so product labels may include other environmental logos or certifications that add to a products 'green' credibility (e.g. Global Green Tag™, GECA, or Cradle to Cradle)

The energy used by any appliance that plugs into a general power outlet can be measured by using an energy monitor. There are many different types of monitors available. They are generally simple to use and cost from $10 upwards. Some local councils have monitors available for loan. Check with your local council or library service to see if they offer this service.

Hot water systems

Approximately 21 percent of the average home's running costs can be due to hot water heating (*Your Home*, 2013). You can reduce hot water usage and associated costs by reducing demand. This is easily achieved through using water efficient showers, tap ware and appliances. Greenhouse gas emissions can be reduced by using renewable energy sources to produce the hot water (i.e. solar, geothermal) or by purchasing green power through your energy retailer.

Hot water systems come in a variety of types and energy sources. Regardless of the type of system you choose, it should be located close to the point of use and all hot water pipes should be insulated to minimise heat loss, particularly in frost prone areas.

Choosing the right hot water system depends very much on your particular situation. Things to consider include household size, budget, available space, location to outlet points, local climate, available energy sources and (if applicable) the existing hot water system.

Check with your local state or territory government for the most up to date information about regulations relating to hot water supply in your area.

The tables following provide a brief summary of the different systems available.

The main types of hot water systems are:

Type	Characteristics
Storage Systems that have a tank and store hot water.	These types of systems contain an insulated storage tank. Under the Australian Standard AS/NZS 3500.4, heated water must be stored at a minimum temperature of 60°C, to inhibit the growth of legionella bacteria. Hot water is limited at any point in time to the size of the storage tank. There are mains pressure systems and gravity fed systems. Storage systems would typically have a sacrificial anode in the tank to reduce corrosion which should be replaced every few years. The water storage unit can be sited internally or externally and can run on electricity, gas or renewable sources (generally solar or geothermal). Storage systems generally have a lifespan of between 10-15 years.
Instantaneous (Continuous flow) No storage tank, heat as they are used.	Instantaneous systems do not store water and only heat it as it is needed so the house will not run out of hot water. These generally cost less to operate as you are only paying to heat the water as you use it, rather than paying to keep water hot in a storage tank all the time. The ideal temperature setting for instantaneous systems is around 50°C. Units can run on electricity or gas (including LPG) and use either electric ignition or a gas pilot light. Instantaneous systems can be sited internally or externally and require less space than storage units. Instantaneous units generally have a lifespan of up to 20 years (depending on the type, water quality, environmental conditions and regular maintenance)

Type	Comments
Electric Systems 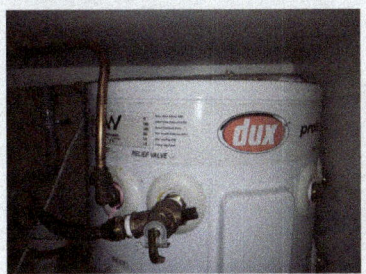 Image: Standard electric hot water unit. 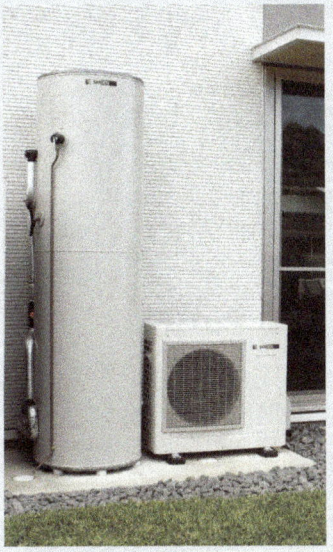 Image: Sanden Heat pump COP 4.5 to 1. (4.5:1) 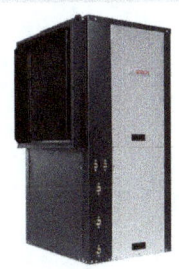 Image: Bosch Geothermal Heat Pump	**Standard electric storage systems** have been used in Australia for many years and are the most expensive to operate. Depending on the size, the unit could contain 1, 2 or 3 heating elements, and could be connected to peak or off peak electricity charges. These units are being phased out in Australia due to their inefficiency, high greenhouse gas emissions and running costs. They are cheap to purchase, but inefficient and expensive to run. To find out more about the government phase-out of this type of water heater see http://ee.ret.gov.au/energy-efficiency/water-heaters/phase-out-greenhouse-intensive-hot-water-heaters Electric heat pumps are a more expensive option to purchase, but are significantly more efficient to run. They work by taking heat from the air which is used to heat a refrigerant that converts to gas, which is then compressed, this generates heat which heats the water. Often described as working 'like a fridge but in reverse', these systems use approximately ¼ to ½ the energy of the old standard electric storage systems noted above. Some units have an electric booster heating element. There is a variety of heat pump units available, so be sure to check the specifications of the product you may be considering and site the unit in an appropriate place. Look for a high co-efficient of performance' (COP) of 4:1 or higher. This means for every 1 kW of energy in, it produces 4 kW of heat output. Choose a quiet model to minimise noise levels. According to the 'Estimated Hot Water Running Costs in Victoria' report (Energy Consult, August 2010) heat pumps can provide between 60 and 71 percent of savings on operating costs when compared to standard electric systems. **Ground Source (Geothermal) heat pumps** are similar to electric heat pumps but don't use the air as a heat source. Instead heat is obtained through water pumped through a deep bore loop (vertical) or a shallow trench (horizontal) ground loop. The water absorbs heat from the earth, warming it. Geothermal heat pumps have a very high COP of 4:1 (outputting 4 kW of energy for every 1 kW used). These systems can be used for producing hot water for general domestic use, hydronic heating and can be used for pool heating. Geothermal heat pumps generally provide an efficient source of heating but can be expensive to install. You can reduce your greenhouse emissions further from running electric hot water systems by purchasing 'green power', installing a solar PV system or using a geothermal system.

Table continued next page.

Type	Comments
Natural (mains) Gas 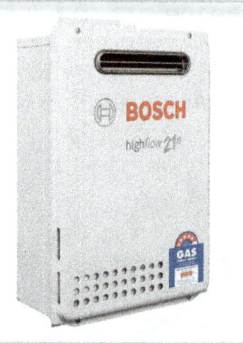 Image: Bosch high efficiency gas instantaneous unit.	Gas can be connected to storage or instantaneous systems and generates lower greenhouse gas emissions than grid electricity. Natural gas systems are generally cheaper to run because gas prices are currently significantly lower than electricity (but this is changing as gas prices are increasing). Standard instantaneous systems can deliver adequate hot water to up to two outlets at the same time which in many situations would generally be sufficient. However if more than this is needed, a high performance unit may be required. These can supply up to several points at a time but may require larger gas pipes. Be sure to obtain expert advice from your plumber to ensure you size the system, and gas pipes correctly. Note that some instantaneous gas systems don't work well with low flow showers and tap ware. Check with the manufacturer or the plumber before you purchase.
Liquefied Petroleum Gas	LPG based systems are more expensive to run than mains supplied natural gas. If you use a lot of hot water this is unlikely to be a cost effective option. Note that instantaneous models, when used with LPG tanks are likely to need a larger gas supply pipe. To minimise frequent replacement/refilling of LPG cylinders choose large storage capacity tanks or bottles.

Table continued next page.

Type	Comments
Solar 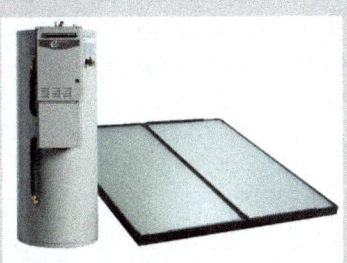 Image: www.insolar.com.au	Solar hot water systems heat the water by collecting and absorbing the energy from the sun into the water and storing it in a storage tank. They come in two types, flat plate and evacuated tube solar collectors. Systems can be gas, electric or solid fuel (wetback) boosted. Boosting can often be turned off in summer months. There are also two different types of configuration, split system (collectors on the roof and storage unit on the ground) or close coupled system (collectors and storage tank on the roof). Solar systems have a high capital outlay but can offer very low running costs, depending on your climate and solar access. They also last significantly longer than other hot water system types and can add value to your home. A solar hot water system can provide up to 90 percent of your hot water needs at no cost and produces very low to zero greenhouse gas emissions (booster type and location-dependant). When considering a solar hot water system, check your local climate and solar access, and obtain expert advice on the right configuration and boosting system for your situation. Solar hot water can provide between 60 and 95 percent savings on operating costs when compared to standard electric systems (Energy Consult, 2013). If you have a solar hot water system, schedule activities that use hot water for the early part of the day so the water can re-heat again before the evening. **Caution:** In some areas the hot water from solar systems can get too hot and there is a need for heat dissipation and/or mixing valves to reduce water temperatures at the output point (tap, shower) to prevent scalding.

© Green Moves Australia 2014.

What's the most efficient type in relation to ongoing operating costs?

1. Solar hot water is the most cost effective, energy efficient and has the lowest greenhouse gas emissions. Particularly when boosted by natural mains gas because mains gas has lower greenhouse gas emissions and is cheaper than electricity, unless you have a solar PV system onsite. If it's boosted by electricity from the grid, depending on use, it may drop to #2.
2. Highly efficient (5 star efficiency rating or more) natural gas instantaneous comes in second place being very cost effective to operate. In greenhouse gas terms LPG is on par with natural mains gas, however the cost to operate is between 2 to 3 times more than mains gas.
3. High efficiency heat pumps come in third place as they generally use electricity and contribute more greenhouse gas emissions than gas. If you don't have mains gas available, and solar is not suitable, heat pump technology (air or geothermal) is the best option.
4. Instantaneous electric hot water comes in at number four and may require a three phase electricity supply.
5. Electric storage units are the least efficient and have been targeted by the government for removal. Regulations in some areas may prevent the installation of electric storage units.

Preventative maintenance

The lifespan of a hot water system can be maximised if the unit is properly maintained during its lifetime. If you are not sure about the requirements for your particular unit, contact the supplier and they will advise you accordingly. The following is a general guide to preventative maintenance servicing.

- Scaling. Some areas have water that is high in mineral content (often called 'hard water'). This can cause build up or scaling of calcium deposits in the heating system components, reducing system performance and potentially causing valve and pump failures. Scaling can be avoided by using water softeners or circulating a mild acidic solution (e.g. vinegar) through the system every 3-5 years or as needed. It's best to use a qualified technician to do this
- Storage systems that have a sacrificial anode will need it replaced every few years. They should also be checked for cracks, leaks or other signs of corrosion at the same time
- Instantaneous units. The in-line screen filter should be checked periodically for debris (time between filter checks will be dependent on water quality). The unit should be flushed periodically (time between flushes will be dependent on water quality) to keep the unit free of scale and lime. This process should be completed by a professional installer
- Solar collectors should be cleaned regularly, checked for cracks in the glazing and that seals are in good condition. Flush out collectors to remove any sludge build up. Check the pressure relief valve is not stuck open or closed. If you are in a frost prone area, ask a qualified technician to check the anti-freeze solutions and for mineral build up in the piping. Some descaling may be required every few years
- Pipes and wiring should be inspected occasionally looking for leaks, damage or degradation of insulation or loose wiring connections

Health implications

Storage tanks should have the temperature set to between 60 and 65°C. Stored water needs to be heated to a minimum of 60°C for at least 35 minutes once a week to ensure that any legionnaire bacterium that may be in the water is killed.

Water temperature for instantaneous systems should be set to approximately 50°C to minimise risk of scalding.

Clause 1.9.2, of AS/NZS 3500.413 stipulates that all new heated water installations shall, at the outlet of all sanitary fixtures used primarily for personal hygiene purposes, deliver heated water not exceeding:

- 43.5°C for childhood centres, primary and secondary schools and nursing homes or similar facilities for the young, aged, sick or people with disabilities; and
- 50°C in all other buildings

Gas systems, particularly those with pilot lights, are best located externally so that if a leak occurs it won't harm those in the home.

Turn off booster units when going away for extended periods, this will save energy. If you have a storage system, remember to wait for the water to reach at least 60°C for a minimum of 35 minutes and flush the hot water pipes before using. Note that it could take several hours to re-heat the tank water.

Further information

Your Home – **www.yourhome.gov.au**

Australian Government, Department of Industry Energy Efficiency – **http://ee.ret.gov.au/energy-efficiency/water-heaters**

Public Health Association of Australia hot tap water temperature and scalds policy – **www.phaa.net.au/documents/130201_Hot%20Tap%20Water%20Temperature%20and%20Scalds%20Policy%20FINAL.pdf**

Regulatory approaches by Australian States and Territories to the Prevention of Legionellosis – **www.health.gov.au/internet/main/publishing.nsf/Content/7FDDB6DADD503805CA257BF0001F985F/$File/legapp1.pdf**

Contact your local government for information on any hot water rebates that may be available. See **www.gov.au**

Contact your local water distributor for information on water saving programs or rebates (refer to your water bill for contact information).

Alternative Technology Association at **www.ata.org.au** has a range of useful buyers guides available, see **www.renew.org.au/buyers-guide**

Australian Consumer Association Choice – **www.choice.com.au**
Hot water systems buyers guide – **www.choice.com.au/reviews-and-tests/household/energy-and-water/saving-water/hot-water-options-buying-guide.aspx**

Appliances in the home

Kitchen appliances

Our kitchens house some of the most frequently used appliances in the home. Most of us have a refrigerator, dishwasher, and cooking equipment, so it's worth giving thought to how to minimise their impact without detracting from their purpose.

In this section we explore considerations for kitchen appliances. Remember the 'Best Practice' points made above - choose the right size for the application, check the energy efficiency label and get the best quality appliance you can afford.

Refrigerators and freezers

An energy rating label is mandatory for these products.

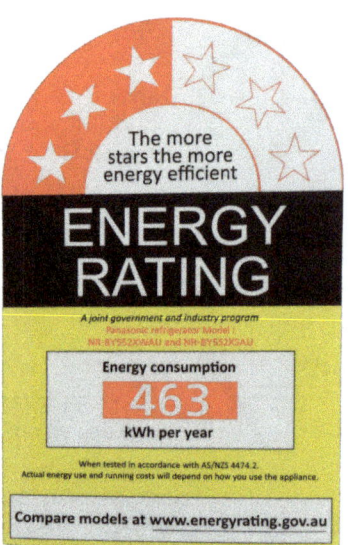

These items are always on and are generally the most used appliance in the home so it is important to choose the most efficient model you can afford. When looking at refrigerators or freezers, the energy efficiency label should tell you everything you need to know. Refer to the sample label which provides the required information for you to calculate the operating costs.

Look at the Energy Consumption figure in the red rectangle box. This shows you the kWh per year.

In this case the refrigerator uses 463 kWh per year.

Look up your energy cost (get this from your latest bill). For the purpose of illustration let's say its .28 cents per kWh.

Then the calculation is:

kWh pa x cents per kWh = cost per year

So the cost to run for this refrigerator/freezer is...

463 kW/pa x 0.28 cents per kWh = $129.64 per year

So a refrigerator that uses 365 kW pa (so just 1 kW per day) at the same kWh billing rate would cost $102.48 per year. This is a useful and simple way to check operating costs.

TIP Look for an annual kWh usage of around 365 or less when purchasing a standard sized refrigerator (that's just 1 kWh per day). It's an easy number to look for on the labels and a very efficient refrigerator!

It is worth noting that some older models (over 10 years old and often used as the beer fridge) can use more than 8 kW per day, which is 2,920 kW pa costing $817.60 a year to run.

Beer fridge tip: if you have a beer fridge that is occasionally used, only turn it on when you need it. Move those odd cans of drink into the kitchen fridge and turn off the beer fridge. When you have a party just turn it back on for use, remembering to turn it off again when the party's over! Alternatively, if you need it on all the time, you might be able to cost justify buying yourself a new, much more efficient model.

You can help your refrigerator operate more efficiently by:

- Ensuring there is at least 5cm of clear space around the appliance (top, bottom and sides) to enable sufficient ventilation for the compressor which contributes to it running more efficiently
- Keeping the right temperature. Food safety laws state that a refrigerator temperature should be set to 4°C. A freezer containing food should be at -18°C
- Check door seals for leaks regularly. There are several ways to check this. Do a visual check and run your hand slowly along the seal and see if you can feel cold escaping. Alternatively you could put a piece of paper in the door and close the door, if the paper falls away or slips then the seals are not sealing properly and should be cleaned or possibly replaced
- Stack food evenly inside the fridge to allow movement of air internally. Fridges work best when around three quarters full

Ovens and cooktops

In Australia there is currently no energy rating label for ovens or cooktops (however, there is a European system). Again, keep in mind the 'Best Practice' considerations above and note that smaller ovens are more efficient because they don't need to heat as much space.

For the cooks among us, there are a few items to remember for cooking appliances.

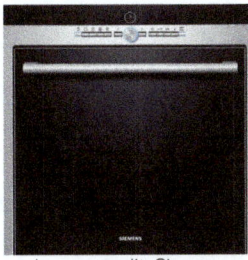

Image credit: Siemens

- Opt for ovens with high levels of insulation and triple glazed, low-e coated windows as they will be safer and more efficient
- Fan forced ovens are about 30 percent more efficient than conventional units.
- Convection microwave ovens are a good option for energy efficient cooking
- Slow cookers are efficient cooking systems (even over several hours), as they are cooking at lower temperatures and lower energy use per hour
- Portable convection ovens are very efficient. They use around two thirds of the power and can cook in half the time and there is no pre-heating needed
- Induction cooktops are the most energy efficient electric type
- Gas cooktops and ovens have a lower greenhouse gas impact. A typical gas oven will use around 3.6 MJ for warm-up and one hour operation – about a third of the GHG impact of a good electric oven. Ensure the kitchen has adequate ventilation and air extraction with gas cookers to maintain good air quality

Some European cookers have energy performance data, usually based on pre heat times and one hour operation at 180°C – the most efficient are those that use around 1 kW per hour.

Induction cooktops use a magnetic field to heat the contents of pans very quickly, however you will need stainless steel or iron based pots to cook with. They are considered to be more energy efficient as they only heat the contact area of the pan on the cooktop.

Ovens are generally internally coated in a type of enamel. When ovens and cooktops are new they should be washed thoroughly to remove any of the factory contaminants before use. Some manufacturers will suggest that ovens are used for the first time without food – this is essential.

The first use of ovens usually releases fumes from the enamel and food should not be cooked in the oven while these fumes are present. Ensure doors and windows are opened and kitchen exhaust fan turned on while completing this process to remove toxic fumes. Wipe surfaces again after fumes have ceased, to remove any residue. Note that this applies to new barbecues too.

A gas flame should burn blue, a lazy yellow flame indicates inadequate combustion which releases toxic gases and means the appliance requires professional attention.

Ovens and cooktops are generally hardwired to the switchboard. When installing a new appliance, consider including a power cut off switch to the oven in a place that's easily accessible. This allows the appliance to be easily turned off for maintenance or to stop standby power wastage. Ensure it is clearly labeled.

Rangehoods

There is no energy rating label in Australia yet for rangehoods.

With homes being much better built these days, it's important not to lose heat and air through the exhaust fans in the kitchen, until you want to. When looking for a rangehood, consider the following:

- Make sure it is externally vented and is self-closing. Models with a heavy filter/damper are best
- Opt for a good air extraction rate
- Ensure filters are easy to remove and clean
- Use LED lights (which are significantly more energy efficient)
- Ideally the rangehood should be the same size or larger than the cooktop size for maximum extraction ability
- Rangehoods with twin fans allow for single side use and reduced noise when in use

Leave the rangehood on for at least five minutes after cooking to remove residual steam and combustion pollutants. Wash the filters regularly for maximum efficiency, some filters can be washed in dishwashers.

Dishwashers

Energy rating and water rating labels are mandatory. Ratings are based on one wash load per day.

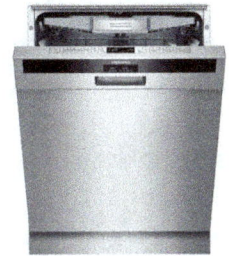
image credit: Siemens

It's important to select the right model for your situation when purchasing a new dishwasher, especially as it is likely to be around for up to 16 years. There are many different types these days, ranging from built in under bench models, drawers and portable compact dishwashers.

What to consider when shopping for a dishwasher:

- Best practice points apply – most energy efficient, right size, good quality
- Ensure it has an 'eco' or 'quick' wash cycle
- Delay start option is useful, especially if you have off peak power options
- Opt for a quiet model to minimise noise levels
- Adjustable racks are useful for dinner party dishes
- Some models allow you to select the drying settings (heat or no heat) for drying cycles
- Newer technology uses heat pump technology which reduces operating costs (by reusing the heat from washing water to dry the dishes later)
- Drawers are generally easier to access and are more suitable for those with mobility limitations

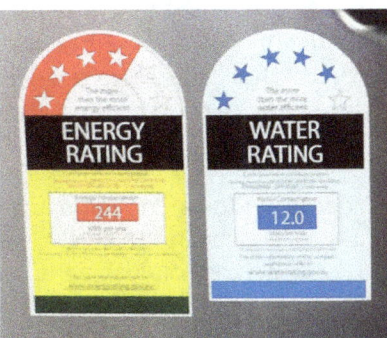
Image credit: Green Moves Aust, 2014.

Note: Always run the dishwasher with a full load and use the quick wash cycles when possible.

TIP Don't wash plastics in the dishwasher, the heat generated during the wash process heats the plastic which causes VOCs inside the dishwasher that can be released into the house when the dishwasher is opened. The heating process of the plastic also makes the plastic deteriorate faster. Switch your household plastics to other alternatives – see the Lifestyle Practices section of this book.

Other kitchen appliances

Energy Rating Labels for other kitchen appliances are not mandatory in Australia.

Many other appliances are only used for a short period of time, e.g. the blender, kettle, toaster etc. The best practice notes above will always apply. Only use appliances when you need to and turn them off at the power point when not in use.

Small kitchen appliances

When choosing small kitchen appliances consider how they are made and the materials that have been used.

We know that it is not ideal to heat plastics, yet plastics are used to make many products and are used in less than ideal circumstances.

Product consideration assessment example:

Product type: Electric kettle

There are many kinds of electric kettles, made from varying combinations of materials in many shapes, sizes and colours. In relation to health it is important to note what the internal surfaces of the kettle are made from as this is what your drinking water is exposed to at boiling point.

The interior of kettles vary significantly. Some are plastic, others may be combinations of plastic and stainless steel, stainless steel and non-stick coatings or plain stainless steel. You may also find plastic plugs holding plastic water level window displays and plastic filter frames. In some instances there may also be a type of rubber or silicone product joining or sealing the base of the unit to the sides. Heating elements may be concealed or exposed (and coated) on the base.

It is interesting to note that labelling does not require material disclosure or any declaration of safety in relation to testing associated with potential migration of chemicals (particularly plasticisers) into the water when used (it is unlikely that such testing has been done).

When shopping for a kettle look for:

- Stainless steel tank - no joins, to avoid joining materials
- No internal plastic in the kettle
- Avoid coating materials inside the kettle (these are often made to look like a stainless steel colour)

The same principles apply for other appliances. Look for options that avoid or minimise the use of plastics where contact is made with food, and options that avoid chemical coatings in contact with food where possible (e.g. stainless steel).

Laundry appliances

The laundry can be a source of high energy use, especially if a clothes dryer is regularly used. Again, the 'Best Practice' comments apply.

Be aware that energy rating conditions differ between washing machines and clothes dryers. Washing machine ratings are based on being used once a day, whereas dryers are rated at being used once a week. If you use the appliance less than this, it will use fewer resources and cost less to run. If you use them more, it will of course, cost more.

Washing machines

Energy rating and water rating labels are mandatory on washing machines.

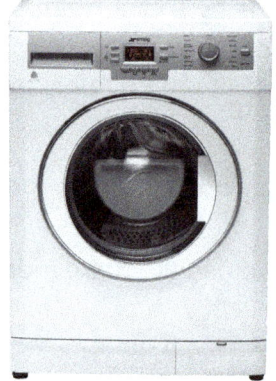
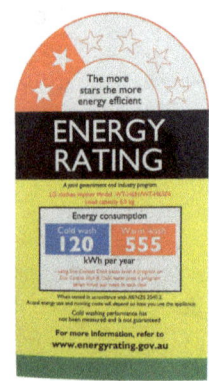
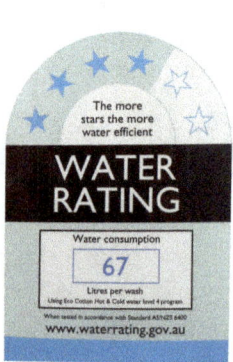

Image credit: Siemens (washing machine) Green Moves Australia, 2014 (labels)

Energy rating labels are based on one wash per day. The lifespan of a washing machine is on average 12 years. The main types are top loaders and front loaders, combination machines are also available that perform both washing and drying functions.

What you choose will depend on your situation and personal preferences, however its worth remembering that front loaders are generally more energy and water efficient than top loaders.

What to look for in a washing machine.

- Best practice points apply – most energy efficient, right size, good quality
- Check with your state, local government and water utilities to see if any rebates are available for water efficient products (there are rebates in some states available to assist with purchasing costs)
- Look for intelligent sensor technology (senses water and load size and adjusts washing time, water level and motor speed to reduce energy)
- Ensure it has an 'eco' or 'quick' wash cycle
- Delay start option is useful, especially if you have off peak power options
- Automatic detergent dispensers are useful, especially for delay start options
- Select one with a water temperature control
- Look for a quiet model
- Opt for wide opening doors (front loader)
- Stainless steel tubs are more efficient as they can take higher speeds and extract more water (which helps the clothes to dry faster).

Here's how to calculate the energy cost of using a washing machine with this label. This washing machine has been rated based on 1 wash load per day (365 days a year).

How many kWh per hot wash does this machine use?

Calculation is 555 kWh pa / 365 days = 1.52 kWh per wash

If I only used it twice a week how many kWh per year would I use?

To find out:

Calculation is 555 kWh / 365 = 1.52 kWh per wash.

1.52 kWh x 104 (twice a week) = 158.08 kWh pa

So 158.08kWh x .30c = $47.42 per year to run (at .30c per kWh).

If .30 cents per kWh that's .46c per wash or $47.24 per year to do the washing (not including washing detergents).

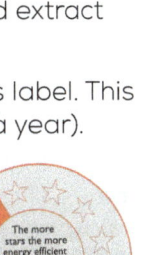

Image: Green Moves Australia, 2014.

The water label (or the technical specifications of the appliance) will tell you how much water a machines uses per wash load.

When considering a new washing machine, front loader models are more energy and water efficient than top loader models. Front loaders can also be built in under benches, maximising bench space, or be built into cabinetry for ergonomic (no bending) use.

Operating considerations

- Always run the washing machine with a full load
- Use cold water washes whenever possible to reduce energy use
- Only wash clothes when they need it, you can often wear clothes twice before they need a wash

Clothes drying

An energy rating label is mandatory, and is based on one drying load per week.

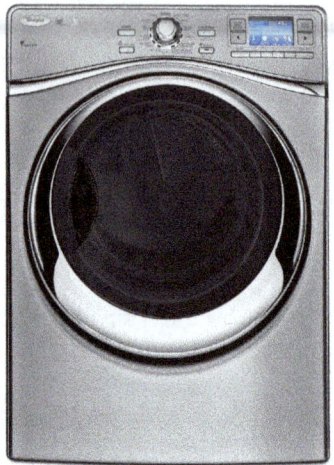 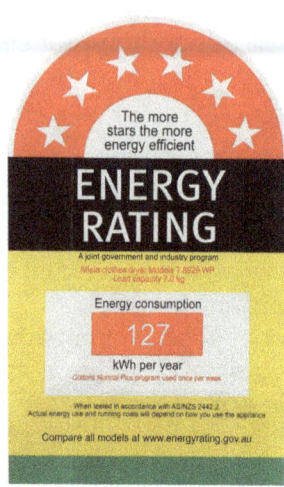

Image credit: Siemens (dryer), Green Moves Australia (energy rating label).

Air drying your washing on an external clothes line is the most efficient and environmentally favourable drying method, unless of course, it's raining.

For days when the external clothes line is not an option, use internal drying racks or airing cupboards (those cupboards near the heating unit). Racks placed near or over ducted heating vents also work well.

The choice of last resort is the clothes dryer. Dryers use a significant amount of energy and should be used sparingly. The two types of dryer units available are electric and gas. The following explores the electric type as this is the most common household dryer.

There is a wide variety of dryers (and drying cupboards) available these days. Standard dryers, as with any item that heats, can use significant amounts of energy. Newer technology (heat pump/inverter) has enabled dryers to improve on their energy efficiency, these heat pump/inverter types can be up to 80 percent more efficient than standard dryers.

What to look for in a dryer:

- Best practice points apply – most energy efficient, right size, good quality
- Delay start option is useful, especially if you have off peak power options
- Moisture sensors are beneficial as they stop the drying cycle when the clothes are ready.
- Lint filter lights are good to remind you to clean the filters for better operation, clean them regularly
- Vent the moist air to the outside
- Express or quick cycles are good for fast drying
- Heat pump types are significantly more efficient than standard dryers

TIP If using a dryer, try getting the clothes/towels half dry on the line first, or use a very high spin cycle before putting them into the dryer. This will reduce the amount of time the dryer needs to operate, saving energy.

Bathroom appliances

Heated towel rails

There is no energy rating label for heated towel rails in Australia at this time.

These appliances can use a lot of energy, especially if left on so be aware of your usage.

If you have a hydronic heating system in the home, install a towel rail type of radiator in the bathroom area so that it provides the bathroom with heat and warm towels.

 **TIP** If you must have an electric heated towel rail, put it on an automatic timer so that it is only on for ½ hour before you use the bathroom, and goes off when you have finished in the bathroom. This allows you to keep the pleasure of a warm towel while minimising the cost.

Heater lamps

There is no energy rating label for heater lamps in Australia at this time.

Heat lamps are often used as a source of light, heat, and sometimes as an exhaust fan.

What to look for:

- Separate switches for heater, fan and lights
- Ensure the switches are clearly labelled
- Opt for one with a LED type light
- Choose a model with a closable exhaust fan
- Position in the unit in the middle of the bathroom or where you would stand to dry off

These types of bathroom heaters generally use a lot of energy but given they are usually only on for a short period it is not as important as having an energy efficient heating system for the whole home.

How to use it:

- Only use the heat lamps when you need to and ensure you turn them off as soon as you don't need them anymore

Bathroom exhaust fans

There are no energy rating labels in Australia for bathroom exhaust fans at this time.

Bathrooms need exhaust fans to extract moisture from the room and minimise the risk of moisture issues such as mould. If exhaust fans cannot seal (close) when not being used they can become a source of heat loss acting as a little chimney in the bathroom. This is not very helpful if you are trying to keep a house warm.

Here's what to look for with bathroom exhaust fans:

- Ensure they are externally vented
- Ensure they are self-closing
- Ideally have them switched separately to lighting*
- Ensure the cover can be removed to be cleaned regularly to ensure optimal performance

*Fans are better if separately switched to give maximum flexibility of use without wasting power. Some lights are switched with exhaust fans (particularly in toilets).

 Exhaust fans are best placed to the outside of the shower entry point, not directly above the shower. This minimises the breeze in the shower area while it is in use and reduces that 'cold breeze' feeling while showering.

Exhaust fans rely on what is called 'make up air' to function properly. Sucking air and moisture out of a bathroom only works well when the 'make up air' comes in at the same rate of extraction. Ensure enough air is able to enter the room as it is being exhausted (i.e. a small opening in a window or leaving the door ajar). If the bathroom is well sealed when the exhaust fan is on, it could prevent moisture from being exhausted which could lead to mould.

When to use the exhaust fan:

- Always use the exhaust fan when showering or bathing to extract moisture from the bathroom. This helps to prevent moisture problems when doing anything that creates steam (i.e. running a hot bath)

 You can also use exhaust fans to help vent the home of hot air by opening doors to nearby rooms (including the bathroom) and switching on the fan. This will create a draught near the area and help to suck out hot air, which should help the home to cool down.

Family room appliances

In most homes the TV and entertainment equipment is regularly used. It's worth knowing how to minimise your energy use and reduce your bills.

Televisions

An energy rating label is mandatory for televisions. The rating is based on 10 hours of active viewing per day.

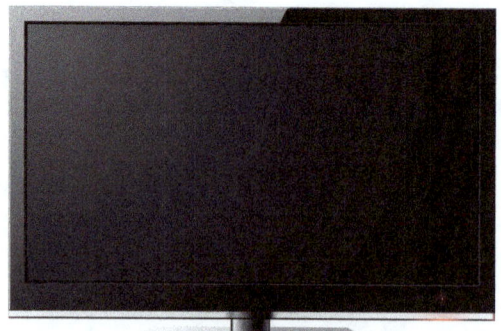
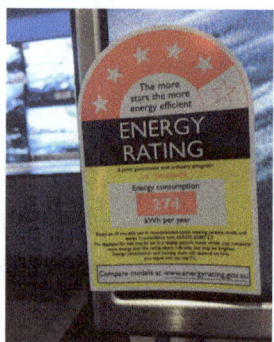

Images: TV, www.ifixit.com. Energy label, Green Moves Aust.

Televisions have become one of the top five energy users in our homes. There are many types ranging from the older cathode ray TV (CRT) screens, plasma, liquid crystal display (LCD) TVs and the latest technology is organic light emitting diode (OLED) TVs.

The most energy efficient models use LCD and OLED technology which can use up to 75 percent less energy than a plasma TV (depending on the size and model). Large televisions also use more energy than smaller TVs.

From an energy perspective, here's what to look for when choosing a new TV:

- Best practice points apply – most energy efficient, right size, good quality
- Opt for a LCD or LED model as they are significantly more efficient
- Get the right size TV for the room, refer to notes below (remember larger TV screens will use more energy)
- Opt for 1080p HD resolution as this gives the most flexibility for content
- A 120Hz refresh rate provides smoother and clearer images, particularly for sports events
- If the TV is in an area with lots of light, opt for high brightness intensity
- Ensure it has a built in tuner
- Ensure it has a few HDMI interface connections to connect the various recording devices and to enable showing of laptop screens if required
- If you intend to use the TV as a media centre include a video graphics adapter (VGA) input
- DVI (digital visual interface) is useful if you want to connect a computer to your TV
- If using the TV for internet, ensure it has an ethernet port or built-in Wi-Fi

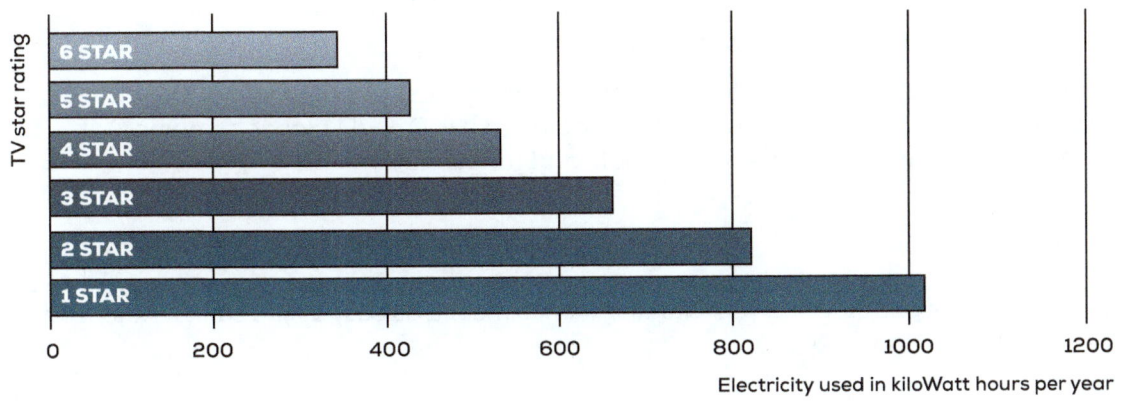

Image credit: Commonwealth of Australia (Department of Industry).

There is a guide to choosing the right TV size on the Amazon website, see www.amazon.com/gp/feature.html?docId=1000021501 .

Manufacturers may also have some recommended distance comments for optimal viewing.

For example according to Toshiba's recommended seating distance for their TVs. If your TV screen size is 100 cm, the minimum viewing distance is 1.2 metres and the maximum viewing distance is 2 metres.

Some models allow you to reduce the energy use even further by turning down the backlight control or engaging a power-saving setting. As light output is the largest contributing factor to energy use, this helps minimise consumption. You will get a slightly dimmer picture if you do this. Check the user manual for further information. Another option is to switch the television off!

Hard disk drives/DVD/Blue-Ray players

Energy rating labels are not used for HDD/DVD or Blue-Ray players in Australia at this time.

These appliances do not tend to use significant amounts of energy, unless you are running it for a significant amount of time (e.g. 10 hours a day).

Items such as hard disk drives tend to come with built in tuners and be always on as they are often used for recording programs for future playback. The energy use while in 'standby' or timer mode is very low particularly in the newer, more efficient models.

It is worth keeping the hard disk drive on a separate 'always on' power point to ensure you don't miss recording items you have programmed. The remainder of the entertainment equipment should be turned off at the power point when not in use.

From an energy perspective, what to look for:

- Best practice points apply – most energy efficient, right size, good quality
- Opt for one appliance that does everything you need (HDD, DVD player combined). It saves space and maximises use of materials and functionality

There is a variety of standby power cut-off switches available so review them all to find the right one that suits your situation. Aim to make it as easy as you can to 'switch off' the standby power.

Gaming equipment

There is a voluntary energy rating label program under consideration for gaming equipment.

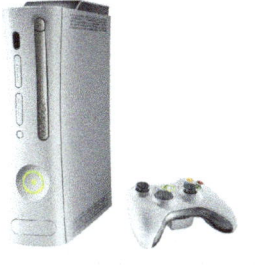
Image: Xbox 360

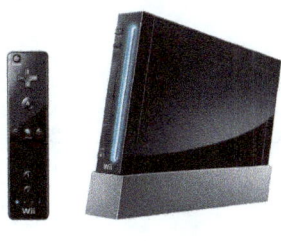
Image: Wii

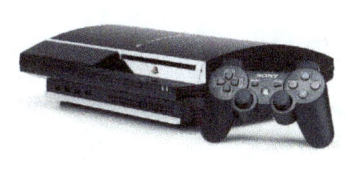
Image: Playstation

Wii, Xbox and Playstation are familiar sights in our family rooms these days and it's important to be aware of their energy usage. As with a TV, energy use depends on how long it's used for and what 'mode' the item is in. Controlling energy consumption of these appliances is possible with a few simple behaviours.

The table below is from a report by Energy Consult Pty Ltd prepared for the Department of Climate Change and Energy Efficiency in 2012 called Video Game Consoles: Energy Efficiency Options.

A study was conducted into the use of video game consoles in the home entertainment area to identify the overall energy consumption from gaming consoles and the impact on household energy usage. Part of that study identified energy use of various systems in a variety of modes. The findings are in the table below.

Mode	MS Xbox 360	Sony PS3	Nintendo Wii	Source
Off	0.67	0.05	10/0.8*	ADT 2011/ Nintendo
Idle (UCI Home Screen)	76.9	67.6	13.0	ADT 2011
Gameplay	81.3	76.6	14.4	ADT 2011
Video Streaming	73.8	61.9	13.3	EPA 2010
Video – DVD	58.9	73.5	n/a	EPA 2010

* Wii power use in standby mode WiiConnect24 enabled/disabled. Table image: Energy Consult, 2012

This shows that the newer models of Xbox and PS3 consoles use under 100W of energy during play, however the Nintendo Wii is still using significant energy even in in standby/off mode (10W when Connect24 is enabled).

It is worth noting that an older Xbox 360 would use between 115 and 200W per hour when in use, and just 0.5W when in standby mode. If you have a 'Kinect Sensor' hooked up, this would draw around 14W per hour. Newer models, as noted in the table above, are much more energy efficient.

The type of gaming experience you are looking for will dictate the type of gaming console purchased. Suggestions below for managing energy wastage are focused on how the console is used.

Energy reduction suggestions:
- Opt for the latest model device (as they are more energy efficient)

- Ensure you can easily turn off the unit at the power source to stop energy wastage when not in use
- Use the device in conjunction with an energy efficient TV (OLED or LCD technology)

TIP If the unit is off, ensure the Kinect sensors/WiiConnect24 sensors are off as well. These continue to draw energy unless the unit it is connected to is off at the power source.

Computers

USA Energy Star ratings are voluntary in Australia. Some computers and monitors carry an energy star rating.

The main types of computers found in a household are desktops and laptops. Desktop computers use more energy than laptops so if replacing any computing equipment, opt for laptops over desktop computers where you can. A desktop computer arrangement can use up to 300W (including screen), whereas a laptop will use around 72W (including screen).

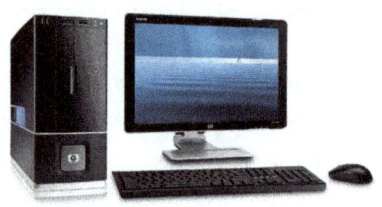

Image: Hewlet Packard

What to look for when choosing a new computer:

- Look for the 'Energy Star' or energy efficiency rating on computers and opt for the most efficient model you can afford
- Opt for LED or LCD screens (which are more energy efficient)
- Choose laptops instead of desktop computers when replacing equipment
- Be clear on the technical specifications you need
- Choose a model that is upgradeable to provide for longevity

When using a computer, the following will help minimise energy use:

- Set up and use the power management options for sleep modes. 'Sleep' mode uses around 10 percent of energy when compared to 'in use'. This is relevant for home computers, laptops and servers on home networks
- Screen savers save screens, not energy. Disable screen savers and enable 'sleep' modes at suitable times to help save energy
- Turn computers off at the power source when not in use, some models have inbuilt transformers which continue to draw energy
- Turn off chargers at the wall when items have finished charging (e.g. mobile device chargers, iPads and tablet computers) as these tend to continue to draw energy, even when nothing is connected to it

TIP If your laptop has a battery, remove it when not in use. Continued charging when fully charged can cause damage and reduce the life of the battery.

Printers and copiers

Energy rating labels for printers, copies and multi-function devices are not in Australia at this time,

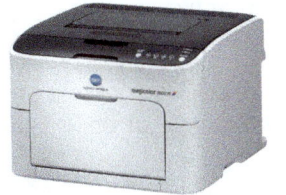

Most desktop printers and copiers use relatively small amounts of energy, but they waste energy through standby and can use large amounts of ink. Many of the newer multi-function devices warm up faster and have very low standby power use.

Image: courtesy of Konica Minolta

When upgrading your printer or multifunction device (MFD), look for:

- One machine that does everything you need (saves space and materials)
- Choose a printer with good resolution and reasonable speed (pages per minute print rate)
- Check the cost of the ink/toner and its availability as often the cost of ink surpasses the cost of the printer very quickly
- Look for a printer that does double sided printing (saves paper)
- Check for energy efficient power saving modes (and use them)
- Ensure it is recyclable at end of life
- Opt for a model that uses refillable ink cartridges

Reduce your environmental footprint by using 100 percent recycled, FSC® certified carbon neutral paper. It really does make a difference.

Appliances – summary

The following is a summary of the key things to remember when shopping for appliances:

- Consider the big energy users and items that are always on or often used
- Choose appliances that are the right size for the purpose
- Check the rating labels and opt for the most efficient appliance you can afford
- Opt for quality appliances which reduces the replacement times
- Ensure adequate ventilation (at least 50mm) around refrigerators.
- Install a clothes line to discourage the use of clothes dryers
- Choose appliances with a high energy star rating, see **www.energyrating.gov.au**
- Choose appliances that do not expose food to plastics or chemical coatings
- Check the Energy All Stars web site for the most efficient products at **www.energyallstars.gov.au**
- Check Ecospecifier or GECA websites for further information on those that may be independently certified
- Ask questions!

Technology

Technology is rapidly advancing and is making its way into our homes in the form of appliances and communication devices. There are global groups which suggest that some of this technology is affecting human health.

For example:

Electric fields – created by differences in voltage. The higher the voltage, stronger the field

Magnetic fields – created when electric current flows. The greater the current, the stronger the magnetic field

Electromagnetic fields – combination of electric field and magnetic field, referred to as EMF

Radiofrequency fields – electromagnetic radiation in the frequency ranges of 3 kilohertz (kHz) to 300 gigahertz (GHz), respectively (ARPANSA, 2013). The primary associated health concern is the heating effect on cells in the body.

Some sources of electromagnetic fields:

- Wiring
- Appliances – fridge, stove, oven, electric cooktop, microwave, alarm clocks, phone chargers, electric fans, televisions, computer equipment, stereo equipment, electric blankets, baby monitors, routers, electric heating, meter box (smart meters)

Some sources of radiofrequency radiation are:

- Mobile phones
- Cordless phones
- Microwave ovens
- Bluetooth
- Communication transmitters

It is interesting to note that there are different views of risk associated with these exposures globally, with some countries taking action and issuing precautionary warnings while others are not.

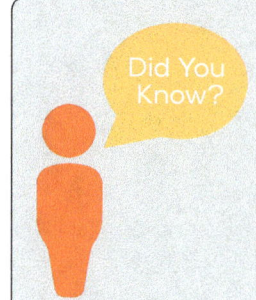

Did You Know?

The International Agency for Research on Cancer issued a press release in May 2011 which stated:

The WHO/International Agency for Research on Cancer (IARC) has classified radiofrequency electromagnetic fields as possible carcinogenic to humans (Group B) based on an increased risk for glioma, a malignant type of brain cancer, associated with wireless phone use. (IARC, 2011)

The Australian Radiation Protection and Nuclear Safety Agency (ARPANSA is the Australian government's primary authority on radiation and nuclear safety. Currently the information available on the ARPANSA website does not subscribe to the same potential risk for radiofrequency electromagnetic fields as outlined by the IARC.

Refer to the ARPANSA website for further information on the Australian assessment of radiofrequency electromagnetic fields **www.apansa.gov.au**

Globally there are different standards as to what is considered safe. It is concerning that precautionary standards issued and initiated in other countries are not always embraced or investigated here in Australia. An example of this is the roll out of Wi-Fi technology into Australian schools despite the IARC caution of this technology being a possible carcinogen.

The argument is poised on the term 'possible', many wanting irrefutable proof of harm before guidelines and standards are changed. Meanwhile countries that are not operating according to a precautionary principle approach (such as Australia) continue the social experiment (using our families) until more evidence is revealed.

TIP As a precautionary measure use hard wired internet access over Wi-Fi where possible.

In the home there are some precautionary strategies to minimise exposure to electromagnetic radiation. Many of these are associated with the bedroom space as this is a zone where we spend around eight hours a day.

Here are some ways you can minimise your exposure:

- Keep appliances out of the bedroom so that your body can rest overnight with minimised exposure
- Use a battery operated alarm clock in the bedroom rather than electric
- Keep mobile phones out of the bedroom
- Avoid electric blankets
- Keep appliances off the walls directly behind the bedhead
- The meter box and switch board should be placed away from spaces frequently used
- Demand switches can be fitted on the switchboard (this requires an electrician) to stop the flow of electricity through cabling when current is not required. These automatically allow current when it's required. This is a good option for bedroom wiring to reduce potential exposures overnight as a precautionary strategy
- Turn off appliances at the power point when not in use
- Use hard wired internet access in the home rather than Wi-Fi
- Restrict time spent on game consoles that use Wi-Fi technology and turn them off when not in use
- Disable Wi-Fi on your computer when internet access is not needed
- Disable the Wi-Fi router at night and keep it located in a place away from areas frequently used
- Put your mobile phone on flight mode when carrying it on your body and turn it back on to get your messages when you can remove it from your body
- For testing of electric and magnetic fields contact a qualified building biologist, ensure they have the relevant equipment prior to engaging services. Some testing equipment can also be hired from ARPANSA for those wishing to check their own home and equipment

Further information

Australian Government Radiation Protection and Nuclear Safety Agency – www.arpansa.gov.au
World Health Organisation – www.who.int/peh-emf/about/WhatisEMF/en/
Dr Magda Havas, PhD – www.magdahavas.com
Council of Europe – Parliamentary Assembly – Resolution 1851 (2011) – The potential dangers of electromagnetic fields and their effect on the environment – www.assembly.coe.int/Mainf.asp?link=/Documents/AdoptedText/ta11/ERES1815.htm

Heating and cooling systems

Heating and cooling systems contribute to the comfort and enjoyment of the home. For people who suffer from allergies or respiratory conditions the type of heating or cooling chosen may contribute to symptoms.

Before choosing a heating or cooling application for your home there are a few issues to be aware of:

- Systems that blow air around the home can cause dry skin and eyes. They also stir up dust around the home and are not recommended for those with respiratory issues
- Gas systems can give off fumes, including the release of carbon monoxide which is poisonous and can kill. Ensure gas heating is always externally flued and install a carbon monoxide detector
- Solid fuel fires tend to produce significant pollution through the burning process and should be well vented through use of chimneys and slightly open window or door to allow a draught to promote extraction. If any occupants have respiratory issues, minimise the use of solid fuels in the home
- Reverse cycle air filters should be regularly cleaned and sanitised to prevent transfer of airborne viruses or bacteria within the home
- Mechanical systems that use fresh air and contain filters for removing pollutants are the best option for healthier indoor air
- Excessive noise levels of appliances can impact on health through disturbed sleep and can increase stress levels. Ensure any system purchased considers noise for both the purchaser and the neighbours. See your local council for regulations covering neighbourhood noise levels in your area

Product considerations

Whatever your climate zone there are likely to be occasions when you'll be looking for some additional warmth or cooling.

There are times when the home is not able to benefit from passive systems, or the passive system needs some help to maintain internal temperatures at a comfortable level. This is when the mechanical heating and cooling systems are needed. How much heating and cooling required is dependent on your home, what temperature you personally are comfortable with and the local climate. In some climates, up to 40 percent of an energy bill can be due to heating and cooling.

Here we provide a guideline for mechanical systems and items for consideration as supplementary heating or cooling in the home.

- Size of the space required to be heated or cooled. Note that the higher the efficiency of the building envelope, the smaller the heating and cooling system that should be needed to be comfortable. See next tip
- Type of unit best suited for particular areas of the home
- Type of unit most suited to occupants needs e.g. asthma or allergies (radiant heat preferred over circulating heat)
- How often you are likely to use it
- What the maintenance requirements are
- Can any filters be easily cleaned?

- If the unit creates mechanical air flow where do you want the outlets, e.g. floor, wall or ceiling
- Check the star rating and choose the most efficient model you can (the more stars the more efficient it is). See the energy rating label description below

Heating and Cooling Energy Rating Labels
Will be together if a reverse cycle unit
Will be separate if only heating or cooling
They all have the same information

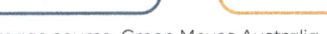

Callouts on the label:
- The more stars the more energy efficient it is.
- The more stars the more energy efficient it is.
- How much cooling OUTPUT
- How much energy INPUT
- The make and model of the appliance
- How much energy INPUT
- How much Heat OUTPUT
- Check operation modes rated

Image source: Green Moves Australia.

TIP: Homes with highly efficient building envelopes (insulation, glazing, draught-proofing) do not need large heating and cooling systems to maintain thermal comfort in the home. This allows the heating/cooling system to be smaller, which is cheaper to purchase and run. Consult your thermal performance rating documentation for the correct size of the system needed, or ask a qualified sustainability assessor to calculate it for you.

The unit that this label belongs to is a very energy efficient unit for both heating and cooling.

For cooling, for every .82 kW of energy put into the unit, you get 4.75 kW of cooling energy out. That's a co-efficient of performance (COP) of approximately 4.5:1 which is very good.

For heating, for every .80 kW of energy in, you get 4.90 kW of energy out. That's a co-efficient of performance of approximately 4.6:1 which is excellent.

You can find out more about the energy efficiency rating of appliances at **www.reg.energyrating.gov.au** Remember, you can reduce the greenhouse gas emissions of your mechanical systems by using renewable energy sources to produce the energy needed (i.e. solar PV, geothermal, purchasing green power).

Passive heating and cooling is free

Where possible always aim to use passive heating and cooling systems first before using your mechanical systems. Passive heating and cooling is free, has minimal environmental impact and tends to provide a better type of heat (radiant heat) and cooling (natural breezes).

Thermal mass - heating and cooling

As discussed in the Build it/Renovate section, building materials that can retain heat have the capacity to contribute to heating a home if used in appropriate places and ways.

To use a thermal mass material for heating it needs to have access to heat to absorb. This is generally provided by solar radiation entering the building, but could also be provided by other sources (such as a mechanical heating system used off peak).

Objects with low thermal mass are good at releasing heat quickly and should be used in hot climates to assist with cooling. To use a thermal mass for cooling, ensure it is protected from summer sun through shading and insulation. Place it in an area where cooling night breezes and air will pass over it to draw out any stored energy.

Utilising the right thermal mass in the correct manner provides for a more comfortable environment and contributes significantly to passive heating and cooling. It's important that thermal mass is sited appropriately, if not it can work against you.

Passive solar heating

Passive solar heating is a form of heating that results from passive design principles and solar access as outlined in the passive house section in the Build it/Renovate section. Homes in climate zones 4-8 would benefit from passive solar heating during cooler months.

For passive solar heating to operate at its best, it needs the following design elements:

- North orientation to primary living areas
- A floor plan that is defined and zoned based on heating requirements
- Appropriate areas of glazing
- Advanced glazing to the northern façade
- Internal thermal mass to store the heat
- Good insulation and draught sealing to the home

How it works:

Passive heating works by capturing the solar radiation entering the home through north facing glazing that is exposed to full sun, often referred to as 'greenhouse principle'. The type of glazing, as well as the framing, affects the efficiency of the process.

Solar radiation enters the home through the glazing and is absorbed and stored within the building by high thermal mass materials such as concrete slab flooring or masonry walls. These must be internal and have access to heat to be most effective.

The absorbed heat is then released back into the home at night where it is used to offset heat loss. Incorporating good thermal mass helps to moderate the internal temperature of a home when temperature variations between day and night are high.

TIP When using high thermal mass materials be sure to also use coatings (paint, varnishes) that are non-toxic and do not off-gas when warmed.

Winter – using thermal mass for heating

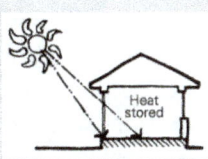

Winter Day
The sun enters the building and warms the thermal mass which absorbs heat during the day.

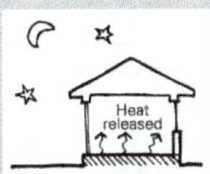

Winter Night
Warmth will be re-radiated back into the room at night. Close window coverings to prevent loss of radiated heat during the evening.

Mechanical heating systems

These come in many types and can be powered by electricity, gas, solid fuels or renewable energy sources. The key to energy efficiency is to only heat the rooms that are being used, and only to a comfortable temperature, so ensure settings are appropriate. There is no point in wasting energy in rooms that are empty. Overheating the home is unhealthy for occupants and results in a higher energy bills.

For heating systems, ducted vents are better placed in the floor or low wall level because the hot air will naturally rise into the rest of the room.

The tables on the following pages provide an overview of the pros and cons for different types of systems. What's best for your situation will depend on a variety of factors. If in doubt consult a heating professional or sustainability consultant to review your situation and needs.

TIP One general rule of thumb is that any type of heating using electricity can be expensive to operate. Another is that the cheaper the appliance, the more expensive it usually is to run. Conclusion: Steer away from small cheap electric heaters.

Common types of heating

Type	Pros	Cons
Ducted Central Heating Works by heating the air and blowing it through the home. Energy source can be gas, electric or renewable.	• Maintains a 'zone' at constant temperature • One system to maintain • Space savings through ceiling or floor ducting • Some inverter systems are very efficient • Many systems provide duct outlet and exchange filters that can be easily removed and cleaned to filter out dust particles Hydronic central heating is the exception and noted separately below	• Expensive to install • Can be expensive to run • Ducting can have substantial heat losses if not well insulated and sealed • When the unit fails, whole home is affected • Zoning baffles can be problematic and result in higher running costs • Ceiling vents allow heat to escape if not sealed, when unit is off • Unoccupied spaces continue to be heated if 'in the zone' • Blows dust particles around the home that may be problematic for those with asthma and allergies
Hydronic Central Heating Works by heating water and passing it through panels to transfer the heat to the rooms. Can be used through wall panels or under floor. Can be solar, gas, electric or solid fuel fired.	• Generally efficient • Easily zoned to a room or area • Minimal heat loss through pipes or zoning • Warms the fabric of the building as well as the space • One system to maintain • More opportunity for renewable heat sources • No hot air blowing dust around (better indoor air quality) • Provides radiant heat (not as drying to the eyes and skin as circulating air) • Low maintenance • Well proven technology • Does not circulate air pollutants when in use, a good option for those with allergies and asthma	• Expensive initial install cost • If using wall panels they can take up wall space

Table continued next page.

Type	Pros	Cons
Under Floor Heating Best installed during the initial build. Uses electric wires or hydronic hot water pipes installed into the concrete slab. The concrete is then heated and releases the heat into the home. Energy source is generally electricity or gas but can be solid fuel fired	• Can be zoned to room or area • No wall or ceiling obstructions • Warms the fabric of the building as well as the space • No hot air blowing around so better indoor quality • Provides radiant heat, an option for those with allergies and asthma as does not circulate dust • Solar, gas or heat pump hydronic heating can be very efficient	• Expensive to install • Electric wire type can be very expensive to run • Slow to respond to changing conditions. (i.e. if heated floor and solar gain combine it can overheat a room, the only way to cool is to open windows) • Unless well insulated, significant heat losses through into the ground or below desired area • Difficult to repair if faults occur in the buried wires/pipes • Electric wire type is generally not recommended by building biologists as some types may emit high magnetic fields that can affect some people's health
Independent room, space heating Works by heating the air and blowing it around the room. Can be gas or electric.	• Maintains a room at a constant temperature • Generally cheaper to run • If failure occurs, only one room is affected • Individual temperature control per room • Reverse cycle inverter systems are very efficient • Natural convection systems can be very efficient • No heat losses from ducting	• Space requirement in each room to site the heater • Gas flues should be flued to the exterior of the house to avoid toxic pollutants accumulating indoors • If using gas, ensure you install a carbon monoxide detector near the unit • Mobile or independent units have a greater chance of causing injury to small children such as burns when touched

Energy sources

Type	Comments
Electric Heaters The key benefit of electricity is that it is readily available and can be provided from renewable sources. Some electric heaters are very efficient, some are not. 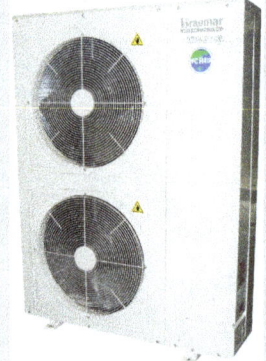 Image: Braemar inverter unit from Seely International 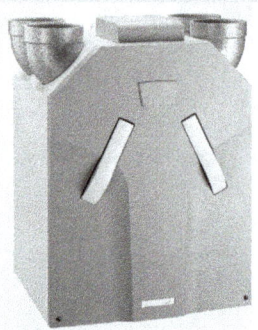 Image: Zehnder ComfoAir	**Types** Older ducted electric heating systems (sometimes called resistance or convection heating) work by converting electricity directly to heat through a heating element. This has air blown over it by a fan and then directs the warmed air to the rooms through ducting. There are not many of these systems around anymore as they were terribly inefficient and expensive to operate. Under floor electric heating can be very expensive to install, maintain (if it fails) and run. Newer technology sees ducted systems using inverter (heat pump) technology, generally a large reverse cycle heating (and cooling) unit. These can be more expensive to buy than gas fired heating units but offer cooling as well so provide a dual purpose. Inverter units are very efficient to run. Similar to heat pump hot water systems, they work by taking heat from the air which is used to heat a refrigerant, which converts to a gas, which is compressed and then generates heat which heats the air. There is a variety of heat pump units available. Be sure to check the specifications of the products. Look for a high co-efficient of performance (COP) – aim for COP of 4:1 or higher (for every 1 kW of energy in, it produces 4 kW of heat energy output). Choose a quiet model to minimise noise levels. These units are generally installed inside the roof space but can also be located outdoors. Units can be zoned and individual room thermostats installed to allow temperature variations. Air is generally recirculated from inside the home. **Heat Recovery Systems** Heat recovery systems work by extracting heat from outgoing air, and reusing it to warm fresh incoming air. It is a key feature of the 'passive house' type of construction, but can be used in any home to assist in providing a healthy and comfortable indoor climate. The system filters dust and allergens from entering the home through the ventilation system and provides for clean fresh air inside the home. The heat recovery systems can recover up to 90 percent of the energy from the extracted air which is reused to warm the incoming fresh air. This significantly reduces pollutants into the home and minimises heating or cooling costs. The units are very energy efficient (they generally run 24 hours a day) and the resultant indoor air quality is excellent, providing a healthier environment for those with allergies.

Table continued next page.

Type	Comments

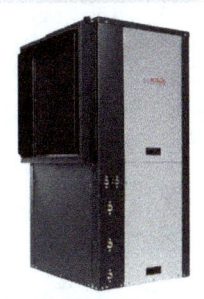

Image: Bosch Geothermal Heat Pump

However using electricity to power a heat source can get very expensive. Unless the electricity is provided from a renewable source it is very greenhouse gas intensive.

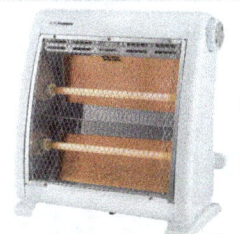

Portable heater
image: www.northerntool.com

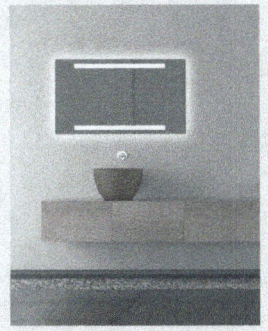

Glass radiant mirror heater
image: Warmer Australia

Ground Source (Geothermal) heat pumps

These are similar to electric heat pumps (also called air source heat pumps) but don't use the air as a heat source or heat sink. Instead heat is transferred to and from the ground by pumping water through a deep bore field loop, called a vertical loop, or a shallow trench, called a horizontal ground loop. The water absorbs heat from the earth, warming it. Geothermal heat pumps have a very high COP at 4:1 (that's outputting 4 kW of energy for every 1 kW used). These systems can be used for producing space heating or cooling, or through hot water use extend to hydronic heating and pool heating.

Electric Space and Portable Heaters

These are designed to heat a smaller room or space. Space heaters are a good way to warm a room without having to heat the whole home. They come in three basic types: radiant, convector and combination heaters. Reverse cycle inverter units are also a good option to heat/cool a single room. Ensure filters are cleaned regularly and fins wiped clean (especially those living in humid conditions to prevent mould growth).

Note that some portable heaters are extremely cheap to buy, but they can be very expensive to run.

All portable heaters should have emergency cut-off switches; some models also have temperature controls and thermostats.

Radiant heaters (generally bar heaters) provide heat directly to your body and objects (not the air) and are very effective in bathrooms and small spaces even with exhaust fans running. These heaters are very effective in short time frames but can be a fire risk if placed too close to anything flammable, or a burn risk to people and animals.

Newer technology has seen infrared radiant heaters embedded into glass in the form of mirrors or even wall pictures. These offer a dual duty appliance and although costly, look and feel good. They get hot to the touch but are much less of a fire and burn risk than the bar heater types. Infrared is a proven efficient heating technology and provides comfortable warmth. They also plug into a standard power socket and can move house with you. The downside is they can be expensive to buy.

 **TIP** Radiant and panel heater types are good options for an asthma friendly household as they do not blow air around.

Fan heaters are simply air being blown over a radiant heating element and are effective at warming a small space relatively quickly, but again can be expensive to run.

Table continued next page.

Type	Comments
	Convector heaters work by air currents passing over an appliances heating element and using natural convection currents. As the air gets hot it rises causing air movement. Convector heaters are quieter because there is no fan. These can also be slower to heat a space as they rely on natural air currents. Examples are water or oil filled heaters and some panel heaters.
	Combination heaters combine convector and radiant attributes into one unit and are suitable for almost anywhere in the home.
	When looking for a space or portable heater, reverse cycle units offer great efficiency. However, smaller convection units, those using around 400W, can be very effective in a small space and cost a lot less to run. Look at the wattage rating on the label. If it says 1500W input, then it is likely to use 1500W (1.5 kW) per hour when operating.
	 For small personal space heating where an electric model is the only option, check the wattage usage on the compliance label and opt for one that uses between 400W to 800W (as opposed to 2000W to 2500W).
	In terms of energy efficiency, most electric space heaters produce one unit of heat for every 1kW of electricity, which means they are 100 percent efficient. It's worth remembering that geothermal heat pumps and inverter reverse cycle units can produce over four units of heat for every 1kW of electricity, which makes them 400 per cent efficient.
	 Models with temperature settings and thermostats are more efficient to run because they know when the temperature is reached and switch off.
Natural (mains) Gas Currently cheaper than electricity but not available everywhere and produces combustion gases. Flues are used to expel gases out of the home. A carbon monoxide detector is highly recommended where gas is used internally.	Ducted gas systems generally have a gas furnace located in the roof, in an internal cupboard or outside. Air is heated by the flame and blown by fans through ducting vents to the rooms. Check the efficiency of the unit (it should have an energy efficiency star rating) and choose the most efficient model you can. These units should also be regularly serviced. **Gas Space and Portable heaters** As with electric space heaters, these are designed to heat a smaller room or space without having to heat the whole home. All gas heaters should be externally flued. Unflued gas heaters can result in water vapour and hot gases (including carbon monoxide) being released into the room and are not suitable for bedrooms, bathrooms or confined areas. There are legal restrictions on their use which differ in each state so check with your local building and plumbing authority to confirm requirements in your area.

Table continued next page.

Type	Comments
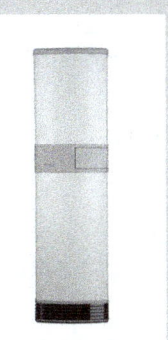 Image: Braemar wall furnace 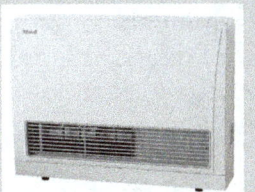 Image: Rinnai Gas heater	Gas space heating units can be very cheap to run and an effective way to heat a space. They are available in various forms such as wall furnace, portable unit or gas fire place configuration. As always, opt for the most energy efficient model you can afford and install an external flue. Always use a licensed gasfitter to install and service and ask for a compliance certificate after installation of new systems. Due to potential gas leakage issues, avoid purchasing second-hand gas heaters. Some units have economy modes, inbuilt thermostats and timers. If you have children, also check for a child lock.  **TIP** Ensuring your gas heater is externally flued is the safest and healthiest way of using it. Asthma Foundation **www.asthmaaustralia.org.au/wood_fire_heaters_addendum.aspx**  **TIP** Where gas heaters are built into brick chimneys or other restricted spaces, be sure to have them tested for carbon monoxide spillage/leaks before each winter. This includes space heaters and decorative log fire type heaters. (source: **www.esv.vic.gov.au**)
Liquefied Petroleum Gas Natural gas supplied in a cylinder to your property. 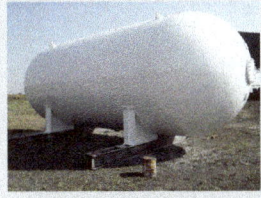 Image: www.funafun.com	LPG based systems are more expensive to run than mains supplied natural gas. If you use a lot of gas for heating (and/or cooking) it is unlikely to be a cost effective option. To minimise frequent replacement/refilling of LPG cylinders, choose large storage capacity tanks or bottles.

Table continued next page.

Type	Comments
Solid fuels (wood, coal) Wood is a renewable fuel, particularly when it's been sustainably sourced. Wood can be quite economical where free access to local wood is available. Solid fuel burning as a fuel source is not generally recommended in urban areas, and may be illegal in some council zones due to the pollution they create. 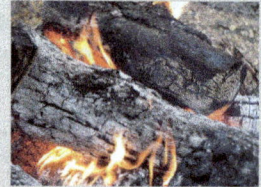 Image: Louis Waweru 2007	In many rural areas solid fuels are used as a fuel source. Slow combustion stoves or solid fuel furnaces heat the air which is then blown by fans through ducting vents to the rooms. Open fireplaces can also use wood or coal and are generally inefficient as most of the heat goes up the chimney. Some of the more recent fire place inserts and designs are more efficient as they pull air from the room, circulate it around the metal fire box and send back into the room. These can warm a room very quickly. They also cool down quickly when the fire is out. Fire places should have a damper which should be closed when the chimney is not in use and open when it is in use. Wood should be very dry (ideally dried out over a summer or longer). Hardwoods tend to have more energy, burn longer and produce less smoke but can be difficult to light. Softwoods are easier to light but can spark in open fires. Always use a guard on open fires to protect from sparks. Do not burn green or damp wood as it causes excess smoke. Do not burn treated wood or composite woods such as mdf, ply or particle board or timbers treated with finishing coats such as paints or stains, as they contain toxic chemicals that will release toxic fumes when burnt. In urban areas residents may be tempted to collect old furniture off the street or debris from building sites to burn. If you know of anyone burning materials that are not raw timber contact the health department at your local council to avoid toxic smoke exposure in the neighbourhood. Coal can be used in most combustion heaters or fire places but can be difficult to light and is messy to handle. It also releases gases and smoke that contribute to pollution. Both wood and coal need to be stored in a dry location. When in use the heating unit needs to be loaded, the fire maintained and the ash cleaned out and disposed of properly.  **TIP** Ensure the room where the fire is, is well ventilated to reduce the build-up of combustion pollutants. Solid fuels are not as energy efficient as gas and electric heating types. They also produce combustion gases, need to be flued (or a chimney) and the smoke produced contributes to pollution. **Health tip:** If you have respiratory issues in the family avoid solid fuel type heaters.

Table continued next page.

Type	Comments
Other fuels (bioethanol, wood pellets) 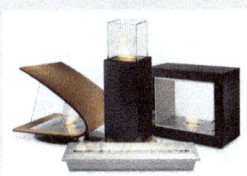 Image: EcoSmart Fire 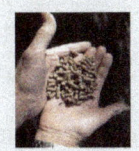 Image: PelletHeaters.com.au Wood Pellets 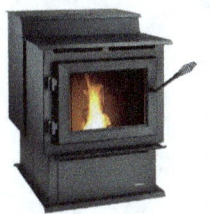 Pellet Fire	**Bioethanol** Bioethanol is an absolute alcohol and considered a renewable fuel that is made from a variety of plant materials. The emissions from burning bioethanol are negligible which allows a bioethanol fireplace to be installed almost anywhere without producing any smoke, sparks or gases that need to be externally vented. As a heat source it is as efficient as any comparably sized open fire place. **Wood Pellets (used in Pellet Fires)** Wood pellets are simply sawdust that has been collected from wood cutting industries, heavily compressed with air to form small dry pellets that look like chicken feed. They contain no chemicals, just recycled sawdust and air. They are around 80 percent efficient, making it up to 350 percent more efficient than open fires (EcoChoice Fires, 2014). Wood pellets are used in pellet fires which are one of the most energy efficient heating devices available. They are also simple to operate. Pellets are poured into the hopper and then automatically fed into a fire pot where a simple electric igniter lights the fire. An external dial or thermostat regulates fuel delivery and actual heat output. Combustion air is drawn through the fire pot by an exhaust fan ensuring perfect air-to-fuel ratios and maximum efficiency. Fresh air is passed through a series of heat exchangers and fan-forced into the living area using a variable speed convection fan. Additionally, heat from the fire pot radiates through the glass door. This dual system ensures an automatic ambience and heat efficiency. (source: Ecochoice Fires, 2014) They produce very little smoke, emit few pollutants, have the lowest emission rate of any wood burner and are considered almost smokeless. However, they do need electricity to feed pellets into the burner and operate the fan. Styles range from traditional stove type (pictured) to modern architectural designs. They are small and compact. **Health tip:** *'Pellet fuel is generally standardised and substantially more uniform in composition than traditional firewood. However, a lack of independent testing and certainty about how much nitrogen dioxide these heaters produce means that this new form of heating cannot be recommended for asthmatics at this time.'* (Asthma Australia, 2014)

Table continued next page.

Type	Comments
Solar Air Heaters	Solar air heaters convert solar radiation into thermal heat, which is carried by air and delivered to a space. 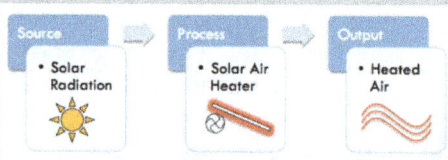 Image: Solar Air Heating Association

Solar air heaters operate on some of the most fundamental and simple thermodynamic principles:

- Absorption of the solar radiation by a solid body results in the body heating up. In broad terms this solid body is known as the 'collector'. Some bodies are better at absorption than others, such as those with black non-reflective surfaces
- Convection of heat from the heated solid body to the air as it passes over the surface. Typically a fan is used to force the air across the heated body, the fan can be solar powered or mains powered

Different types of solar air heater technology achieve this process using the same basic principles but through the use of different solid bodies acting as the collector. The fan that transfers the air across the heated surface is also used as part of a ducting system to direct the heated air into the dwelling space. In addition to heating the air within that space, the heat can further be absorbed by thermal mass such as walls, flooring, furniture and other contents. Such heat is effectively 'stored' and slowly dissipates beyond sunlight hours.

Night time cooling

Many solar air heating systems also have cooling capabilities by transferring cooler outside air into a house, or transferring hot air out of a house or roof cavity. This is particularly effective after sunset on hot summer days.

Most systems utilise a thermostat or other means of automatically controlling the airflow, so that a house isn't over-heated or over-cooled.

While they are not a replacement for mechanical heating systems, they supplement standard internal heating by providing a supplementary passive heat source. Benefits include a higher level of comfort, lower carbon emissions and lower power bills.

These heaters are directly affected by cloud cover and should be sited to maximise solar access. They can be fixed to walls or roofs.

| **Heat shifting** 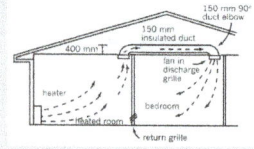 Image: Your Home | Heat shifting involves a low energy method of moving warm air from one part of the home to another using vents, ducts and fans. The vent should be closable for when heat shifting is not needed. |

Operational considerations

You can maximise the efficiency of your heating when it's running by:

- Zoning off areas by closing doors between heated and non-heated spaces
- Close all windows in the room to prevent heat loss (unless using a gas or solid fuel system that needs the ventilation)
- If the sun is directly hitting any of the glazing let it into the room, it will assist to warm the space
- Set the thermostat to a reasonable temperature and wear a jumper. For each degree less you have to heat, up to 10 percent of running costs can be saved
- Unless you have double glazing, close blinds or curtains to help retain heat in the room and minimise heat loss through the glass, especially at night
- Only heat the rooms that are occupied and in use
- If you have high ceilings, a low speed ceiling fan can help to push the warm air back down
- Turn the system off or reduce the heat setting at night to save energy
- Use automated timers if they suit your lifestyle to provide warmth when you need it, and to turn the system off when you are not home

Preventative maintenance

The lifespan of mechanical systems can be maximised when the unit is properly maintained during its lifetime. If you are not sure about the requirements for your system contact the supplier and they will advise you accordingly. The following is a general guide to preventative maintenance servicing.

- For ducted and split system units, clean the air intake grates and filters every 6-12 months to ensure good air flow into the system. This is particularly important if the unit is well used. Check with your supplier, some can be DIY jobs, others will require a service technician. Your supplier can advise
- Service the units in line with the manufacturer's recommendations. This will ensure that it operates at optimal efficiency and minimises the risk of failures
- If any gas appliances are in the home, install a carbon monoxide detector near the unit. They are cheap to buy, easy to install and could save lives if a leak occurs
- Gas systems, particularly those with pilot lights, are best located externally so that if a leak occurs it won't harm those in the home
- Fire places with chimneys should have the chimney cleaned and inspected annually

---

Further Information

Your Home – www.yourhome.gov.au

Better Health website - www.betterhealth.vic.gov.au/bhcv2/bhcarticles.nsf/pages/Gas_heating_health_and_safety_issues

Asthma Australia – www.asthmaaustralia.org.au/wood_fire_heaters_addendum.aspx

Solar Air Heating – www.solarairheating.org.au

Energy Safe Victoria website – www.esv.vic.gov.au

Passive cooling

As with heating, when it comes to cooling opt for passive methods first. Open windows, shade areas of glazing where the sun directly hits and let the breezes through the home. When that is not enough, then consider using a mechanical cooling source.

Every home in Australia can benefit from passive cooling at various times of the year and it is applicable to all climate zones. Passive cooling works by utilising a combined approach to reducing heat gain and cooling breezes into the home. The contributing factors are a highly efficient building envelope, facilitating heat loss through access to cooling breezes, air movement, earth coupling and evaporation.

The main design elements are:

- Orientation to capture cooling breezes
- Increase internal natural ventilation by providing unobstructed air flow paths through the home,
- Use of fans to provide air movement on still days/nights
- Include exit points for warm air, ideally high windows or vents
- Window types and glazing that enable capture and direction of cooling breezes into the home (i.e. louvers, casement types)
- Appropriate shading (through eaves, pergolas, shade blinds or planting)
- Appropriate insulation types (reflective and bulk) and levels (e.g. correct R value for climate zone) within the home
- Use high thermal mass structural materials when building for housing in locations where day/night temperatures have a high variance
- Use low thermal mass construction materials when building in locations where there is a low day/night temperature range (i.e. tropical zones)
- Use of light coloured building structure and roofs to reflect heat and minimise heat gain through the structure

Some examples of these points are below.

Summer – using thermal mass for cooling	
	Summer Day Thermal mass protected from the sun by shading. This keeps the thermal mass cool.
	Summer Night Cool breezes and convection currents pass over the thermal mass drawing out stored energy (flushing) and cooling the building.

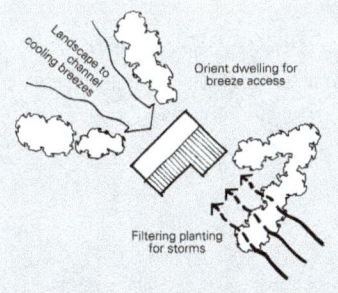

Image source: Passive Cooling, Your Home

In this example the cooling breezes are directed into the home through landscape.

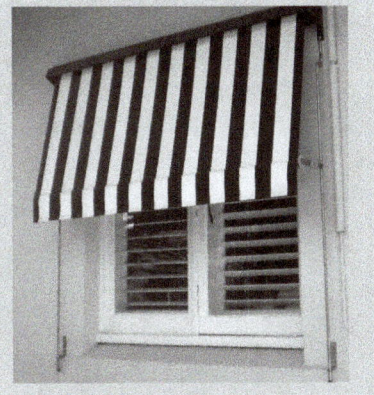

Image: rainsfords.com.au

Removable or adjustable shade devices such as blinds or external shutters can help to reduce heat into the home.

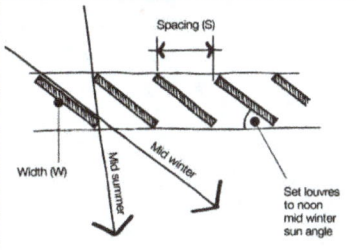

Fixed shading such as pergolas with appropriately angled louvers can let the sun in during winter months and provide shade in summer.

This facilitates passive solar heating and cooling for the home.

Note that angles will change depending on location.

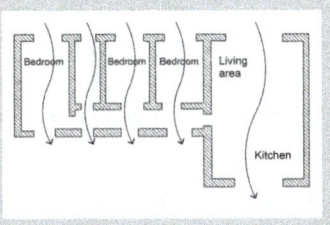

Image source: Passive Cooling, Your Home

Internal layout. This type of internal floor plan facilitates cooling breezes to flow through the internal structure and cool the home.

Table continued next page.

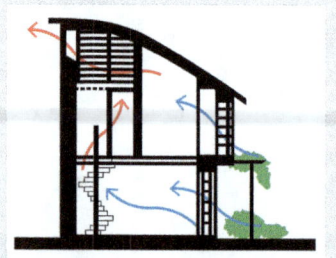

Image source: Passive Cooling, Your Home

Stack ventilation. In this diagram, cooler air enters at the lower levels, as the air warms up it rises and can exit through vents/windows located high in the structure. This causes convective air movement and improves cross ventilation.

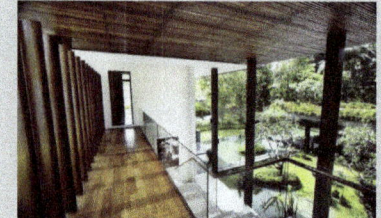

Image: Marvel Building www.marvelbuilding.com/big-house-beautiful-ponds-cooling-elements-sun-house.html

A form of passive evaporative cooling can be obtained by placing water in the form of ponds or pools to the north side of the home near window openings. As the hot air travels over the water it cools and then enters the home.

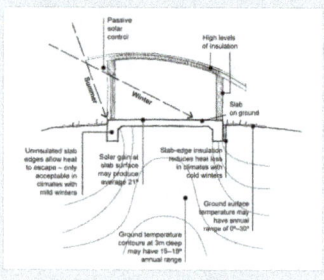

Image source: Passive Cooling, Your Home

Earth coupling uses the cooler ground temperatures to stabilise household heat gains.

Ensure areas around an earth coupled slab are well shaded.

Passive cooling and health

Good ventilation flushes fresh air through a home and takes older, stale air out which improves indoor air quality.

Natural ventilation can introduce allergens into the home such as pollens, therefore for those suffering from allergies and respiratory complaints, consideration needs to be given to appropriate times for natural ventilation to be used. For example:

- Still days when no wind is present to minimise pollens or allergens throughout the house
- Avoid times when lawns are being or have been recently cut
- Avoid days when smoke is present such as from neighbours burning open fires, burn offs and local fires
- Avoid opening windows and doors when neighbouring construction work is occurring

Mechanical cooling

Mechanical cooling tends to be powered by electricity. How greenhouse gas intensive the unit will be depends on the electricity source operating the unit. If you are using your own on-site generated electricity from a renewable source (solar, wind or geothermal), then greenhouse emissions will be low to zero. If you are using electricity from the mains grid, it will be highly greenhouse gas intensive and expensive.

The most popular methods of cooling are fans, air conditioners and evaporative cooling systems. Solar air conditioners and geothermal cooling units are growing in popularity as confidence in the technology, and pricing, improves.

The humble fan

One of the most effective methods of cooling is by using fans. These are available in a variety of types, from ceiling fans, portable (pedestal), wall and even floor fans. They are a very economical method of cooling a home and are the cheapest of all mechanical cooling devices to operate. Fans do not actually lower the temperature or remove humidity from the air, they simply circulate air which provides a cooling effect of around 3°C.

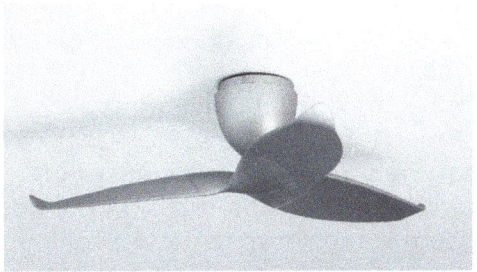

Image: Aeratron fans

Ceiling fans come in a wide variety of sizes and designs with varying features such as lights, decorative blades, and reversible use (for use in winter). To optimise the efficiency and aesthetics of a ceiling fan consider the following:

- Where the best location is (generally the centre of the ceiling)
- Room size is used to determine what size of fan to select (blade span)
- Check ceiling height. Low ceilings are often not suitable for ceiling fans, minimum ceiling height should be between 2.1m and 2.4m and is dependent on the model chosen. All fans should be at least 2.4m from the floor to the blades and ideally 300mm from the ceiling
- Choose a fan that has an efficient motor for the attached blades and blade pitch, and is quiet to run. Most fans operate at a top speed of 200 RPM (repetitions per minute)
- Blade pitch (angle of the blades relative to the fan) determines how much air is pushed around. Aim for a blade pitch of between 10 and 20 degrees. The larger the pitch, the stronger the motor needs to be (due to air resistance). A good rule of thumb is to aim for around 14 degrees
- Fan control could be through a remote controller, a pull cord or a wall switch
- Fans should run clockwise in winter (to move warm air off of the ceiling) and counter clockwise in summer (to create a cool breeze)
- Ensure you do not install a fan between a ceiling light source and the floor as this can result in a light strobing effect when the fan is in use. This could potentially trigger headaches, epileptic seizure or other similar issues
- Good quality fans tend to be quieter and more stable

TIP If you have a remote control for your fan, use double sided velcro to stick it to the wall or door frame where you mainly turn it on/off. Having it stuck to a wall/frame should ensure that it won't get lost so easily.

Free standing, portable fans (pedestal, floor fans)

These fans are generally cheap to buy and you can position them wherever you like, move them around as needed and put them away for winter. Most have variable speeds, some have remote controls and timers. They can be very useful for pushing air through a home and providing efficient cooling.

When choosing a portable fan, consider:

- Where you are likely to use it, choose an appropriate style and size
- A bladeless fan is more expensive but very safe around small children
- What's the maximum airflow? Check cubic feet per minute (CFM) notation to identify low and high air flow fans
- Do you need an oscillating feature?
- Look for a fan with slip resistant feet so it stays put on smooth surfaces
- Check the cord length. Is it sufficient for your needs? (some are very short)
- Where there is a 'cage' around the blades for protection, check that it can be easily opened and replaced to allow cleaning of the blades, but not so easily opened that a child could do it

Whole of house fans

A whole of house fan is one large, strong fan built into the ceiling and vented through the roof space. These units consist of a fan, ceiling vent (that should close when not in use) and external roof vents to expel the air. It works by creating an up-draught that moves the air in the home, pulling it upwards towards the fan and into the roof space. Roof space air is then flushed outside through vents in the eaves. Windows must be open in the home when the fan is on.

A whole house fan brings cooler outside air into the home (assuming it is cooler outside) and reduces heat load in the ceiling. They are relatively cheap to operate and create a cooling breeze through the home.

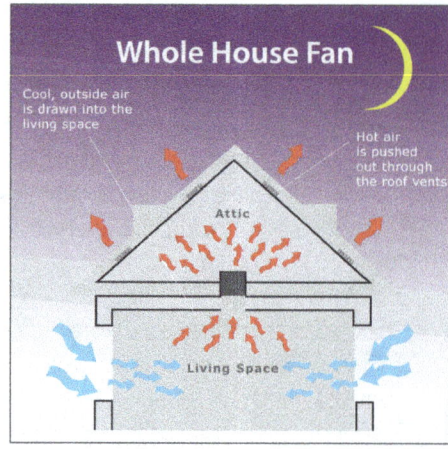

Image: http://dollenselectric.com/whole-house-fan-installers-san-jose-ca

Note that windows and internal doors must be open in the home when the fan is running. Similar to exhaust fans, enough 'make up air' must be able to enter the home to vent it properly.

Product considerations

- Size the unit appropriately (dependent on cubic metre area of home)
- Check the noise level of the fan is low when in operation
- Ensure internal ceiling vent closes when fan is off (and ideally have one that is insulated, particularly if the house is in a cool climate zone)
- Check if there are any restrictions with your local council before installing

Fan maintenance

Ensure the fan is completely switched off before carrying out any maintenance or cleaning.

- Clean the blades regularly as per manufacturer's instructions

Evaporative coolers

Evaporative cooling systems are very effective in dry climates, but not in humid climates. They can be a very energy efficient unit to run (basically just a fan and some water) and come in both whole of house ducted systems and portable models. The lifespan of evaporative coolers is generally 20 years.

Evaporative cooling systems work by drawing outside air through moist filter pads. The air temperature drops as the water evaporates into the air moving through the cooling pads. The image below demonstrates how the process works.

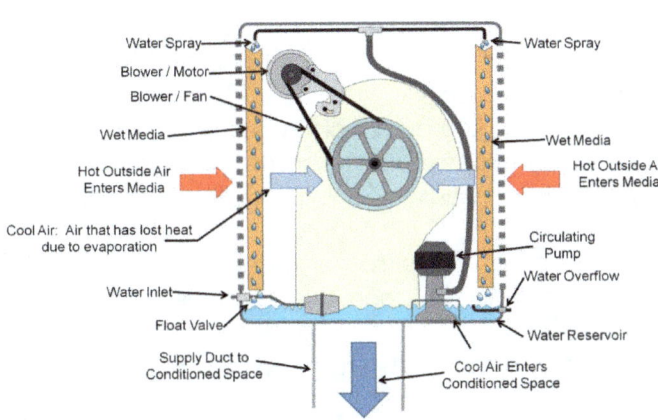

Image credit: https://basc.pnnl.gov/sites/default/files/HVAC122_Evapcooler2_DS_5-7-14.jpg

If using an evaporative system you must ensure you follow the manufacturer's operating instructions, which in many cases require windows and doors to be open in rooms throughout the house to allow the warmer air to leave the home. Evaporative coolers can bring a home temperature down to around 27°C (refer to Origin Energy's FAQ on Evaporative Coolers at **www.originenergy.com.au/3281/FAQs**).

Evaporative units use water through pad evaporation (up to 60-100 litres per hour) and non-evaporative water purge of between five and 30 litres per hour, so they can be water use intensive. The amount of water a unit uses depends on the salinity control, water management and installer settings.

A pilot study conducted by the Australian Institute of Refrigeration, Airconditioning and Heating (AIRAH) on water use in evaporative coolers (funded by the DSE and Smarter Water Fund in 2011) found in residential systems that water bleed or dump rates were set at levels much higher than those required. The study also found that significant water savings could be achieved if these processes were optimised.

The report concluded that

'by operating evaporative units without bleed, but rather dumping the full system once per 24 hours of operating during the summer months, non-evaporative savings of around 95 percent could be made.'

Portable units need the water levels checked regularly to ensure the unit doesn't run dry.

Product considerations:
- Size the unit appropriately to the space to be cooled (note that if you have a highly insulated home, cooling requirements will be reduced)
- Choose a unit that is as energy and water efficient as you can afford
- Consider noise levels (if not for you, for your neighbours) and opt for a quiet model
- For allergy sufferers consider that the requirement of leaving doors or windows open allows dusts and pollens to enter the home

Additionally, for ducted systems

- Look for a high evaporation efficiency rating
- Rain water can be used for evaporative coolers as long as it is clean (potable) and not open to contamination. Do not use recycled water as water quality varies significantly
- Choose a model that has a 'ventilation only' mode for when outdoor temperatures are suitable and ventilation only is needed. This can potentially provide some comfort when humidity is high
- Select ducting that is insulated to at least R1.5 or R2 to help the system deliver the cool air to the areas
- Select a system that has variable speeds to give more flexibility in cooling
- Automatic controls (thermostat, timer and speed) are helpful at maintaining internal temperatures and switch the unit on and off as necessary
- Automatic shutoff (winter seal) dampers are flaps in the duct which open when on, and close when off. This is a necessary feature if you want to keep the home warm in winter months. Vent covers are another alternative but will require manual installation and removal
- Ensure the system is set to dump the water every 24 hours (rather than bleed) during summer months, this can save up to 95 percent of non-evaporative water use (AIRAH, 2011)
- Water drainage pipes can be directed to pools or plants but may have high salt content so ensure plants species are salt tolerant
- Choose a system that manages water automatically and that uses conductivity sensors to control water bleed or dump of water volumes as they provide the best water efficiency. Others tend to waste lots of water if not correctly commissioned
- If in a bushfire prone zone, install ember protection screens or if installing a new unit, ensure it meets the new BAL requirements (AIRAH, 2011)

Evaporative cooler maintenance

- Service the unit and clean the filters in line with the manufacturer's recommendations (generally every two years)
- AIRAH states that it is best to carry out maintenance at the beginning and end of each cooling season. Ensure you use a reputable maintenance service provider
- The AIRAH report of 2011 states that older evaporative coolers can be modified and improved and outlines a standard process for retro commissioning evaporative cooling systems to operate more efficiently

Bushfire zone considerations:

The new laws bought into the National Construction Code (NCC) include the new Bushfire Attack Level (BAL) standard 3959-2009.

Evaporative coolers are noted in the new BAL requirements. The standard prescribes that:

...evaporative cooling units shall be fitted with butterfly closers at or near the ceiling level or, the unit shall be fitted with non-combustible covers with a mesh or perforated sheet with a maximum aperture of 2mm, made of corrosion-resistant steel, bronze or aluminium.

These are often referred to as BAL 29 compliant units.

When there is a fire in the area, run the unit to wet the pads (or wet them with a hose) then turn it off as soon as smoke is over the home or ash starts to fall. This will minimise the risk of fire entering the home through the evaporative cooling unit.

Health considerations

- Check noise levels are acceptable
- Evaporative cooling tends to increase indoor humidity and could increase levels of mould. To minimise the potential of this occurring, ensure units are operated in weather conditions considered suitable by the manufacturer and operated in a manner in line with manufacturer's instructions

Refrigerated air conditioners

Refrigerated air conditioners work the same way as a refrigerator and can reduce internal temperatures and humidity in a space. Air conditioners use refrigerants to convert gas to a liquid and back again to transfer heat from inside the home to outside. Units consist of a compressor and a condenser (generally located outside) and an evaporator/fan unit on the inside.

Types of refrigerated air conditioners:

Window air conditioners

These are systems that sit in a window with interior controls. They work by pulling in air from the room, removing heat and dehumidifying it and expelling the hot air externally and the cooler air internally. These are generally low cost, easy to install and plug into existing general power outlets in the home.

Wall air conditioners

These are systems that are built into a wall opening with interior controls. They work the same as window air conditioners. These are generally low cost and plug into existing general power outlets, however they can be expensive to install if you need to make a hole in the wall.

Portable air conditioners

These are generally freestanding, on wheels and easily transported and can be evaporative or refrigerated types. They work in the same way as window/wall air conditioners and need to have the exhaust externally vented to provide effective cooling inside. Prices range from cheap to quite expensive depending on what you buy. They do tend to take up floor space but are easy to move out of the way and store when no longer needed.

Ductless split systems

Effectively in two parts, the heat exchanger and fan is separated from the condensing unit. These units can be highly energy efficient and can provide quiet cooling for an area (room or a zone). They comprise of a condenser unit which is generally installed outside and one or more wall or ceiling mountable blower units placed in the areas to be cooled. Each internal unit can be controlled independently. There is no ducting which helps to increase the unit's efficiency. They are more expensive but can offer cooling for larger spaces and higher rates of efficiency.

Reverse cycle air-conditioners

Sometimes referred to as 'heat pumps' or 'inverter' technology, reverse cycle air conditioners are effectively a refrigerated air conditioner with a valve that enables it to switch between operating as an air conditioner or a heater through reversing the flow of the refrigerant. They can be particularly energy efficient with a co-efficient of performance up to 5 kW of output to 1 kW of energy. Most are around the 4.5 kW output to 1 kW of energy input.

Ducted or central air conditioning systems

Ensure the ducting is well insulated, sealed, zoned and self-closing when not in use.

Product considerations:

- Size the unit appropriately to the space to be cooled (note if you have a highly insulated home, cooling requirements will be reduced). See www.fairair.com.au to help with selecting and calculating cooling requirements
- Ensure the unit has a thermostat so you can control temperature
- Opt for the most energy efficient model you can (look for the stars)
- Check the cooling capacity suits the space you want to cool
- Check the noise levels and ensure they will meet local regulations
- Check if filters are easy to remove, clean and replace
- Check the cost and accessibility of new filters when they are required
- Look for airflow settings so you have flexibility on air direction
- Consider a unit with a timer so you can set it to go off at night
- Remote control units make it convenient to operate the unit
- Check if the unit has a 'dehumidifier' to help control moisture in the home

Operational considerations

- For refrigerated units, install the condenser on a shaded side of the home
- Locate the internal unit high in the room (ceiling or high wall position)
- Use a fan in conjunction with an air conditioner for a better cooling effect
- Close windows and doors in the space being cooled when the air conditioner is on (not applicable to evaporative cooling)
- Set summer temperatures at around 25-26°C
- Always turn off the unit when leaving the home for more than half an hour
- If the unit is heavily used, clean the filters monthly
- If the unit is only used for cooling turn it off at the main power switch before winter. Some systems have a sump heater which can use up to 400W per day in standby mode

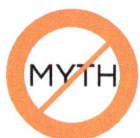

MYTH BUSTER:
Leaving the AC running all day is cheaper than turning it off when I go to work and back on later when I return. This is a myth – it is cheaper to turn the unit off and have it come on (possibly using a timer) half an hour before you get home.

Refrigerated cooling is best suited for those allergic to dust, moulds and pollens.

Maintenance:

- Service the ducted air conditioner in line with the manufacturer's recommendations and use a qualified technician. They should check the refrigerant, and clean the condenser coils, evaporator, fan blades, fan motors and filters
- Clean or replace the filters at least once a year to prevent bacteria and allergens being recycled into the house

Refrigerated ducted cooling health considerations:

Ducted air conditioning systems:

- If not well maintained, promote the growth and spread of microorganisms
- If not well maintained, contribute to decreased indoor air quality, particularly if the unit and any filters are not kept clean
- In humid conditions refrigerated air conditioners help to reduce moisture content in the indoor air that can contribute to mould growth (dehumidifying as they cool)
- Tend to dry out skin and eyes and can contribute to dehydration
- Can assist to filter the indoor air which is beneficial if the unit's filters are kept clean

A note about refrigerants

For many years the primary refrigerant in air conditioners was R22 (Freon). However, R22 is now a prohibited substance. This is because R22 is a hydro chlorofluorocarbon (HCFC) which contains ozone depleting chlorine. In accordance with the Montreal Protocol, from 2010 the manufacture of systems using R22 is now prohibited, and production of R22 itself is scheduled to cease by 2020. As a result, R22 is likely to become difficult to replace in the future and systems with alternative refrigerants should be sought. It has a high global warming potential (GWP) of 1,810 (USA EPA, 2010).

Global warming potential (GWP) is a measurement (usually measured over a 100-year period) of how much effect the refrigerant will have on global warming in relation to carbon dioxide (CO_2). CO_2 has a GWP = 1. The lower the value of GWP, the better the refrigerant is for the environment.

R410A (often called Puron) does not contain chlorine so does not contribute to ozone depletion. R410A is becoming more widely used but must be used in systems that are designed to use it. R410A allows for higher system efficiencies and lower overall impact on global warming. R410A cannot be substituted into existing systems that currently use R22 refrigerant. While R410A does not contribute to ozone layer depletion, it has a high global warming potential (GWP) of 2,088. (USA EPA, 2010).

HFC32 (or R-32) has a higher capacity and efficiency than R410A. It reduces the amount of refrigerant needed in an air conditioning unit and is suitable for refrigerant recycling (expected to be achievable in the near future). However, there are concerns on the flammability of this substance which are still being investigated. HFC32 has a low global warming potential of 675, when compared to R22 and R410A refrigerant types. (USA EPA, 2010).

It's wise to plan ahead and choose a unit that uses R410A or HFC32, not only because of the reduced environmental impact, but also for future availability. Refrigerants can leak from the closed loop system they operate within, which results in 're-gassing' being required. Ensure any leaks are found and fixed before re-gassing. Many refrigerants are toxic, some are also flammable. Ensure the compressor unit is well vented or externally located to minimise any potential health risks.

Solar air conditioning

There are two main types of solar cooling. The first is through the use of solar energy to provide electricity or heat energy to a refrigerated air conditioning unit (referred to as a solar air conditioner). The other is solar powered roof space ventilation systems that remove heat build-up in the ceiling space.

First let's look at solar air conditioning. There are two types of solar air conditioners on the market in Australia; units that offer the ability to run your air conditioner from solar power and a system called solar thermal which uses the sun's heat.

Solar powered air conditioners are simply conventional air conditioners that are powered directly through photovoltaic (PV) panels. These units provide the ability to 'load shift' energy use during peak periods, offer reduced energy costs and lower greenhouse gas emissions. Some hybrid systems have PVs and a battery which is charged when the unit is not in use. These systems can run on DC (direct current) or AC (alternating current). The main difference is that the unit uses the sun (or a solar charged battery) to provide the power to operate.

Solar thermal air conditioning is considered the next generation of solar air conditioners. They work by absorbing solar energy through a thermal collector (a process called 'sorption'). Air is pulled over coils containing a sorbent material. The sorbent material (usually a silica gel) pulls the moisture and heat from the air which results in cool air. The cool air is then fed into the home.

Image: Kingtecsolar

Solar ventilation on the other hand is focused on removing hot air from a home's roof cavity and replacing it with external ambient air (cooler air).

Roof spaces, particularly those with dark roof tiles and little reflective insulation (sarking) can get extremely hot during summer months. This can result in heat being absorbed into the home (especially if there is inadequate insulation at ceiling level) making internal temperatures higher than external ambient temperature. Solar roof ventilation units use a solar powered fan to expel the hot air from the room and drag in fresh, lower temperature ambient air. They are also good for allowing moisture that migrates through the ceiling to escape the building, reducing condensation and mould issues.

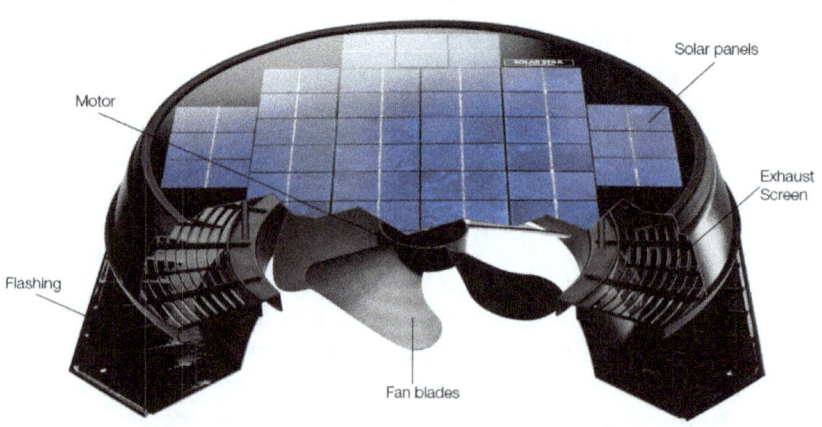

Image: www.roofventilationblog.com.au/commercial-roof-ventilation-chart-alternatives/266/

Once installed they cost nothing to run and can reduce significant heat build-up in the roof space and the living areas. They are very quiet and generally will only operate when the sun is shining.

There are several types of solar ventilation systems available in Australia. Obtain professional advice to determine which product is most suited to your home.

Look for a unit that has a temperature sensor and switches on/off as required, and is UV and weather resistant. Ensure the roof structure enables air to enter from under the eaves or elsewhere to stop pressure build up.

Systems that heat and cool

Reverse cycle units

As described earlier, reverse cycle units using inverter technology are very energy efficient. Look for the COP, the higher the ratio (e.g. 5:1) the more energy efficient it is. All units should offer at least 4.5:1 COP values.

Geothermal

Geothermal (often called ground source heat pumps) systems utilise the ground temperatures to provide heat, cooling, and hot water to a home. Direct heating and cooling works by pumping water in a closed loop system through a deep bore (for heating) or a shallow trench (for cooling). For heating, the water absorbs the heat from the surrounding warm earth. For cooling the system works in reverse. Heat pumps are attached to circulate and extract the heat/cool from the water and direct it into the home.

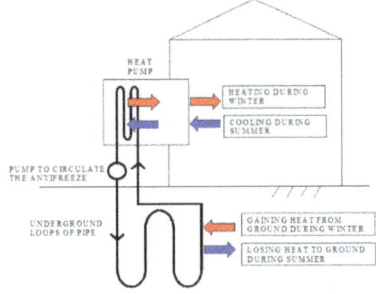

Image source: Berkley Heat and Cool

Geothermal is a highly efficient, well proven and environmentally sound method for providing heating and cooling (and even hot water) to a home. Geothermal systems are gaining popularity in Australia, and are well used internationally. Installation costs can be high but running costs are minimal.

See the Australian Geothermal Energy Association for more information
www.agea.org.au/geothermal-energy/australian-projects-overview/

Solar heating, cooling and hot water

The CSIRO has invented and are currently testing a concept model solar heating, cooling and hot water system for residential properties. Testing is progressing in Australian residences and the product may be available to the public within a few years. This technology solution will reduce greenhouse gas emissions, energy bills and demand for grid electricity. It is an innovative three-in-one technology that provides hot water, cooling and heating.

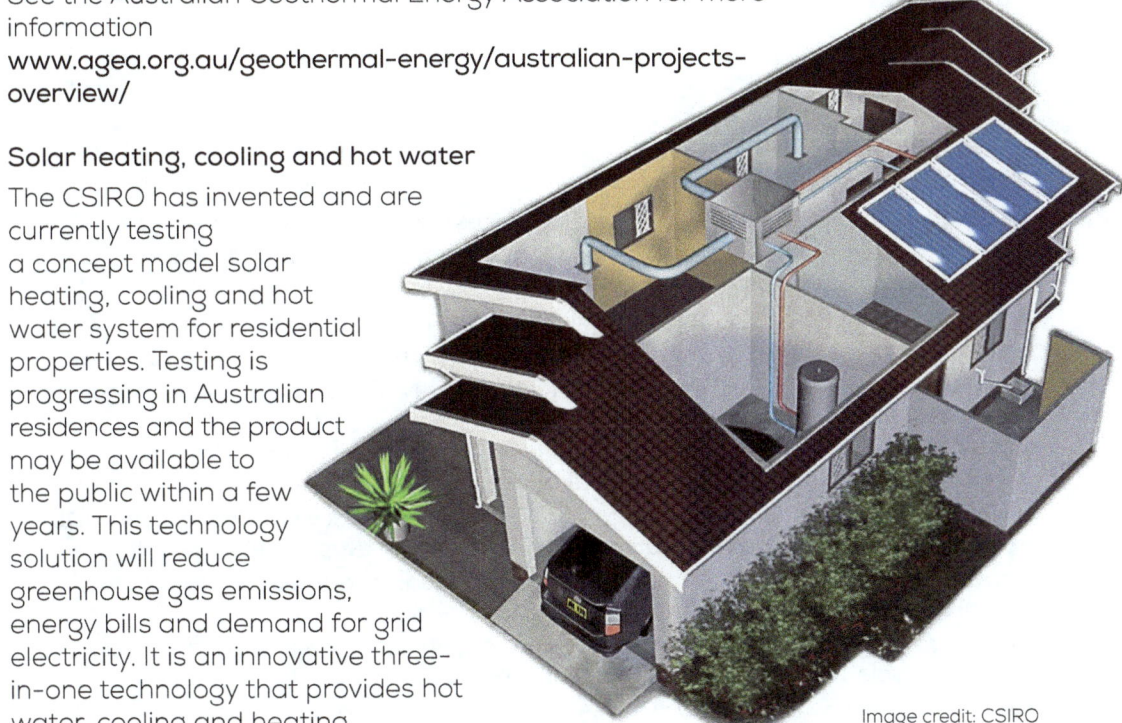

Image credit: CSIRO

It works by using heat from the sun and employs both desiccant and evaporative cooling technologies.

Solar heat is first collected and stored as hot water, which can be used directly in the house. A portion of the hot water is diverted into the solar air-conditioning unit, which is used to either heat or cool the air coming into the building.

See www.csiro.au/solar-cooling for more information.

Summary:

In order to get the best out of your mechanical heating or cooling systems and have them operate as efficiently as possible, before you install a system ensure you:

- Draught-proof the home (or room) to minimise heat/cooling loss when the system is used
- Insulate the ceiling appropriately to minimise heat loss and heat gain
- Only heat and cool areas you need to
- If using ducting, ensure it is insulated to at least R1.5 and well-sealed at joints; where possible include vents that can be closed when not in use
- Install external shading where needed
- Get the correct size unit for the area. Note: homes that have been built to 6 Star (or higher) thermal performance rating should be able to install smaller sized units due to the efficiency of the building

The Choice website has an online calculator that helps you calculate the requirements for heating and cooling a space. See it here at www.choice.com.au

The Fair Air website also has a free online calculator to help calculate cooling requirements, see www.fairair.com.au/

Further information

Your Home – www.yourhome.gov.au
CSIRO – www.csiro.au
Government Energy Efficiency Rating of appliances – www.reg.energyrating.gov.au
Osman P, Ashworth P, CSIRO, 2009. *The CSIRO Home Energy Saving Handbook*, Sydney, Pan McMillan Australia Pty Ltd.
Asthma Australia – www.asthmaaustralia.org.au/
Solar Air Heating Association – http://solarairheating.org.au
Australian Government, Department of Industry. Energy Efficiency – www.ee.ret.gov.au/energy-efficiency/water-heaters
Australian Institute of Refrigeration, Air Conditioning and Heating AIRAH – www.airah.org.au and AIRAH's Fair Air site www.fairair.com.au/
Download the 'Water efficiency for Evaporative Air Coolers' report at www.airah.org.au/imis15_prod/Content_Files/TechnicalPublications/AIRAH_residential_evap_cooling_bpg.pdf
Australian Geothermal Energy Association – www.agea.org.au/geothermal-energy/australian-projects-overview/
Alternative Technology Association at www.ata.org.au has a range of useful buyers guides available, see www.renew.org.au/buyers-guide
Australian Consumer Association Choice – www.choice.com.au

Indoor plants

Indoor pants are a functional furnishing accessory. Choosing a plant for aesthetic value and its potential to clean indoor air can assist in creating a healthy home.

In 1980 NASA's John C. Stennis Space Center discovered that household plants could remove VOCs from sealed test chambers. The results of their investigation suggested that one potted plant per 100 square feet of indoor space in an average home or office was sufficient to cleanse the air of pollutants (Brethour et,al, 2007).

Further studies have since been undertaken and the ability of plants to improve the quality of air we breathe is now accepted and promoted within corporate commercial building developments.

In 1990 the Plants for Clean Air Council (PCAC) and Wolverton Environmental Services Inc began to cosponsor research to build upon earlier NASA findings. Given that numerous sources of formaldehyde were present in the modern home, the removal of this pollutant was studied.

According to the publication *How to Grow Fresh Air* by Dr B.C Wolverton (1996), the following top twelve indoor plants to remove the toxic gas formaldehyde from indoor air are:

1. Boston Fern
2. Florists Mum
3. Gerbera Daisy
4. Dwarf Date Palm
5. Janet Craig
6. Bamboo Palm
7. Kimberly Queen Fern
8. Rubber Plant
9. English Ivy
10. Weeping Fig
11. Peace Lily
12. Areca Palm

The top ten plants identified by Dr B.C Wolverton that have ease of growth, maintenance, resistance to pests and efficiency of removing a variety of chemical vapours are:

1. Areca Palm – Chrysalidocarpus lutescens
2. Lady Palm – Rhapis excelsa
3. Bamboo Palm – Chamaedorea seifrizii
4. Rubber Plant – Ficus robusta
5. Dracaena deremensis 'Janet Craig'
6. English Ivy – Hedera helix
7. Dwarf Date Palm – Phoenix roebelenii
8. Ficus maclellandii – 'Alii'
9. Boston Fern – Nephrolepis exaltata
10. Peace Lily – Spathiphyllum

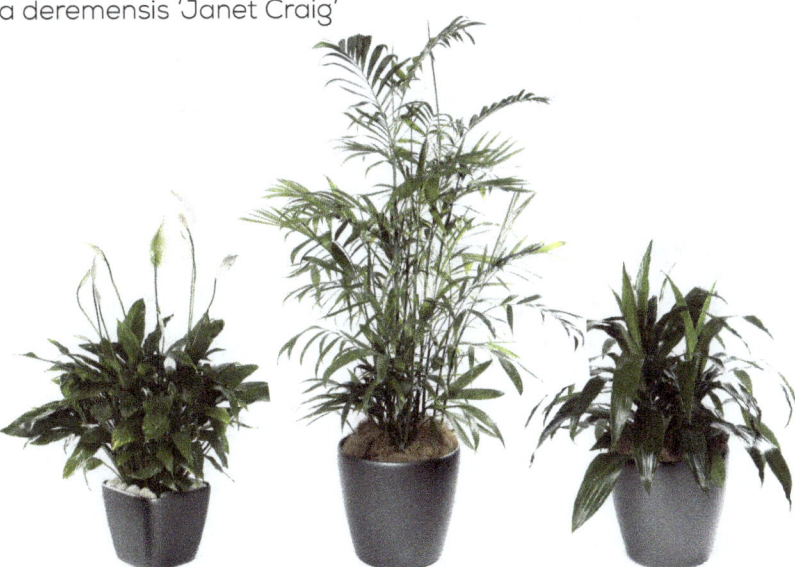

Image supplied by TLC Indoor Gardens. Left – right: Spathyphillum Peace Lily, Large Bamboo Palm and Large Janet Craig.

Section resource summary:

Alternative Technology Association - www.ata.org.au

Australian Building Codes Board (ABCB) at www.abcb.gov.au The ABCB has some very useful free booklets online. These include:

- Condensation in Buildings (2011)
- Construction of buildings in Flood Hazard areas (2012)
- Using on-site renewable and reclaimed energy sources (2011)
- Sound Insulation (2004)
- Various Energy Efficiency Provisions

Australian Government, Department of Industry, Energy Efficiency website has some useful energy efficiency information at www.ee.ret.gov.au/energy-efficiency

Australian Government Energy Rating website: www.energyrating.gov.au has good information on energy ratings for appliances.

Australian Windows Association has a useful glazing calculator at www.efficientglazing.net

Building Products Life Cycle Inventory - www.bpic.asn.au

Carpet Institute of Australia - www.carpetinstitute.com.au

Choice - www.choice.com.au

Ecospecifier Global - www.ecospecifier.com.au

Equipment Energy Efficiency - reg.energyrating.gov.au

Good Environmental Choice Australia (GECA) - www.geca.org.au

Green Moves Australia - www.greenmoves.com.au

Green Painters - www.greenpainters.org.au

Green Guard Certification – USA - www.greenguard.org
(Some products available in Australia with this certification)

Guide to Greener Electronics - www.greenpeace.org/international

What's wrong with PVC? – The science behind a phase out of polyvinyl chloride plastics – www.greenpeace.org.uk/MultimediaFiles/Live/FullReport/5575.pdf

Healthy Interiors – www.healthyinteriors.com.au

Oeko-Tex - www.oekotex.com

Living Greener website – www.livinggreener.gov.au

Water Efficiency Labelling Standards – www.waterrating.gov.au

Your Home – Australia's guide to environmentally sustainable homes – www.yourhome.gov.au

Step 3
Our behaviour – consumer choice

> Before reading this chapter visit **www.storyofstuff.org** and watch the 'Story of Stuff' video collection for an entertaining insight into the reality and consequences of modern life.

Look at the list of personal products below.

How many of these products do you use in your home?

How many of the products listed below have ingredients you don't understand?

How many chemicals from this list of products below are you being exposed to through inhalation, absorption or ingestion?

Have you stopped to think about the number of pollutants you may be exposed to from product choices every day?

- Air freshener
- Bath soap or body wash
- Hair shampoo
- Hair conditioner
- Shaving cream/gel
- Aftershave lotion
- Skin products – cleanser, toner, creams
- Moisturiser
- Antiperspirant
- Perfume/cologne
- Toothpaste
- Bath products
- Mouthwash
- Hairspray/gels
- Cosmetics
- Nail polish
- Sanitary products – toilet paper/sanitary napkins
- Laundry detergent
- Fabric softeners
- Toilet cleaner
- Floor cleaner
- Bench/surface cleaner
- Oven cleaner
- Window cleaner
- Pest sprays/products
- Scented candles/plug in products
- Deodoriser products for shoes, cupboards, soft furnishings
- Stain repellent or stain remover products
- Crease free/ironing products
- Dry cleaned textiles
- Hair dye/colouring products
- Speciality hair products – lice treatments
- Sunscreen
- Plasticised fabrics
- Plasticised or chemically treated furniture
- Plastic food storage
- Tinned foods (others)
- New renovation – new materials

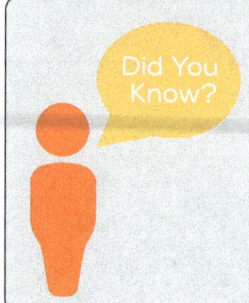

Did You Know?

Imported candles may contain lead wicks.

A ban on candles with lead wicks came into effect in 2002, however it is impossible to police all importers. The ACCC website states 'candles containing more than 0.06 percent of lead when burned in an enclosed area for a long time can release high levels of lead into the atmosphere and cause lead poisoning'.

Source: ACCC

The health of our home environment is constantly changing and is directly affected by the choices we make as consumers. The products we choose to buy have an impact on industry demand and subsequent manufacturing (associated pollution), the health of our home environment and the health of our community i.e. impact on community air, water and food.

Choosing products that have reduced toxicity reduces the potential for pollutant exposure through inhalation, absorption or ingestion which is a healthy approach for long term wellbeing. This also supports demand for environmentally sensitive products that will result in healthier communities.

Healthy home strategies:

- Minimise the use of products that contain harmful ingredients
- Read product labels and check the ingredients against a consumer database. See the 'Shop Wise' resources section
- Eliminate products that are not essential to use
- For necessary products seek natural, nontoxic alternatives
- Avoid sprays, opt for topical products to avoid inhalation or ingestion of products
- Use products in accordance with their use instructions to avoid unnecessary exposures
- Look for household consumables that are independently verified as being organic by certifiers such as (not limited to):
    – Australian Certified Organic - www.aco.net.au
    – Australian Certified Organic Pty Ltd - www.austorganic.com
    – Australian and International Organic Certifier (NASSA) - www.nasaa.com.au

Where organic product options are not available, look for product certification from an organisation that evaluates toxicity and environmental credentials, such as:

GECA - www.geca.org.au
Ecospecifier – www.ecospecifier.com.au

Toxic chemicals are in your home

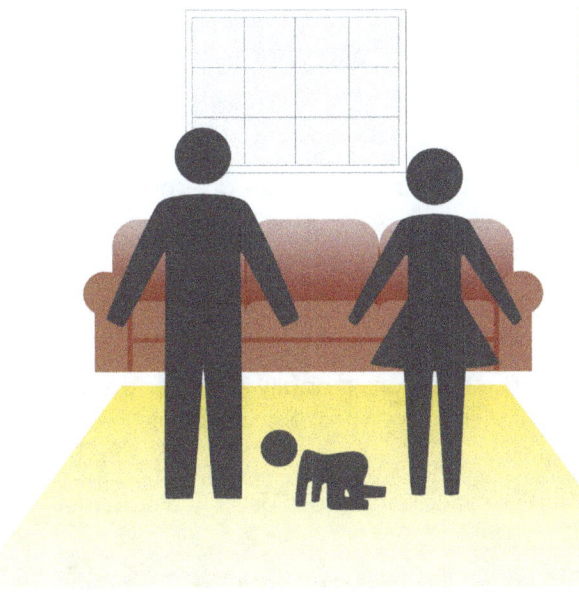

PFCs (perfluorinated compounds)
Used in:
- clothing
- cookware
- food containers
- carpets

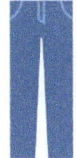
BPA (bisphenol A)
Used in:
- food can linings
- baby bottles
- receipt paper
- CDs and DVDs

Formaldehyde
Used in:
- carpeting
- soaps and detergents
- cabinetry
- glues and adhesives

Phthalates
Used in:
- air fresheners
- paper
- vinyl tile
- wood varnishes and lacquers

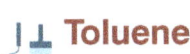
Toluene
Used in:
- paints
- flooring adhesives
- plumbing adhesives
- adhesive removers

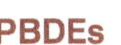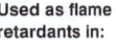
PBDEs (polybrominated diphenyl ethers)
Used as flame retardants in:
- furniture
- electrical equipment
- TVs and computers

Toxic chemicals are in your body

BPA is found in **9** out of **10** Americans

PFCs, PBDEs and **phthalates** are in **99%** of pregnant women

232 toxic chemicals were found in umbilical cord blood from U.S. newborns

They're putting your health at risk

Fertility problems are linked to **PFCs, PBDEs** and **phthalates**

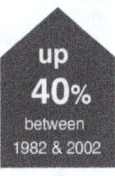
up **40%** between 1982 & 2002

Asthma is linked to **toluene** and **formaldehyde**

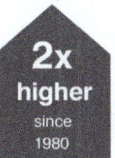
2x higher since 1980

Parkinson's disease is linked to **trichloroethylene** and other chemicals

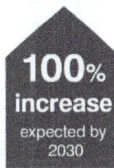
100% increase expected by 2030

©2012 Environmental Defense Fund

Copyright © Environmental Defense Fund. Used by permission. The original material is available at www.edf.org/health/where-are-toxic-chemicals-your-home

Shop wise - resources

Certification schemes

Certification schemes offer the value of independent verification of product claims.

Each certification body has its own unique assessment criteria that investigates different qualities of a product.

Not all environmentally endorsed products are necessarily healthy product alternatives. There are many issues associated with a product that can be explored to verify its appeal for environmental endorsement and healthy choice endorsement.

It's important to understand a certification body's assessment criteria to be able to gauge the value of their certification logo found on product labelling.

There are many certification bodies across many product sectors globally. Certifications of a product are done at considerable cost to the producer. They are often very expensive due to the investigation and audits required on a product.

If a product is certified by an independent group the certification logo is usually displayed prominently on the label.

The following are examples of the main 'eco' certification scheme logos that can found on building and furnishing related product labels in Australia.

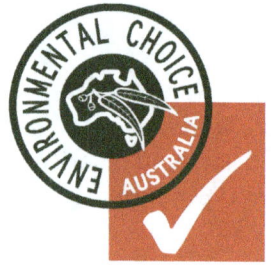

Good Environmental Choice (GECA) – www.geca.org.au
Good Environmental Choice Australia (GECA) is an independent, not-for-profit organisation that runs the internationally recognised Environmental Choice Australia Eco labelling Program.

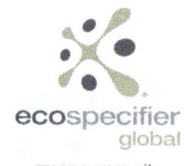

Ecospecifier - www.ecospecifier.com.au
Ecospecifier is home to leading certified and verified sustainable products with over 6,700 sustainable products. Ecospecifier also does the research for you delivering innovative sustainable product solutions based on your specific needs.

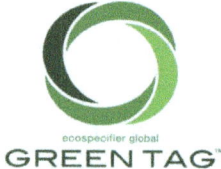

Global Green Tag www.ecospecifier.com.au
Global GreenTag is a unique, green product rating/certification program that provides a single point of reference for green consumers, professionals and procurement processes with world-leading global reach and relevance.

Table continued next page.

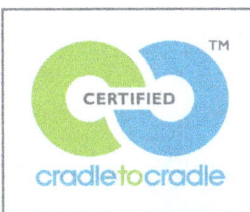

Cradle to Cradle (C2C) – www.c2ccertified.org

The Cradle to Cradle Products Innovation Institute is a non-profit organisation created to bring about a large scale transformation in the way we make things. The basic premise is that waste = food and all products can be designed with materials that are safe for humans and the environment in their given use, and can be recycled, up-cycled, or safely biodegrade into the environment.

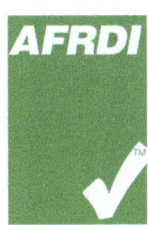

AFRDI – Australasian Furnishing Research & Development Institute – www.furntech.org.au

AFRDI is an independent not-for-profit technical organisation providing standards, testing, product certification and research for buyers and sellers of furniture. AFRDI's commercial furniture sustainability certification scheme, AFRDI Green Tick, is based on the product meeting the requirements of AFRDI 150 Sustainability Standard - Commercial Furniture at either the Silver, Gold, or Platinum Level. AFRDI Green Tick is recognised by the Green Building Council of Australia (GBCA) and corresponds with furniture and assemblies related Material Calculators in Green Star rating tools. Critically, AFRDI's sustainability standard seeks to influence the culture of future furniture design, so that in time, it can be more easily refurbished or recycled, reducing waste. AFRDI for many years has operated a system of quality certification for furniture and furniture components known and widely recognised as AFRDI Blue Tick, based on the performance of a product to the functionality, strength, durability, and safety test criteria carried out to the applicable Standard.

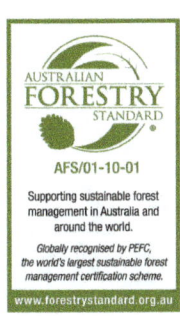

Australian Forestry Standard (AFS) – www.forestrystandard.org.au

Australian Forestry Standard Limited is a not-for-profit public company and an accredited standards development organisation which manages the Australian Forest Certification Scheme (AFCS). The AFCS provides a mechanism for recognising and encouraging good forest management in Australia and tracing wood from certified products along the supply chain into wood and paper products.

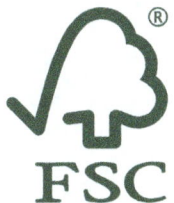

Forest Stewardship Council® (FSC®) http://au.fsc.org

The Forest Stewardship Council® (FSC®) is an international, membership based, non-profit organisation founded in 1993 by environmentalists, social interest groups, indigenous peoples' organisations, responsible retailers and leading forest management companies to develop standards based on the '10 Principles for Forest Stewardship' by which responsible forest practice can be measured.

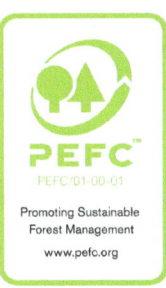

Programme for the Endorsement of Forest Certification – PEFC – www.pefc.org

PEFC is an international non-profit, non-governmental organization dedicated to promoting sustainable forest management, the Programme for the Endorsement of Forest Certification is the certification system of choice for small forest owners.

Table source: © Green Moves Aust. 2014.

Other international certification schemes occasionally seen in Australia include Green Guard (USA) and Blue Angel (Europe).

If a product does not have independent certification, look for:

- Environmental Policies. These are often publically available online
- Environmental Management Systems certification through ISO 14001:2012 – look for the logo and certification
- Label claims of environmental and/or health attributes of the product
- Is the product sold in Europe? Europe tends to have higher standards generally in relation to environmental and health attributes of products.

Be wary

Be aware that many products create logos for their labels that look like a certified symbol to give the illusion of independent endorsement. Certification bodies usually have a website where products they have certified are listed so that label claims can be checked.

Many certification bodies issue a certification number that can be verified as current with the certification body. Products that have been assessed are usually subject to renewal audits. Given the cost of certification, some companies have been known to continue using a certification logo despite renewal audits not being done and certification not being current.

Get to know the certification assessment criteria for products that you use regularly so that you understand what the certification body has endorsed and what they have not assessed.

Beware of 'green wash'

Green wash is defined by the Oxford English Dictionary as 'Disinformation disseminated by an organisation so as to present an environmentally responsible public image.' It means an organisation is telling you it's green when it's not.

Ways to spot green wash

Below are the 10 key signs of green wash. When you are next looking at a 'green' product or service, think about doing the following:

Ask exactly what is 'green' and/or healthy about this product, what is it made of, where and how is it made, are the materials used 'green'. Is there any health risk associated with the product through toxins and chemicals? At end of life, is it recyclable (or preferably 'up-cyclable'), or is it bio degradable, does it provide food for another living thing?

Look at what the whole company is doing about being environmentally responsible. Does it employ locals; have a corporate sustainability policy or a fair trade policy? Are its policies public, does it include environmental sustainable processes and does it measure its social, economic and environmental footprint? Sustainability should also be mentioned in the company's annual report.

So here's what to look for...

1. Vague or 'fluffy' language, using words with no clear meaning (e.g. eco-friendly)
2. Green products vs. dirty company – e.g. energy efficient light bulbs that are made in a factory that pollutes rivers and uses child labour
3. Suggestive pictures – images that indicate an unjustified green impact (e.g. flowers blooming from exhaust pipes)
4. Irrelevant claims – emphasising one tiny green attribute when the rest of the product and how it is made is not 'green'
5. Best in class - declaring they are slightly greener than the rest, even if the rest are pretty terrible
6. Just not credible – eco-friendly cigarettes? Greening a dangerous product doesn't make it safe
7. Gobbledygook – jargon and information that only a scientist could check or understand
8. Imaginary friends – a 'label' that looks like a third party endorsement, except it's made up
9. No proof – you could be right but where's the evidence?
10. Outright lying – totally fabricated claims or data

Source: These 10 green wash points have been summarised from the Futerra Greenwash Guide at www.futerra.co.uk

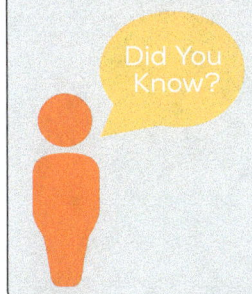

Did You Know? The use of celebrities to promote products is another way to lull consumers into being comfortable with products that may not necessarily be green. Be especially wary of 'sponsored' blogs or adverts, this indicates the writer has been financially rewarded by way of free or discounted product or paid to endorse a product. Many blog sites (some celebrity sites) seek payment to display article content where a product is mentioned.

Shop wise tools

Most people have very little time to research products beyond labels, even though in many instances we would like to know more about a product. Research can be time consuming. These sites will help you quickly delve deeper into products that can be found around the home.

Product Safety

The Australian Competition and Consumer Commission recall app

www.accc.gov.au/about-us/tools-resources/recalls-app

The app enables you to search the national recalls database by product name or category. For website recall information visit www.recalls.gov.au

The Chemical Maze app and book

www.chemicalmaze.com

Know what food additives and cosmetic ingredients to avoid

The Chemical Maze makes it easy to recognise additives and ingredients in foods and cosmetics having the potential to cause discomfort and ill-health. A pocket-sized version is also available.

Choice

www.choice.com.au

Choice provides consumers with product purchase and testing information. Choice is Australia's independent consumer advocacy and advice organisation testing and reporting on product quality and claims.

Healthy and efficient sustainable home

Australian Government Energy Rating website

www.energyrating.gov.au

Information on energy ratings for appliances

Australian Windows Association

www.efficientglazing.net

Useful glazing calculator

C2C Certification

www.c2ccertified.org

Database of 'cradle to cradle' certified products.

Ecospecifier

www.ecospecifier.com.au

Database of certified and verified sustainable products.

Environmental Protection Authority – EPA Victoria

www.epa.vic.gov.au/Ecologicalfootprint/calculators/default.asp

Ecological Footprint Calculator

Equipment Energy Efficiency -

www. reg.energyrating.gov.au

Good Environmental Choice Australia – GECCA

www.geca.org.au

Eco labelling program with database of certified products and services.

Green Guard Certification

USA - www.greenguard.org

(Some products with this certification are available in Australia)

Green Moves Australia

www.greenmoves.com.au

Sustainability resources, useful checklists, relevant articles, consultancy and training

Green Painters

www.greenpainters.org.au

Guide to Greener Electronics

www.greenpeace.org/international

The Healthy Home app

www.itunes.apple.com/au/app/healthy-home

The Healthy Home app helps families worldwide assess and create a nontoxic home environment that prevents illness and promotes wellbeing. Use your healthy home app to assess each room in your home to determine assets and challenges that can potentially impact on family health. Create a checklist for one or multiple houses. Walk through your home and take the quiz that provides tips for every question and gain insights from the global links. Take notes and collect photos for your reference. Create your asset and challenges report to get started in making changes to suit your budget.

Healthy Interiors

www.healthyinteriors.com.au

Features healthy option products and a healthy home resource library

Shop Ethical

www.ethical.org.au/get-involved/resources/shop-ethical-app

The Shop Ethical app provides consumers access to over 4,000 products with related company information so that consumers can make informed and ethical decision whenever they shop.'

Water Efficiency Labelling Standards
www.waterrating.gov.au

Your Home – Australia's guide to environmentally sustainable homes
www.yourhome.gov.au

Personal care products

Environmental Working Group (EWG)
www.ewg.org/skindeep/app

Environmental Working Group (EWG) has created an app from the Skin Deep Cosmetics database into the Skin Deep mobile app. Access safety info about products, brands, and ingredients on your phone. Scan the barcode of your products and receive a rating about the product toxicity assessment.

Environmental Working group – Sunscreen Buyers Guide
www.itunes.apple.com/us/app/id378866183?mt=8

'EWG's guide helps consumers find products that get high ratings for providing broad-spectrum, long-lasting protection and that are made with ingredients that pose fewer health concerns.'

National Library of Medicine – Household Products Database
www.hpd.nlm.nih.gov

The US Department of Health & Human Services database contains information on thousands of consumer brands with details about health effects from material safety data sheets (MSDS), allowing consumers to research products based on chemical ingredients.

Safe Cosmetics Australia
www.safecosmeticsaustralia.com.au

'Our mission is to raise toxic-free awareness, promoting companies that formulate products based on natural plant and mineral ingredients. Safe Cosmetics Australia assists consumers who wish to exclude harmful chemicals from the products they choose by delivering a toxic free list of companies who have been independently reviewed.'

Pesticides in and around the home

Beyond Pesticides
www.beyondpesticides.org

Non-profit organisation based in Washington, DC, 'which works with allies in protecting public health and the environment to lead the transition to a world free of toxic pesticides.' Provides a range of online resources and fact sheets.

National Pesticide Information Centre (NPIC)

www.npic.orst.edu

'NPIC provides objective, science-based information about pesticides and pesticide-related topics to enable people to make informed decisions about pesticides and their use. NPIC is a cooperative agreement between Oregon State University and the US Environmental Protection Agency.'

NRDC Smarter Living – GreenPaws Flea and Tick Products Directory

www.simplesteps.org/greenpaws-products

A listing of products that have been reviewed by the NRDC highlighting chemicals contained in products and the level of risk they may pose.

Pesticide Action Network Database (PAN)

www.pesticideinfo.org

'The Pesticide Action Network (PAN) database provides toxicity and regulatory information for pesticides.'

Pesticides, Food and You – The Dose Makes The Poison?

Friends of the Earth Report, 2012

www.foe.org.au/sites/default/files/TheDoseMakesThePoisonFeb2012_0.pdf

Informed consumer resources

Agency for Toxic Substances & Disease Registry – USA

www.atsdr.cdc.gov/substances/index.asp

Toxic substances and how they affect health, providing an A-Z substances database and substance profiles with details about health issues.

Environmental Health Perspectives

www.ehp.niehs.nih.gov

This is a peer reviewed journal containing research and news on topics concerning human health and the environment. The journal is published with support from the National Institute of Environmental Health Sciences, National Institutes of Health, US Department of Health and Human Services.

Environmental Working Group

www.ewg.org

USA based advocacy organisations of professionals who research and report on health and environmental concerns.

European Chemicals Agency – ECHA

www.echa.europa.eu/en/web/guest/support/documents-library

Document library of information related to chemical fact sheets and European chemicals legislation. (It is interesting to compare chemicals approved in Europe compared with Australia)

Healthy Child Healthy World

www.healthychild.org

California-based non-profit organisation that promotes industry accountability and community engagement to advocate for safe products and policy.

International Agency for Research on Cancer

www.iarc.fr

A World Health Organisation agency that conducts global research on cancer. The IARC provides reference publications and resources for the development of cancer prevention strategies.

National Geographic Interactive - Our Toxic Homes

http://ngm.nationalgeographic.com/2006/10/toxic-people/multimedia-interactive

Interactive display of rooms throughout a home environment and known health hazards.

National Industrial Chemical Notification & Assessment Scheme (NICNAS)

www.nicnas.gov.au

Department of Health chemicals regulatory body.

Chemical fact sheets are available - **www.nicnas.gov.au/communications/publications/information-sheets/existing-chemical-info-sheets**

National Institute of Environmental Health Sciences

www.niehs.nih.gov

Research facility that explores how the environment affects people.

National Pollutant Inventory

www.npi.gov.au

The National Pollutant Inventory tracks pollution across Australia.

'The NPI is an internet-based database that provides free information to the community, government and industry on the emissions and transfers of substances to our environment.' Providing substance fact sheets and emission source summaries.

Our Stolen Future

www.ourstolenfuture.org

Information about the emerging science and issues surrounding endocrine disrupting chemicals and health concerns.

Safer Chemicals, Healthy Families

www.saferchemicals.org

Coalition of organisations, researchers, professionals and individuals researching and lobbying for safer chemicals, protective laws and public education.

TEDX – The Endocrine Disruption Exchange

www.endocrinedisruption.org/endocrine-disruption/tedx-list-of-potential-endocrine-disruptors/chemicalsearch

This database logs chemicals which have the potential to affect the endocrine system. 'Endocrine effects include not only direct effects on traditional endocrine glands, their hormones and receptors (such as estrogens, anti-androgens, and thyroid hormones), but also all other hormones and signalling cascades that affect the body's systems and processes, including reproductive function and fetal development, the nervous system and behaviour, the immune and metabolic systems, gene expression, the liver, bones, and many other organs, glands and tissues.'

United States Environmental Protection Agency

www.epa.gov

Extensive source of information relating to environmental factors affecting the indoor and outdoor environment. Provides specific information as to indoor environmental hazards in the home.

Washington Toxics Coalition

www.watoxics.org

Non-profit organisation that collates consumer interest information on products, chemicals, practices and children's health.

Material safety data sheets

ChemSupply

www.chemsupply.com.au

Chemical supplier to the Australian industry has a database of material safety data sheets (MSDS). Visit the documentation section to access the database.

MSDSXchange

www.msdsxchange.com/english/index.cfm

International collection of material safety data sheets.

TOXNET – United States National Library of Medicine

www.toxnet.nlm.nih.gov

Database on toxicology, hazardous chemicals, environmental health and toxic releases.

Navigating Plastics

	Recycling number	Abbreviation	Polymer name	User	
✓	1 PETE	PETE or PET	Polyethylene Terephthalate	Soft drink & juice bottles, pillow fill, textile fibres, carpet, laminated sheets, clothing	Repeated use of same bottle or container could cause leaching of DEHP, an endocrine disrupting phthalate and probable human carcinogen. Single use only
✓	2 HDPE	HDPE	High-Density Polyethylene	various bottles - milk, water, juice, shampoo, detergent, pipe, cups, playground equipment, toys	Can be white or opaque
✗	3 V	PVC or V	Polyvinyl Chloride	Pipes, windows, toys, gumboots, raincoats, shower curtains, hose, furniture, flooring, vinyl wrap in kitchens/bathrooms	Considered the most damaging of plastics to environment, releases carcinogenic dioxins when manufactured or incinerated and can leach phthalates when in use. **May contain BPA**
✓	4 LDPE	LDPE	Low-Density Polyethylene	plastic bags, various squeeze bottles, shrink film, garbage bins	
✓	5 PP	PP	Polypropylene	Crates, toys, housewares, kitchenware, caps and closures, pot plants, carpet fibre, film, appliance parts	Can be clear, coloured or cloudy in finish
✗	6 PS	PS	Polystyrene	Medical disposables, meat trays, disposable cups, packaging, office accessories, yogurt & dairy containers, waffle pods for buildings, insulation	There has been concerns that this may leach toxins
?	7 OTHER	OTHER	Other plastics, including all other resins and multi materials (eg laminates) eg acrylonitrile butadiene styrene (ABS) acrylic, nylon, polyurethane (PU), polycarbonates (PC) and phenolics	Furniture, electrical, medical, boating, automative sector items – floor coatings, computer equipment, signs, textiles, cabinetry, lining boards	Note Polycarbonate contains BPA Select with caution.

Refer to :
http://healthychild.org/easy-steps/know-your-plastics
www.pacia.org.au - Plastics Identification Code
www.ecocycle.org/files/pdfs/pocket_guide_singleprint.pdf
© Healthy Interiors 2014

Image source: © Healthy Interiors 2014.

Step 4
Lifestyle practices

Beyond building or renovating a home to minimise potential allergens, there are many daily decisions and household practices that also contribute to the health of a home, particularly for those with allergies and those who value their health.

Use this list to give your home a health makeover and start implementing practices that minimise pollutants to support good health.

A healthier sustainable home

Steps to creating a healthier sustainable home:	
Ventilation	To reduce indoor humidity and flush out built up VOCs, regularly open doors and windows to encourage air circulation. <ul><li>Ensure you use exhaust extraction fans when cooking, using the bathroom or using appliances that create humidity in the laundry.</li><li>Regularly clean exhaust fan covers for efficient performance</li></ul> **TIP** If building a new home, plan to move in at the beginning of summer. Then open all windows and doors as often as possible. This will help dry out the house.
Waterproofing	Minimise moisture around the home. Ensure gutters are cleaned regularly to prevent backflow into the roof/ceiling where mould can grow. <ul><li>Repair any leaks from taps and pipes inside the home quickly to prevent moisture and mould growth.</li><li>Ensure that extraction fans are vented to the exterior of the home and not into the ceiling space, to prevent pollutants, moisture and mould in the roof space.</li></ul>
Storage of products	<ul><li>Don't keep chemicals, paints, fuel and pesticides in the house as these can continue to release emissions/fumes while stored.</li></ul>
Appliances	<ul><li>For new food related appliances, use without food until fumes cease</li><li>Always choose good quality, correctly sized, energy and water efficient appliances</li><li>Clean filters in appliances regularly – such as washing machines, dryers, air conditioners and heaters to minimise pollutant circulation and maintain efficiency.</li></ul>

Table continued next page.

Steps to creating a healthier sustainable home	
Appliances (cont...)	• Use appliances such as dishwashers and washing machines with a full load. • Service heating and cooling units in line with manufacturer's recommendations to maintain efficiency. • Check refrigerator temperatures are at 4°C for the fridge, and 18°C for the freezer • Don't place plastics into the microwave or dishwasher. Plastics when heated can encourage chemicals to migrate into food. When plastic is heated in the dishwasher it increases off-gassing. • Cover gimble downlight fittings with a product-approved cover to prevent heat loss and ceiling debris and pests accessing the house from the cut out void. Better still, replace them with sealed lighting units which will allow more effective insulation of ceiling spaces. • Keep electrical equipment out of bedrooms and away from bedroom adjoining walls where possible. People with suspected electromagnetic sensitivities should seek an assessment from a building biologist. • Use a water filter for drinking water • Dust appliances with a damp cloth to remove polluted dust, and wash after use • Turn appliances off at the switch when not in use.
Daily practices	• Take shoes off at the front door to prevent pollutants being walked through the house. • Keep indoor moisture low to minimise condensation. Relative humidity should be below 60 percent (ideally 30 - 50 percent). This can be measured with a humidity meter available from the hardware store. Refer to the graph in the Your Air Matters section. • For hayfever sufferers - to minimise the spread of pollens indoors, place worn clothes in the laundry, rather than the bedroom, straight after wearing them outside. • Avoid 'crease free' textiles as formaldehyde is used to achieve this attribute and is a known irritant to the skin and can cause allergic reactions (carcinogenic properties). • Turn on heating or cooling systems only when you need them.
Fragrances	• Avoid fragranced products indoors e.g. air fresheners, scented candles, perfumes, essential oils, colognes, aerosol deodorants and hair spray products as these release VOCs into indoor air, contribute to poor indoor air quality and can trigger asthma and allergies.
Bedding and bedroom	• Wash bedding in hot water to kill dust mites • Opt for a mattress free from chemical treatments and petrochemical derived foams • Beds elevated off the floor designed to allow air flow reduce the risk of microbial growth in the mattress or flooring. • Air mattresses and pillows regularly in direct sunlight (indoors for hayfever allergy sufferers)

Table continued next page.

Steps to creating a healthier sustainable home	
Bedding and bedroom (cont...)	<ul><li>Opt for natural fibres for bedding such as wool blankets & organic cotton sheeting</li><li>Avoid PVC and plasticised mattress protectors – opt for natural fibre textiles such as organic cotton, hemp, linen, wool or blends.</li><li>Vacuum mattresses in the home regularly (with a clean vacuum attachment)</li><li>Keep wet items out of the bedroom e.g. wet towels</li><li>Avoid furniture in the bedroom that contains plastics or synthetic materials such as bedheads, side tables and storage boxes.</li><li>Opt for hardwood bedding furniture free from upholstery to minimise dust</li><li>Remove clutter that collects dust in the bedroom</li><li>Avoid plastic decorator items such as plasticised wall papers, wall decals, plastic lamp shades and plasticised storage items.</li><li>Keep mobile phones out of the bedroom when sleeping</li><li>Use a battery operated alarm clock in the bedroom rather than a phone or electric clock radio – this is precautionary minimisation of electromagnetic radiation levels while sleeping (use a hot water bottle rather than an electric blanket).</li><li>For kids' rooms, keep out any toys, bags, scented stationery or accessories that have an odour (VOCs).</li></ul>
Window treatments	<ul><li>Blinds and shades are preferable for allergy suffers rather than drapes/curtains as blinds accumulate less dust and allergens. Opt for natural fibre materials free from chemical treatments such as stain resistant chemicals and flame retardant chemicals. Blinds are available or can be custom made from metal, timber or fibres such as organic cotton, hemp, jute, wool blends or sea grass. Avoid PVC and plasticised backings that contain phthalate chemicals. These heat up in the window and release VOCs</li><li>Gently vacuum window coverings regularly to remove dust</li><li>Where blinds are used, opt for heavy linings to assist with keeping heating in the room during winter</li><li>Use external blinds to shade glazing in summer months to reduce heat build-up in the home</li><li>Close the window coverings at night when heat needs to be retained in the home</li><li>If using curtains install a pelmet cover at the top of the curtains to reduce heat loss during winter months</li><li>Avoid window furnishing with chemical treatments, especially topical treatments that may migrate into household dust</li></ul>

Table continued next page.

Steps to creating a healthier sustainable home

Flooring	• Vacuum flooring regularly with a vacuum containing a HEPA filter or ducted vacuum system. • Have carpets professionally cleaned with steam (no chemicals) every two years in warm weather (only when they will dry quickly). A carpet dry-clean without using toxic chemicals would be a better option. • Avoid toxic cleaners when cleaning surfaces as these can leave a residue on surfaces that may be absorbed or inadvertently ingested • Replace any damaged flooring with sustainably sourced materials.
Soft furnishings	• Regularly vacuum soft furnishings such as lounge suites and upholstered chairs (with clean attachments) • Minimise the use of foam furniture – opt for certified options free from flame retardants where possible • If you have foam in products ensure it is not exposed. Replace or repair damaged upholstery to minimise exposure • Avoid textiles with chemicals added such as stain resistant, crease resistant, flame resistant treatments • Opt for textiles that are independently certified as free from toxic substances
Windows and doors	• Ensure any condensation on windows and frames is wiped quickly to avoid mould growth. • Ensure flyscreens are in good working order to prevent access by pests • Draught-seal all external doors and windows with appropriate seals to minimise draughts and increase comfort • Open windows and doors regularly to dissipate built up VOCs and improve indoor air quality
Furniture	• Opt for furniture made from low emission materials such as solid timber (with low VOC sealer/coatings), rather than particle board or composite boards that can contain formaldehyde and adhesive VOCs • Avoid furniture made from plastics as these can release fumes/VOCs, contain phthalate chemicals and at end of life contribute to toxic landfill • Use sustainably sourced or recycled furniture where possible
Cleaning	• Dust can contain mites, chemical pollutants, pollens, fungi and bacteria. To minimise the spread of these potential allergy triggers use a damp cloth to dust to prevent particles becoming airborne • Use a HEPA filter vacuum with a bag system so that the sealed bag can be removed easily without rereleasing dust • Keep family members with allergies out of freshly vacuumed rooms for up to an hour after vacuuming to allow any airborne dust to settle • Use nontoxic cleaners to avoid chemical residue throughout the house that can be inadvertently ingested or absorbed. This will also minimise VOCs for better indoor air quality

Table continued next page.

Steps to creating a healthier sustainable home	
Cleaning (cont...)	• Avoid opening the dishwasher before it has cooled to prevent the release of steam filled with detergent vapour • Have a separate washing basket for work clothes, this is particularly important if a family member works in the trade sector. This will minimise the spread of industry pollutants to family clothing • Wash work clothes separately from other family clothing to minimise the spread of occupational pollutants. • Use a 'sensitive' washing powder free from artificial fragrances, optical brighteners, phosphates, and petrochemical surfactants (opt for plant based – biodegradable). Some enzymes (although natural, are made from selected strains of bacteria) are known to cause allergic reactions such as asthma and skin reactions. If you suffer from either, avoid enzyme detergents, opt for plain soap powder instead and rinse well. • Mould is a fungal growth that thrives in dampness, darkness and spaces with poor ventilation. Mould can trigger allergy and/or respiratory symptoms. Clean/remove any mould as it appears and establish the cause to prevent reoccurrence – use an N-95 mask when cleaning mould. Wash hair and clothes when complete to discard of any spores. • Always wash new clothing or linen before use to remove any manufacturing chemical residue • Avoid dry cleaning where possible due to toxic chemicals used. If it is unavoidable, request minimal chemical use if possible e.g. steam and ensure that garments are hung outside for a few hours to release VOCs from solvents used before taking dry cleaning into the house. Seek out non-toxic dry cleaning businesses
Children's toys	• Regularly place children's toys (excluding plastic items) in direct sunlight to help kill dust mites and germs • Washable toys to be washed in hot soapy water – if washing is not possible place favourite soft toys in the freezer for 24hrs regularly to help kill dust mites, mite eggs and bacteria (ensure dried properly before using) or place in hot sun (not plastics) • Avoid soft plastic items as these may contain phthalate chemicals that have been linked to a range of health concerns • Keep children's toys away from pets • Buy toys from reputable brands. Avoid cheap imported toys that may not have had compliance checks • Choose toys made with nontoxic glues, paints, colours. This will normally be proudly displayed on the label if applicable. • Opt for toys made from natural materials such as solid timber, organic cotton, wool, hemp, sisal, rattan, sea grasses

Table continued next page.

Steps to creating a healthier sustainable home

Garden	- Make informed choices for plants around the home to minimise allergy irritants
- Avoid the use of toxic gardening products such as pesticides, fungicides and weed killer. Products used in the garden can be inhaled and absorbed, or residues may enter the house via shoes. Opt for nontoxic and natural pesticide management
- Don't use grey water on edible plants
- Ensure grey water does not 'pool' or form a 'mud' area around the home. If it does, keep children away until it is fully absorbed by the ground as it can carry bacteria which can be transferred and create illness
- Locate the compost zone away from the house to keep associated pests away
- Use mulch to maintain healthy soil to retain moisture and reduce weeds
- Where possible install a sub-surface irrigation system to minimise evaporation and put the water where it is needed, at the roots of the plant
- Use rain water tanks where possible, to store gardening water
Managing pests	- Opt for physical pest management rather than chemicals
- Ensure flyscreens are on doors and windows
- Clean spilt food sources quickly to prevent attracting pests
- Ensure windows and doors and any gaps are sealed around the house to minimise pest access
- Consider plants around the house (but not directly against the house) that repel insects and pests. If using a pest product opt for traps or contained liquids/powders rather than chemical sprays.
- Have the house inspected by pest specialists every year to identify any issues early and minimise potential problems/treatments.
- Remove stagnant water sources around the home as these can be breeding grounds for insects
Pets	- Cat and dog dander (loose scales, feathers or hair from animal skins) can trigger asthma and allergies. If pets must be in the house keep them in well ventilated areas. Do not allow pets into the bedrooms (especially those of allergy sufferers) as dander is food for dust mites
- Wash pets with nontoxic, natural cleaners to prevent residue being inadvertently ingested from hand to mouth action after members of the family have been affectionate with pets. This is also healthier for your pet!
- Wash and groom pets outdoors
- For families with allergies, opt for non-shedding or low shedding pet species
- Clean/wash pet bedding area regularly
- Draught-proof pet doors

Table continued next page.

	Steps to creating a healthier sustainable home
Food	- Avoid food packaged in plastics due to health concerns linked to Bisphenol A and phthalate chemicals migrating onto or into food
- Avoid tinned foods that contain plasticised linings – e.g. BPA (Bisphenol A)
- Avoid cooking in or with plastics
- Opt for stainless steel cooking utensils. Avoid plastics
- Opt for stainless steel, glass or ceramic pots/pans rather than chemically coated products e.g. non-stick items
- Store food items in glass, stainless steel or ceramic
- Always wash fresh fruit and vegetables prior to consuming
- Opt for organically certified food to reduce consumption of agricultural chemicals
- Opt for a filter on drinking water
- Opt for a water filter to remove chlorine from shower and bath water that can be an irritant for the skin and respiratory system
Guests	- Ask guests to take shoes off at the front door
- No smoking in the house or near the doors and windows
- For those with sensitivities - ask guests (or hang a sign) not to wear strong fragrances when visiting

Copyright © Healthy Interiors 2014.

Creating a healthy child's space

Children are one of the most vulnerable groups to the potential pollutants lurking in the home. Their smaller bodies mean they cannot metabolise chemical exposure as efficiently as adults. They also breathe more rapidly than adults and are therefore particularly vulnerable to vapours.

The excitement of creating and decorating a child's space is one of the joys of parenthood. As parents we try to create spaces for our children that have elements of fun, comfort and safety. As parents it seems we never have enough time in a day, yet there is a mountain of information from global organisations and scientists about our home environments that we need to know about.

With childhood allergies and asthma rates rising, it makes good sense to explore our home environment for potential triggers. For those who don't suffer from ill health a healthy home is a preventative measure for expectant parents.

The toxic materials that many children's products are made from are worrying and should be a national health concern. A child doesn't have to eat their bedroom furniture for potential pollutants to get into their body. What is in a child's air is inhaled. Pollutants in and around the home can also be inadvertently ingested through hand to mouth action or absorbed by the skin.

With the plethora of decor product choices on the market it is easy to become overwhelmed by the options. The experience of shopping for children's products can be likened to the experience of being a kid in a candy store: plenty of colour, texture and the potential for harm.

Children spend a significant amount of time indoors. Further to nutrition and exercise, the home environment plays a significant role in the health of children and families. As parents we consider safety a priority for spaces that children are in but the health of a room is often forgotten.

The following is a checklist and tips for minimising pollutants in spaces for kids.

Kids space – minimising pollutants

Item	Opt for	Tip
Furniture	Hardwood, cane/rattan.	Low emission finish - oil, wax or paint finish if required
Flooring	Hardwood flooring.	Low emission oil, wax finish
	Carpet – natural fibre.	100 percent wool or sisal with low emission backing and underlay.
Floor rug	Wool, sisal, seagrass, cotton, jute.	Ask if the product has been chemically treated – e.g. flame retardant, or stain resistance. Imported products may have been fumigated.

Table continued next page.

Item	Opt for	Tip
Soft furnishings	Natural fibres. Wool, organic cotton, hemp	Avoid textile chemical treatments e.g. stain resistance. Organic options where possible. Use Oeko-Tex certified fabrics where possible.
Window furnishings	Natural fibre – seagrass, bamboo, cotton, timber, rattan	Low emission blockout or finishing coatings where required. Avoid plastics.
Wall decoration	Framed prints, photos, timber artwork, paper or textile artworks	Avoid PVC wall decals and plasticised wallpapers
Paints	Naturally derived paints where possible. Only use low/zero VOC paints	Try to avoid painting during pregnancy and with small children. If painting is necessary, ideally air the space during painting and for a few weeks before use.
Storage	Timber boxes, woven baskets – jute, cane	Avoid plastics – phthalate chemicals (endocrine disruptors)
Light fittings / lamps	Fabric on metal frame, cane, timber, jute or for ceiling lamp – glass or metal (only where out of reach of children).	Avoid plasticised lamp shades as the plastic can be heated with extended use making it volatile to off-gassing.
Toys	Solid timber, fabric.	Avoid plastics especially PVC
Heating	Radiant heat rather than ducted e.g. hydronic	If using ducted, install filters. Avoid sources that can inflict burns.
Cooling	Refrigerant cooling	Avoid moisture generating cooling sources or fans with blades not suitable for children.

Copyright © Healthy Interiors 2014.

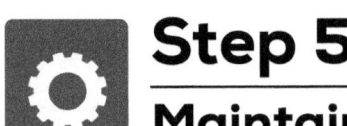

Step 5
Maintaining a home for efficiency & health

Maintenance summary checklist

Spring	Can do	Done it
Repair screens		
Clean cooling unit filters		
Cooling serviced in accordance with manufacturers recommendations if required		
Clean exhaust covers – bathroom, kitchen & laundry		
Remove stagnant water sources from around the home		
Clear gutters and downpipes		
Vacuum under and around fridge		
Replenish deteriorating surface coatings		
Clean lighting (some types need dust removed that can get blown around by cooling and fans		
Vacuum soft furnishings (soft setting) – drapes, upholstered chairs with a HEPA filter vacuum		
Test smoke detectors and carbon monoxide detectors		

Summer	Can do	Done it
Clean flyscreens		
Carpets cleaned (bi annually) – no toxic cleaners		
Air pillows and bedding in hot sun (inside for hay fever sufferers)		
Clean exhaust covers – bathroom, kitchen and laundry		
Remove stagnant water sources from around the home		
Clear gutters and downpipes		
Vacuum under and around fridge		
Vacuum soft furnishings – drapes, upholstered chairs		
Check the refrigerator seal		

Table continued next page.

Autumn	Can do	Done it
Check door and window seals and replace as needed		
Clean exhaust covers – bathroom, kitchen & laundry		
Clean lighting (some types need dust removed), that can get blown around by heating sources		
Remove excess leaves and foliage from around the home that may cause moisture and attract insects		
Vacuum soft furnishings – drapes, upholstered chairs		
Clear gutters and downpipes		
Vacuum under and around fridge		
Replace batteries in smoke alarms		
Replace batteries in carbon monoxide detectors		
Have any heating appliances serviced in accordance with manufacturers recommendations		
Clean heating filters		

Winter	Can do	Done it
Clear gutters and downpipes		
Clean exhaust covers – bathroom, kitchen & laundry exhaust covers		
Vacuum soft furnishings – drapes, upholstered chairs		
Vacuum under and around fridge		

Table continued next page.

Periodic	Can do	Done it
Clean washing machine filter		
Clean dishwasher filter		
Replace water filters in line with manufacturer recommendations		
Wipe out fridge regularly		
Clean dryer filter		
Clear gutters and downpipes		
Repair any damaged surfaces		
Fix any leaks, check tap ware, garden taps, toilets and any water using appliance		
Maintain healthy soil for indoor plants (not too wet to avoid mould growth)		
Water mains to house turned off when away to check for leaks (unless using automated watering systems)		
Clean floor rugs		
Replace shower and bath water filters in accordance with manufacturers recommendations		
Clean door mats		
Use pest baits or nontoxic deterrents as needed to avoid pest issues		
Run hot water and baking soda through the drains		
Put 1 cup of vinegar through the dishwasher to descale		
Descale the washing machine regularly using 3-4 cups of white vinegar and ½ cup of baking soda on a hot wash		
Dust throughout the house with a damp cloth		
Vacuum floors regularly with a HEPA filter vacuum		

Copyright © Healthy Interiors 2014.

Specialty equipment periodic maintenance

For your solar hot water system, clean and check panels (if flat panel), check connections and tank for corrosion. For instantaneous systems, clean inline screen filters. If high mineral content water descale if necessary every three-five years. Use a qualified professional to ensure system warranties aren't voided.

Have your wind power equipment serviced annually by a qualified professional. Check guy wires if used.

Renewable Energy storage batteries – check that the battery terminals are clean and tight and that electrolyte levels are above the minimum levels. Batteries may also need to be fully charged/discharged at regular intervals dependent on manufacturer recommendations.

Ensure the filters for air purifiers or house ventilation systems are cleaned in line with manufacturer recommendations.

Removing mould

Western Australia's Department of Health outlines the following steps and solutions for removal of mould.

1. Eradicate mould when it occurs and establish the cause to fix the issue
2. Do not dry brush the area as this can release mould spores into the air which spreads the mould further and can cause an allergic reaction in some people.
3. There are several treatments for mould. Do not use bleach as it has a high pH which makes it ineffective to kill mould. It only bleaches the colour to make it disappear.
4. When cleaning mould wear gloves, glasses or goggles and a P-95 face mask to protect yourself from mould spores.

Option 1 – tea tree oil

A 3 percent solution or 2 teaspoons in a spray bottle with two cups of water. Shake and use.

Option 2 – fermented vinegar

Use 80 percent white fermented vinegar solution (available from the supermarket) with water. After applying the mixture leave for at least 20 minutes and then lightly sponge with clean water for removal.

Low allergen and sustainable gardening

Getting the most from your outdoor space

Professional Contribution – Belinda Thackeray

The way we live in Australia, with our mostly temperate climate, gardens really are an extension of the home and living space. We aspire for these outdoor areas to be used for recreation, relaxation and enjoyment of all, whatever the season. From vertical walls on balconies to large display gardens in backyards, green space and gardening are wonderful ways of connecting with nature.

According to the Asthma Foundation NSW, more than 2 million people in Australia suffer from asthma. This is a serious breathing disorder affecting about 20 percent of children and 10 percent of adults. Gardens and some plants can trigger problems for people living with asthma, allergies (swelling, rashes, wheezing and itching) and hay fever (sneezing, running nose, itchy eyes and blocked nose). Triggers include: pollen, mould spores and contact allergens. This chapter explores simple and practical ideas to help you create an allergy and asthma friendly garden space of your own. Managing your personal health and the growth of your garden is possible, and requires some planning in design, plant selection and management.

Getting started – plants and soil

It's important to have an understanding of how plants grow so you can provide them with the best care. These basics can save you a lot of effort and in time money by selecting the most appropriate plants for your garden design and knowing how to make them thrive.

Healthy soil is the key to strong healthy plants that are more able to resist disease and survive attack from many pests. Soil provides plants with air, water, nutrients and support. Most plants take up water and nutrients via their roots, so this is where water and fertiliser needs to be applied. Light (usually sunlight) is also necessary for healthy plant growth.

Garden soil and potting mix are two different things. Soil is made up of solid mineral (inorganic) matter, dead and living organisms (organic matter), air, water and nutrients. Potting mix is predominately a bark based product with a range of additives depending on the type.

Garden plants usually have their feeder roots growing in the top 20 – 30cm of soil. Improvement and enrichment of this top soil area prior to planting can really assist with structure, water holding capacity and can

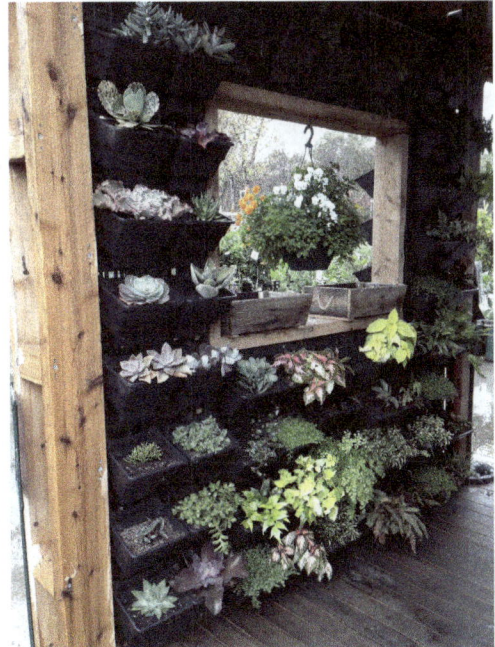

Vertical gardens are a great way to create a garden feature, especially where space is limited, such as on balconies and in courtyards. Image supplied by Belinda Thackeray

introduce essential nutrients for healthy plant growth. Depending on the soil type, different levels of improvement may be needed. Common soil types are (a) clay with sticky particles and a fine texture which provides poor drainage and aeration, (b) loam with medium round particles, usually suitable for most plants, and (c) sand with large angular particles which provides poor water holding capacity.

Organic matter like peat, mushroom compost, manure, straw, sugar cane, lucerne hay, organic mulch, compost and combinations of these are fantastic soil conditioners. They can be dug/forked through the soil before putting in new plants. These products can be purchased in bags from garden centres and also in bulk (trailer and truck loads) from landscape suppliers. Some people may have access to animal manure from farm and stable environments. It is usually a good idea to rot down or compost the manure prior to applying to gardens. Fresh manure can quickly turn into a mass of weeds and may burn some plants. Good compost will reach an amazing 70°C it breaks down, which is usually a high enough temperature to kill any weed seeds. For the most benefit, soil improvement should be an on-going process, with routine additions of organic matter whenever new plants are added to gardens. Organic mulch like lucerne and sugar cane can also be used as a form of soil conditioner.

As these products often contain mould spores, micro-organisms and bacteria, people living with asthma or allergies should take adequate precautions when using. Depending on the degree of the problem it may be suitable to just wear a mask (see Personal Protective Equipment) and apply on a still day, or you may need to get someone from your family who isn't affected by asthma or allergies to do this gardening job, or pay for a garden maintenance professional to do it for you. The Asthma Foundation of Victoria also suggests ensuring that the windows and doors of your home are securely shut while gardening as mould spores, micro-organisms and bacteria may be stirred up in the air. It can be best to leave them closed for several hours after soil improvement activity.

In pots, always use good quality potting mix. Don't ever dig up garden soil and put into pots as it is usually too dense and difficult for plants roots to grow through it. Potting mix is usually very barky and loose to allow easy growth of plant roots and for water to drain freely. Depending on the type of potting mix that you select, there are a lot of different options available for different plant and pot types; the mix will have certain amounts and types of control (slow) release fertiliser added.

Mixes may also contain water crystals which look like jelly crystals and swell/fill up with water. This is then slowly released where the plants need it, at their root zone. Having these crystals in the mix means that plants can go for longer between watering. Potting mixes designed specifically for terracotta pots usually have more water crystals whereas potting mixes designed specifically for growth of cacti and succulents will not contain any water crystals. Water crystals can be purchased separately from garden centres and added to your own potting mix if you are repotting or mixing your own. If you are using these, it can be a good idea to pre-hydrate prior to use, so as to avoid pots overflowing as crystals in the mix expand.

Soil wetters are also often found in potting mixes which can help with hydrophobic or water repellent soils. These are like detergents that break down waxy coatings that can form on soil particles. Soil wetters can also be purchased in granular and liquid form, and applied to increase soil water penetration.

When selecting potting mix, always make sure that it is an Australian Standard Certified product. You can tell this by looking for the five tick, Australian standard symbol. This potting mix has to maintain certain air and moisture holding levels and have a stable pH to meet the standard. All potting mixes have a safety warning on the packet which is important to follow. Most mixes and many mulch products recommend to avoid breathing dust or mist; wear a mask if dusty; wear gloves; keep product moist when handling; and wash hands immediately after use. These warnings should be closely followed, particularly by people living with asthma or allergies. Always use in a well-ventilated environment and store any leftover potting mix, after gardening in cool, dry conditions like in a sealed plastic container or airtight garbage bin in a garage or garden shed. When opening a bag of potting mix, always do this away from your face.

Pollination is an important process in plant growth and is required for flowers to set fruit and produce seeds. Basically, it involves transfer of pollen from a flowers anther to a flowers stigma so fertilisation can occur. Plants can be self-pollinating or cross pollinating. Some plants require wind, bees, birds or other vectors for pollination to occur. As widely noted, most plants that cause sensitivity for people living with asthma or allergies, are those requiring airborne pollination. Pollen is usually produced by the male plants and only travels short distances. Asthma NSW reports an increase in air borne pollen being measured from August to March in Australia.

Designing and planning your garden

If you're keen to start a new garden or update your existing one, the best way to work out which plants are suitable for growing in your area is to go for a walk around your local neighbourhood and look at gardens. Check out garden styles, and how different gardens look within the overall yard setting, and with different styles and shapes of houses. You will quickly start to see elements that you like and could imagine in your garden and work out what you find appealing or unappealing. Investing a little time for this research early in your garden design planning will help you to set a clear direction of the outdoor space that you would like to create.

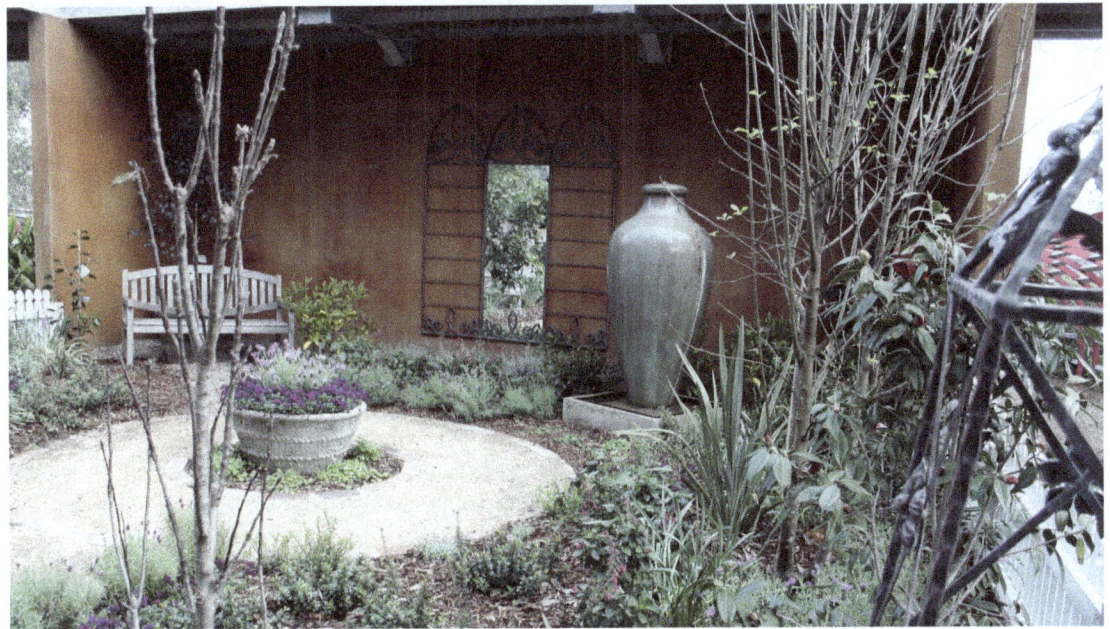

Eden Gardens at Macquarie Park in Sydney has a dedicated Asthma and Allergy show garden, developed in conjunction with Asthma Foundation NSW, to inform, educate and support people living with asthma and allergies. Image supplied by Belinda Thackeray

Take note of colour schemes, plant types, and other garden features from hard surfaces like paving, edging and mulches to focal points like water features, sculptures, garden furniture and specimen plants. Botanic Gardens, local parks, display gardens in large garden centres and private gardens opened as part of Open Garden schemes can also provide great inspiration.

Consider the wind pollination process. Pollen is a trigger for many allergy and asthma problems and should be a key consideration in initial planning decisions for your garden, especially gardens close to windows and doors where concentrated high pollen sources could enter the house.

When choosing plants for a new garden consider the following:

- How severe is the medical condition?
- Are garden areas positioned near windows and doors or in the direction of usual breezes?
- Is a person suffering from allergies or asthma required to care for the garden?
- Are pets living in the garden (e.g. dog) that may bring pollens into the house?

If you are planning a makeover of an existing garden area, you may decide to revamp the space to make it more asthma and allergy friendly. Plants that are high wind pollen producers could be replaced with more suitable plant species. If there is a particular high allergy plant that you like, design techniques used may include planting potentially problematic wind pollinated plants down wind, away from your house, windows and high traffic areas like along driveways and paths.

Mark Ragg in *The Low Allergy Garden* (Sydney 1996) suggests planting a screening, thick layer of shrubs and small trees (5-10m thick) to minimise pollen from other areas entering your garden. It may also be possible to select plants that flower and produce pollen at times of year when you are less likely to be spending a lot of time in the garden. Wind pollinated plants and grass can also be pruned or mowed prior to flowering and therefore before the release of pollen.

Creating a large new garden from scratch can be a costly activity. If budget is a constraint, you may wish to plan the overall garden space but develop, construct and plant the garden in manageable stages. Try starting with either the front or backyard or by creating garden rooms. Budget may also dictate if you DIY or use garden design and construction professionals.

For allergy and asthma sufferers who cannot change their surrounding garden, you may like to consider professional garden care services to avoid exposure to pollens in the garden. This may include lawns being mowed, trees pruned, mulch spread and compost turned. Spending money for a professional to undertake this regular garden care service may be a priority investment if your potential discomfort/trigger of other problems is significant. This is a personal decision based on individual circumstances.

Site and needs analysis

Start your design by closely looking at your garden and outdoor space. A great way to record information about your site is to measure it out and creating a very simple bubble diagram on a piece of paper. You need to map out where your house and any existing features, trees and gardens are located. Look at the sun path (the sun will rise in the east and set in the west, having a much lower arch during the cooler winter months in Australia), soil type (clay, sand or loam) and pH (the acidity or alkalinity of the water contained in growing mediums which influences the availability of nutrients).

Next you need to think about your use of the garden space. Are you creating something for display, such as large lawn areas with seasonal bloomers or are you creating something to use, like edible herbs, vegetables and fruit? Do you need areas of grass for recreation, for use by children or animals? Do you need other functional features like a clothes line and storage shed? When will you predominately be using the outdoor space – for summer entertainment or for winter vegetable production? Is there particular views that you would like to change, like a plain brick wall you see from your kitchen or a neighbouring road? All of these personal garden requirements should be noted down and solutions thought through as part of the garden design process.

For example if you want to screen off a functional garbage bin area in your outdoor space, you may consider growing a flowering climber or espaliering a citrus or camellia over a screening frame. Alternatively you may like to install a slatted screening wall which is painted a feature colour or has a water feature or mirror attached.

There are many different garden styles that can be created using different lines and shapes, hardscapes, focal points (like fountains, sculptures and specimen trees), plants and mulches. The combination of these elements creates a certain style of garden. For example a typical cottage style garden has curvy paths and garden beds, planted with a rambling and informal mixture of bright-flowering annuals, perennials, edible plants, bulbs and trees, chosen for seasonal flowering and form. From roses and agapanthus to grevillea and lavender, a diversity of different plants are featured and usually planted in odd numbered drifts. Timber fences, stone, brickwork, wrought iron and garden seat, arches and arbours are often incorporated.

A typical Asian garden features symbolic elements like gravel, stones, rocks, water together with clipped shrubs and trees to recreate the natural environment. Scale, form and texture are very important elements. Usually only a limited range of plants are featured, and in repetition including bamboo, azaleas, wisteria and nandinas.

Plant selection

Plant selection is usually the last stage in garden design, once all the basics shapes, lines, styles, features and hardscapes have been planned. Consider plant form and height, texture, colour (leaves and flowers), flowering season, and whether it is evergreen, deciduous or classified as low pollen producing.

Always read plant labels and only select species which suit your position and requirements. If the label states that a plant grows in full sun, this means it will withstand direct sunlight all day, including hot afternoon sun. If the label states that the plant grows in part shade, this means it is able to grow in a combination of sun and shade, with morning sun usually being best. If the label states that a plant will grow to 30m high, it will eventually in 5, 10 or 30 years be a very large tree and thus dominant garden feature, shading out areas below. The size may be able to be controlled to some extent by selecting a dwarf variety of the plant or via pruning but this type of plant cannot be kept small. You may be better off selecting a smaller growing plant species. Plant labels also contain information about the individual plant growth including amount of light, water, soil type, and fertiliser needed for optimum growing conditions.

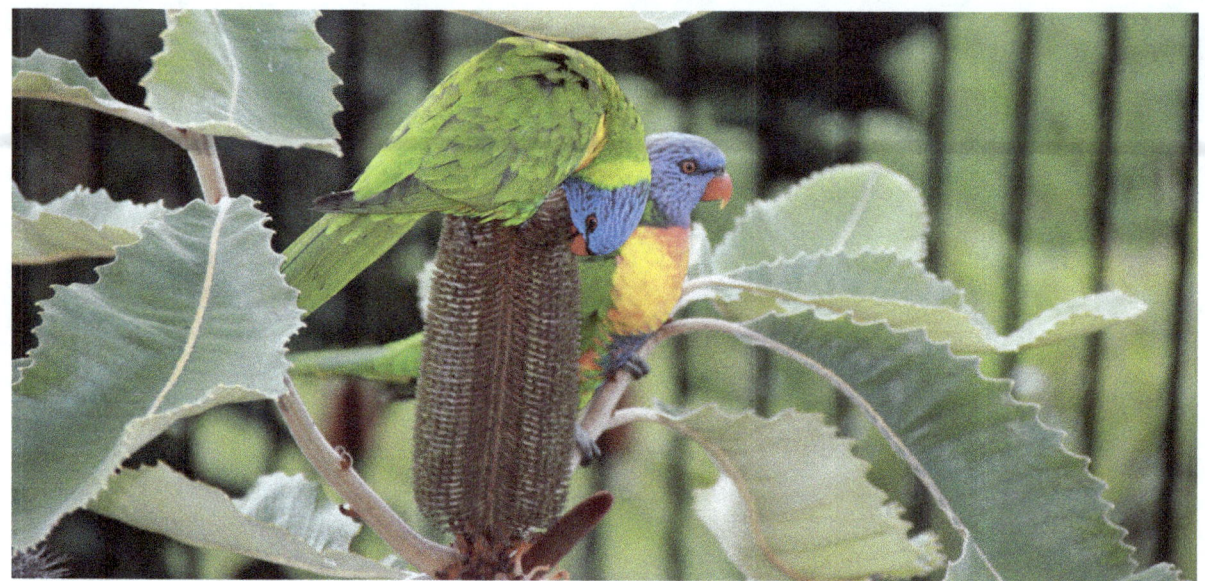

Banksia are Australian native plants that are mostly pollinated by birds. They attract birds with their stunning flower spikes that usually appear through winter and spring. Image supplied by Belinda Thackeray

There is such a great variety of plant species and cultivars now available. Electronic plant selector tools can assist with picking the best plants for your own garden situation. You can input information about sunlight, moisture and soil type for your local area; and select size, shape and colour of desired plant. Tools are available that make suggestions about suitable plants and provide basic growth information with photographs.

With plant positioning, it can be beneficial to group plants with similar requirements – pH, water, soil type and fertiliser together. You may also consider planting a variety of plants that will flower over an extended period and over several seasons. Always follow size information on the plant label and position to allow space for growth, planting more densely if creating hedges. Plants are sold by the size of the pot in garden centres, so savvy consumers can often select more advanced plant stock at a good price. Some plants can also be grown from seed which usually take about 4-6 weeks to get to size of seedlings. Large garden centres usually offer year-long plant guarantees on perennial plants which can provide you with confidence in the quality of the plants that you are purchasing and planting.

Planting in a pot

1. Water the plant thoroughly and allow excess water to drain.
2. Select a pot slightly larger than the one the plant is currently growing in. Ensure there is a drainage hole.
3. Gently remove plant from the pot and loosen the soil slightly.
4. Using a premium potting mix, place a layer of potting mix in the base of the new pot to bring the plant to the required height.
5. Position the plant so the existing soil level is 2cm below the rim of the pot and infill the gap around the roots with more potting mix
6. Tap the pot to settle the mix, adding more as required.
7. Water thoroughly and allow excess water to drain.
8. Water and feed as required.

Source: Eden Gardens

Planting in the ground

1. Water the plant thoroughly and allow excess water to drain.
2. Dig a hole in the garden bed twice as wide and twice as deep as the pot size.
3. Mix some soil conditioner with the existing soil. A plant in a pot measuring 200mm across the top will require a bucket full of soil conditioner.
4. Add water saving crystals according to instructions and mix with soil/soil conditioner mix.
5. Remove the plant from its pot and loosen the soil slightly. Position the plant in the hole, at the required height.
6. Infill around the plant with soil/soil conditioner, taking care not to cover the stem beyond the previous soil level.
7. Gently firm the soil and water thoroughly.
8. Place a 5-7cm layer of mulch on the soil surface leaving a gap around the stem.
9. Water regularly until the plant is established.
10. Water and feed as required.

Source: Eden Gardens

Seeds, berries, leaves, stems and saps of some plants can be poisonous. Westmead Children's Hospital (NSW) poisonous plant list includes Angels' trumpet (Brugmaisia sp.), cycads and oleander (Nerium sp.). Other plants can cause irritation and intolerances to individuals, which build up over time. For example the fine hairs on some grevillea plants can irritate the skin causing contact dermatitis, after repeat exposure. Try to avoid these problem plants in your plant selection.

If looking to avoid high pollen plants choose items for the garden from lists produced by state asthma organisations for people living with asthma or allergies. As mentioned, plants that rely on birds and insects for pollination rather than wind, generally don't release pollen into the air. These may have large, colourful flowers to attract pollinators, including: abelia, azalea, tibouchina, lavender, banksia, citrus, petunia and pansy. Asthma Foundation NSW recommends avoiding plants from Asteraceae family (daisies, chrysanthemums and chamomile) and trees (wattle, casuarina, elm, eucalyptus, melaleuca, oak, cypress and pine). Other common features of plants that can cause problems for people living with asthma or allergies include strongly scented plants and plants labelled as seedless or fruitless, which are males, as they may produce large amounts of allergenic wind borne pollen.

Recommended plants for asthma and allergy friendly gardens include:

Herbs – basil, chives, dill, fennel, horseradish, marjoram, mint, oregano, parsley, rosemary, sage and thyme.
Groundcovers – native violet, rosemary, tea tree, thyme, pratia, kidney weed and snow in summer.
Grasses – buffalo, kangaroo, greenless couch and weeping grass.
Flowers – alyssum, anemone, begonia, coleus, cornflower, foxglove, glossy abelia, impatiens, lobelia, nasturtium, nemesia, pansy, petunia, phlox, snapdragon, verbena, viola and bulbs.

Climbers – ivy leaf geranium, star jasmine, banksia rose, kiwifruit, trumpet vine, passionfruit and pandorea.
Shrubs – azalea, banksia, bottlebrush, camellia, callistemon, cistus, escallonia, flax, gardenias, kunzea, lavender, leptospermum, melaleuca, myrtle, plumbago, rhododendron, weigelia, westringia and yucca.
Trees – citrus, flowering crab apple, old man banksia, peppermint gum, bay laurel, coastal banksia, lillypilly, silky oak, most prunus, cabbage palm, magnolia, paperbark and scribbly gum.

Source: Asthma Foundation NSW

Edible gardens

Home grown vegies, herbs and fruit are healthy, convenient, easy to grow and often taste better than shop-bought produce. Growing your own can reduce food security concerns and allows you peace of mind about how the produce has been grown and what fertilisers and pest control products, or lack thereof, have been applied. Before launching into full scale edible gardening, think about things that you and your family like to eat and start with growing them. There is no point putting months of time and effort into growing a certain crop if you are not going to use and enjoy the produce.

Many edible plants can be grown in pots or in gardens. For best results you need a warm, sunny, open position with four to five hours of direct sunlight each day and protection from

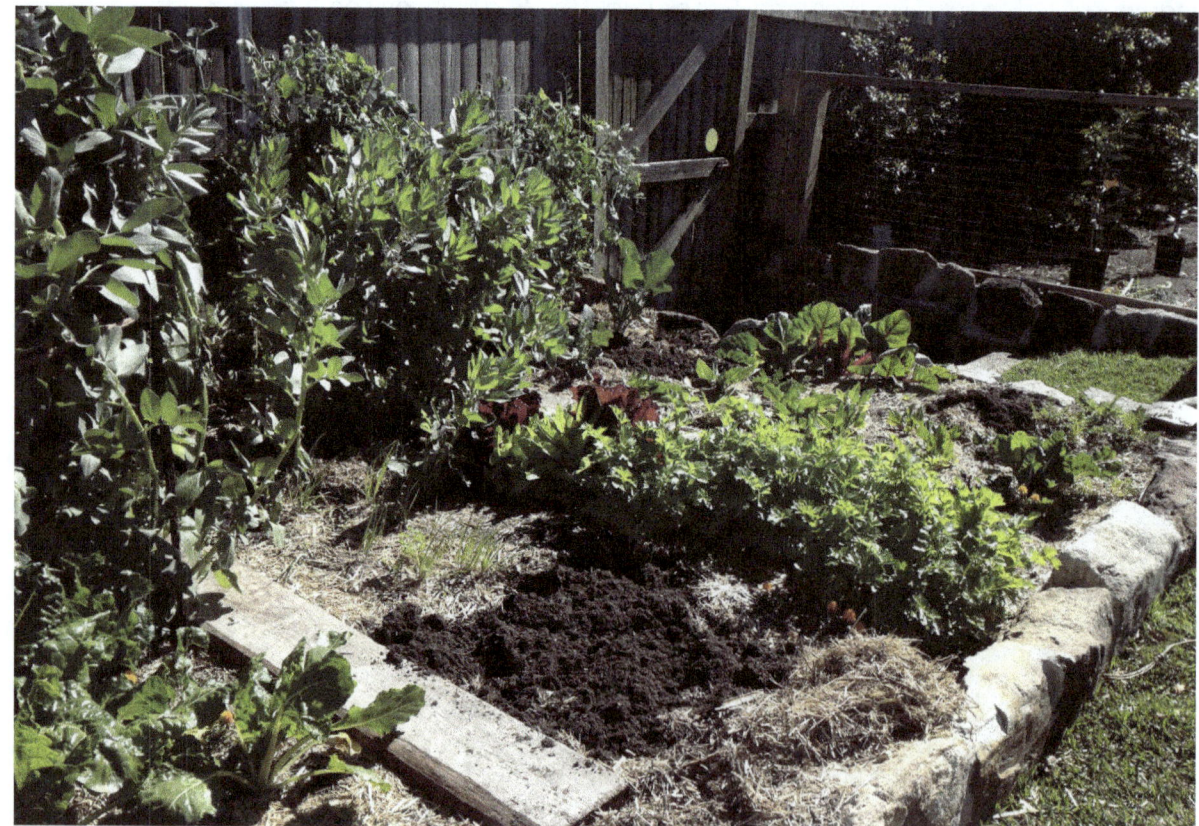

Growing your own produce in a backyard vegetable garden can be a rewarding experience for gardeners.
Image supplied by Belinda Thackeray

strong winds. Edibles usually don't cause specific problems for people living with asthma and allergies. Mark Ragg in *The Low Allergy Garden* suggests avoiding English spinach and corn which produce a lot of pollen. Hairy tomato plants can also cause contact allergies for some individuals.

Most vegetables are annuals which need to be replaced every six months, for warm and cool seasons. In temperate Australia, warm season varieties are usually grown from September onwards and include tomatoes, capsicums, sweetcorn, eggplants, cucumbers, pumpkin and squash. Cool season varieties include Asian greens, broad beans, potatoes and broccoli, which are usually grown from around March. Lettuces, carrots, silverbeet and beetroot can be grown year round in temperate areas. As most vegetables grow quickly they require regular applications of water and fertiliser.

If you are new to growing vegetables, it can often be wise to start off with a few plants and after success plant more. In warm periods after the danger of frost has passed, why not try growing tomatoes? 'Sweet Bite' is a vigorous growing variety which produces loads of small cherry tomato fruit, 'Apollo' is an early fruiting tomato variety which has good disease resistance, 'Roma' has medium size oval fruit which are great for sandwiches, and 'Pot Prize' is a compact tomato variety perfect for growing in pots. Other vegie favourites especially with the kids are round 'Rolypoly' carrots, fast-growing snowpeas and peas, and miniature vegetable varieties such as mini cos lettuces and mini beetroot.

Seed and seedlings can be planted successively over a few weeks to prolong the garden's produce season. This is especially important for fast growing vegies such as the non-heart forming lettuces like 'Tuscan mix' and baby spinach leaf that can be harvested after about a month and are great for salads and sandwiches.

If you have an established vegetable garden, it is a good idea to practice crop rotation. Plant different types of plants each season to avoid build-up of any crop's particular pests and diseases and to prevent depletion of specific nutrients from the soil. For example, rotating from a seasonal leaf crop like spinach to a seasonal fruiting crop like tomatoes to a seasonal root crop like radishes.

Herbs grow in similar conditions to vegetables, and in both pots and in gardens. Many are perennial plants that grow into attractive shrubs and groundcovers in time. These include thyme, rosemary, oregano and chives. Mint is another perennial but can grow rampantly. Plant mint separately or in a pot so it doesn't take over other plants you are trying to grow. Annual herbs may be planted seasonally like basil, dill and parsley in the warm season and coriander in the cool season. Herbs should be harvested (which is a form of tip pruning) often to encourage bushy new growth, and ideally picked in the morning when plant water content is high.

With fruit, most are perennial plants that crop once a year, usually during the warm season. Most varieties prefer sunny positions and many can be grown in pots or in the ground. Depending on varieties, some need cross pollination to produce fruit which means you may need two plants, a male and a female.

In temperate areas, fruit that is easily and commonly grown in home gardens is citrus which thrive in sunny positions in pots and in gardens. Many varieties are grafted which means they are hardy and produce masses of fruit, once established. For lemons try cultivars 'Eureka' which has rough skin but fruits year round or 'Meyer' which is thin skinned. For oranges try 'Valencia' which ripens in summer or 'Navels' which ripen in winter. For limes try 'Tahitian' with seedless juicy fruit or 'Kaffir' which are less juicy (and the leaves are good for use in Asian cooking). For other easy to grow fruits, blueberries are small shrubs that can do well in cool and temperate areas, producing masses of fruit over a season. Olives produce fruit after about three years, which need to be soaked, salted and preserved in oil before eating. Passionfruit grown on climbing vines, fruit after about 18 months and should be replaced every four to five years. Strawberries can be grown in pots and gardens, fruiting over several months.

There is something very rewarding about being able to feed your friends and family with things that you have grown yourself, especially if produced organically. Whether it is the passionfruit in a cheesecake, the lettuce in a salad or the chilli in a sauce, the options are limitless.

Creating a biodiverse garden

Biodiversity is the variety of all living things from plants and animals to micro-organisms. Gardens for biodiversity can be easily created in backyards

Australian native plants are usually insect or bird pollinated, producing only small amounts of pollen, so they are suitable for growing in gardens of people living with asthma or allergies. Plants can be selected that flower at different times of the year, to cater for a diversity of birdlife. Other ways to encourage birdlife in gardens include minimising disturbance, providing water and food, and providing habitat/shelter.

Basic garden design ideas for biodiversity can include, layering a diversity of Australian native plants from tall and medium trees like banksia, bottlebrush and lilypilly through shrubs/grasses like kangaroo grass and grevillea, to groundcovers like brachycome and scaevola.

Lawns

Lawns can be an attractive and functional part of any outdoor space. They are wonderful for dogs to run around on and for children to play. When selecting the variety of lawn to plant it's important to consider level of traffic, climate and light conditions. Certain lawn varieties like couch and kikuyu grow in full sun, while others like buffalo and zoysia grow in shade. Some grass varieties can also be high pollen producers once they flower, which can cause problems for people living with asthma or allergies. The Asthma Foundation of WA lists fescue, perennial rye and Bermuda grass as potential problem varieties. If these lawn varieties are used they should be kept short through frequent mowing so flowering and pollen is minimised.

The Asthma Foundation of Victoria recommends planting low pollen producing grasses like hybrid couch, Santa Ana and Windsor Green, and the Asthma Foundation of WA recommends planting Greenlees couch and buffalo grass.

Mark Ragg in *The Low Allergy Garden* advises that most pollen is released a couple of hours after sunrise and the pollen rises and sits in a layer 50cm to 2m off the ground. This supports the suggestion that people living with asthma or allergies should mow lawns early while still covered in dew, and to always wear appropriate personal protective equipment like masks and wrap-around glasses.

Buffalo grass and other coarse textured varieties can cause irritation and contact allergies with some individuals. It may be best to avoid direct exposure to skin, or take an antihistamine product prior to exposure.

Lawns can be planted from turf or from seed. It is cheaper to grow from seed but can take a period of time to become established while the area needs to be kept free of foot traffic. Planting from turf, although initially more expensive, provides an instant effect and if watered frequently can start to grow roots in a few weeks.

Australia native grasses like kangaroo grass, may not provide the traditional rolling green effect, being coarser, tufty and brown/grey coloured, but native grasses usually don't produce much pollen and don't need mowing/cutting back very often. If you do not have constant foot traffic, other low groundcover plants like pennyroyal or native violets may provide an alternative to lawns.

Garden management

When to garden

It's important to consider time of day to do your gardening jobs to minimise problems that may occur from pollen exposure. Checking the weather forecast is a great start. Often cool, cloudy, damp, still days are better for gardening than dry, hot, windy days. Weatherzone Australia has a four day pollen count with a pollen index that measures potential for pollen to trigger allergic reactions in susceptible individuals and gives one of five different rating levels. This is calculated for every capital city in Australia, except Darwin, on a daily basis from September to January. The rating is then listed at low for the rest of the year. As a general rule, Weatherzone suggests 'pollen levels in the atmosphere will be highest on hot days and on days where a dry wind is blowing'.

The rating on these pollen levels ranges from extreme for sufferers of pollen allergies which is 'typical on days with high temperatures and dry/hot winds where recommended precaution is to stay indoors', through to low for sufferers of pollen allergies which is 'typical on cold, wet days where there is likely to be little pollen released into the atmosphere'.

Accordingly to the Asthma Foundation of NSW, peak pollen season for trees is from September to October, and peak pollen season for grasses is from November to January. When gardening during this peak pollen period, it can be beneficial to get up early and out into the garden while there is still dew on plants which means there is less likely to be wind-borne pollen around. Before going out into the garden to undertake gardening tasks, make sure that you close your house windows and doors and keep them closed for several hours.

Personal protective equipment

The use of personal protective equipment when gardening can assist to minimise exposure to potential allergens. Always read and follow warning labels on all potting mixes, mulches, fertilisers and insecticides. Just because these products are available so commonly, even often in supermarkets alongside everyday food and household items, don't become complacent about these warnings.

General precautions to take in the garden include physical covering of skin by wearing long-sleeved tops and gloves, long pants and enclosed shoes. This is to avoid sun exposure and any contact allergies. Depending on your individual situation and the gardening jobs being undertaken, it can be advisable to also wear a mask, hat, wraparound sunglasses and gloves. Try to avoid touching your face and eyes while you are gardening, and always wash your hands well after gardening, even if you have been wearing gloves.

Remove all gardening clothes once you finish and before going into your house, as they may have pollen attached to them. Have a shower to wash off any potential asthma or allergy triggers, especially from your hair. It may also be a good idea to wash these clothes separately.

Soil improvement, compost and fertilising

Soil improvement is an ongoing process and can be achieved by adding organic matter regularly. This results in improved soil structure which then permits free passage of water, air and plant roots. Soil improvers include peat, mushroom compost, manure, straw, lucerne, compost, vermipost and combinations of these.

Compost is partly decomposed organic matter which is usually made in a compost bin or heap. This is a great way of recycling organic kitchen scraps and garden waste into a rich product that can improve soil structure and water holding capacity while acting as a fertiliser. Mould spores and micro-organisms in compost may trigger problems for some people living with asthma or allergies, so it is always important to use appropriate personal protective equipment, especially when turning and spreading compost. Making compost is simple, you just need to layer. Start with carbon rich waste like dry leaves, twigs, paper, straw, dry grass and wood ash, then with nitrogen rich waste like vegetable scraps, fruit peels, fresh lawn clippings, animal manure and green foliar trimmings. This is in a ratio of about five parts carbon to two parts nitrogen. The compost needs to be kept damp but not wet, and turned regularly to add air which aids the breakdown process.

Depending on the time of year and conditions, NSW Environment and Heritage suggests that it usually takes about 8-10 weeks for turned compost systems to produce good compost. This can then be added to pots and gardens as a soil conditioner for most plants.

If you live in a unit or mostly produce kitchen scraps, not garden waste, a worm farm may suit you better. Worm farms are boxes that contain compost worms, which are a special breed of earthworm that convert organic waste into 'vermipost' and 'worm tea'.

These worms need moist conditions and a constant supply of food. They eat most kitchen scraps except dairy, meat, citrus, garlic, onions, and will not survive in the garden. Both vermipost (granular worm waste) and worm tea (liquid worm waste) are nutrient rich by products that once diluted, can be added to pots and gardens as a fertiliser.

It is important to fertilise plants to ensure healthy growth. Fertilising provides the essential nutrients for plant growth including nitrogen, phosphorous, potassium and various macro nutrients in different ratios. It's a personal choice whether organic or inorganic fertiliser is used. Organic fertiliser usually assists to improve soil structure while inorganic fertiliser is manufactured to a chemical formula, allowing an exact amount of specified elements to be provided.

Fertilisers come in various different forms. Control (slow) release fertilisers are tiny polymer coated balls that release small quantities of nutrients over an extended period of time, usually 6-9 months. Soluble fertilisers (from liquid or powder) are mixed with water, usually in a watering can and provide an instant release of nutrients. Granular fertilisers provide a short-term concentrated dose of nutrients.

It's a good idea to water plants thoroughly before and after applying fertilisers. Fertilisers should always be applied at soil level and in accordance with label instructions. Over-fertilising can kill plants and cause environmental problems. Australian native plants only require low levels of phosphorous so use fertiliser specific to natives.

Soluble seaweed based plant tonics can also be diluted and applied to help stimulate root growth. This can beneficial for all plants, especially those that have recently been planted.

Mulch

Mulch is a material spread over the soil surface which can create a certain garden style or look, and helps to conserve soil moisture, which means you have to water less often. It also keeps soil and plant roots cool, and can help to suppress the growth of pesky weeds. There are two categories of mulch - organic and inorganic.

Organic mulches including bark, straw, lucerne and sugar cane, add nutrients to the soil as they break down. They may also contain dust and mould spores which can cause problems for people living with asthma and allergies, especially when digging and spreading. Always read the label on the mulch bags; it is often recommended to wear a mask and to wet slightly before handling. These mulches need to be topped up and replaced periodically. For example a fine bark mulch spread 7cm deep may need to be topped up at least every two years.

Inorganic mulches including pebbles, gravel, scoria, crushed gravel and polished glass are permanent mulches that do not need replacing. As these do not decompose, they don't add any nutrients to the soil. These mulch options may be more suitable for people living with asthma or allergies, and suit many garden styles.

Mulch can be bought in bags from garden centres or from landscape companies in bulk, either by trailer load or can be delivered by tipper truck, which is usually more

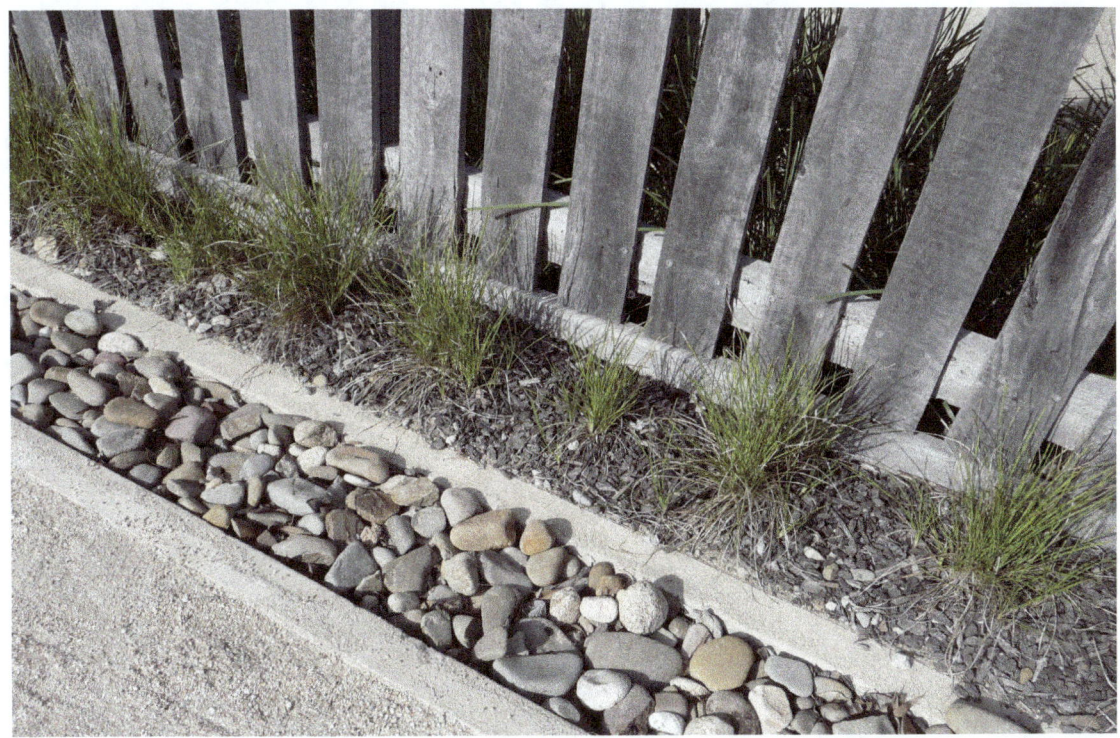

Mulching a garden can help to conserve soil moisture and create a particular garden style.
Image supplied by Belinda Thackeray

economical. It is often advised to spread sheets of newspaper, thick cardboard or weed mat over damp soil prior to spreading mulch. This inhibits the growth of weeds by blocking out the sunlight they need to thrive. Spread evenly over the soil surface, about 5-7cm deep, taking care to not spread mulch too close to plant stems as it can cause fungal disease problems.

Managing pests and diseases in the garden

Pests and diseases can cause problems in the garden when they start to inhibit the growth and health of a plant. Some plant diseases like black spot and mildew have spores which can also affect those living with asthma or allergies.

Many people choose to control garden pests and diseases organically, meaning without the use of synthetic chemicals. This may involve biological, cultural, mechanical and physical management strategies. You may also select disease resistant plant varieties. There are now cultivars available in many flowering plants that are disease resistant like psyllid resistant lilly-pillies.

A pest and disease management system called integrated pest management can also be used to manage pests and diseases successfully in gardens. In this system, management does not necessarily mean the complete elimination or eradication of a pest. It can mean controlling pest numbers before they build up to a point at which they can cause significant problems in the garden. It usually follows a series of steps and can include the use of some chemical products, however to achieve a garden with minimised pollutants, chemicals need to be avoided where possible.

If you do use pesticides, always follow label instructions and use appropriate personal protective equipment.

Steps in an integrated pest management system include:

- Pest identification – needs to be correct
- Pest monitoring – early detection
- Determination of critical damage level – when to take action
- Pest control strategies include:
  - plant selection – diversification of species, local native plants are more resilient
  - physical removal of pests and their residues
  - biological control (predators)
  - cultural practices (for strong, healthy plants)
  - 'natural' pesticides / suggested controls

Source: Eden Gardens

Not all bugs are bad

Insects in the garden are necessary and 'good bugs' help with:

- Pollinating fruit trees
- Eating plant waste and creating fertiliser
- Providing food for birds and animals essential to a healthy eco system
- Improving soil condition
- Eating other pests that harm plants

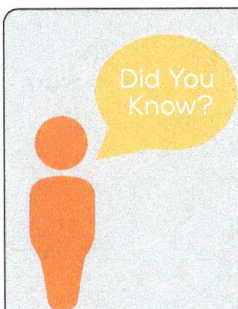

Did You Know? Honey bees are in trouble! Bee numbers in some countries are declining. Bees are essential to pollinate gardens and many food production plants. The use of some pesticides has been suggested as contributing to their decline.

An example of how the integrated pest management system works, could involve snails attacking lettuce seedlings growing in your garden. You have seen the snails so you know they are causing the problem. You need to decide if you want to lose your lettuces (or some of them to snail damage) or whether you want to control the snails. Putting a ring of crushed eggshell or sawdust around each seedling, which slugs and snails are unlikely to pass over due to the rough texture, may be enough to stop the snails. If this doesn't give you the result you are after, you could put on gloves and hand remove the snails from garden areas, which can be easily done, especially during the evening or after rain when the snails are often active. The collected snails would then need to be squashed or put in the freezer to kill. If you are still experiencing problems with snail damage, you may want to sprinkle a pelletised iron complex slug and snail control pellet (select one that is also pet friendly) around the lettuces. This would be effective in controlling the problem, while not affecting worms and other beneficial insects in the soil.

Watering

All plants need to be watered regularly until established. As mentioned, plants take up water via their roots, so it's usually best to apply water directly to the soil not the foliage. Wet foliage can lead to disease problems with some plants, especially if they have been watered in the evening and the weather is humid. It is best to water in the morning if possible. Drip irrigation watering systems are usually much more efficient than overhead sprinkling systems, as water is applied directly to plants roots where it is needed. This assists with preventing black spot on roses and powdery mildew on cucurbits like zucchini and cucumber, as can increasing air circulation around plants through routine thinning and pruning of dense foliage areas.

Use water crystals and soil wetters to assist with soil water penetration and retention. Always remember gardens and pots need to be watered more often during warm weather.

Weeds

Weeds can be a problem in any garden situation. Weed plants are basically any plant that competes with more desired plants for light, water, nutrients and space. It's important to keep on top of weed control. Remove by hand or change their growing conditions. For example, shading out weeds, applying boiling water and steam, or by applying a nontoxic weedicide are effective methods. Many weeds are prolific wind pollen producers and should be monitored and managed in the garden and in surrounding outdoor areas of allergy or asthma sufferers. If you do not have time to remove weeds, you can cut off flowers as they are forming, to avoid seed being set. Bagged flowers/seeds should be thrown away, not composted.

Asthma weed/Pellitory (Parietaria judaica) is of particular concern to people living with asthma. Asthma weed is a common, perennial weed. It has sticky leaves and small green flowers that produce pollen year round that can cause serious allergic reaction. To reduce potential exposure to pollen you may need to revert to using a carefully chosen product to control weeds, rather than by hand. Many councils in urban areas are working to control weeds like asthma weed and privet in common recreation spaces so as to lessen potential problems from wind borne pollen.

Tips to minimising chemical use in the garden

1. Create healthy soil and compost mulch
2. Weed minimisation – a thick layer of mulch helps to minimise weed growth while providing nutrients and water retention attributes for plants. Keep mulch a few centimetres away from stems to prevent moisture related diseases.
3. Weed regularly while weeds are easy to remove, this will also minimise the spread of any seeds and reduce the need for chemical intervention. Boiling water or hot steam is helpful to kill weeds.
4. Plants natives to your location and types of plants that are suitable for site conditions e.g. wet or dry soil, sun or shade. Opt for plants that are resistant to insects and disease.
5. Appropriate watering – excess watering can create unhealthy soil. Systems that water the roots allow the soil to partly dry which assists to keep soil healthy.
6. Not all insects are bad for the garden – many bugs in the garden are helpful. Using pesticides often kills the bad and beneficial bugs. Creating a garden system that provides conditions for good bugs helps to keep others low.
7. Garden maintenance – remove hiding places that encourage harmful pests e.g. remove old pots or debris around the garden where snails or slugs may accumulate.
8. Regularly inspect the garden identifying a problem early helps with minimal intervention.
9. Early identification of pests in the garden may result in pest eradication success from hand picking out pests or setting garden traps such as beer traps (container placed into the soil with a small amount of beer to attract snails and slugs).
10. If a problem arises get expert assistance to identify an issues and identify options before reaching for chemicals. Correct identification can minimise incorrect chemical treatments.
11. If chemical intervention is required, choose the least hazardous products and only apply when rain is not expected to avoid run-off into the garden.
12. Avoid combination products so that only minimal product is used for specific purpose.
13. If using products in the garden only treat specific areas. Avoid a broad approach as this may be detrimental to the garden's natural balance.

© Healthy Interiors 2014.

 **TIP** Don't place garden beds up against the house as it keeps moisture around the footings of the home moist and moisture may attract termites. If garden beds are near the foundation of the home ensure the garden beds are not higher than the foundation of the building.

The insights above are some basics to consider in the garden. As many gardeners will confess, gardening is a journey of knowledge. Creating a healthy, sustainable, productive garden has many benefits to both human health and the environment. The level of pleasure derived from a garden is proportionate to the level of care we give to our natural surroundings. Designing the home environment to have minimal impact on nature provides many opportunities for reward, be it an uplifting view, home grown produce or the enjoyment of visiting wildlife.

Further information

- To find out more about asthma, allergies and low allergy sustainable gardening visit or read:
  Asthma Australia – www.asthmaaustralia.org.au
  Asthma Foundation of Victoria – www.asthma.org.au
  Asthma Foundation NSW – www.asthmansw.org.au
  Asthma Foundation WA – www.asthmawa.org.au
  Weatherzone Australia – www.weatherzone.com.au – for air borne pollen index
  Westmead Children's Hospital – www.chw.edu.au – for a list of poisonous plants
  Mark Ragg – *The Low Allergy Garden*, Hodder & Stoughton, Sydney, 1996

- To find out more about sustainable gardening visit or read:
  Australian Organic – www.austorganic.com.au – for information on organic gardening and organic certification of growers and producers in Australia
  NSW Environment and Heritage – www.environment.nsw.gov.au – for composting information
  Sustainable Gardening Australia – www.sgaonline.org.au – for sustainable gardening information
  NSW Environment Protection Authority – www.epa.nsw.gov.au – for details on integrated pest management
  Permaculture Australia group – http://permacultureaustralia.org.au

- For garden inspiration and design ideas visit or read:
  Eden Gardens – www.edengardens.com.au – lifestyle horticulture centre in Sydney's Macquarie Park, with asthma and allergy friendly display garden
  Open Gardens – www.opengarden.org.au – for information on Australia wide open gardens
  Plant This – www.plantthis.com.au – for plant selector tool

Investment sense

Building or renovating a property involves significant financial investment. Whether you are building or renovating to live in a premises, or place it on the rental market, there are many reasons why investing in healthy and sustainable attributes are of value. The world is moving in an environmentally conscious direction and living costs are rising. Beyond these two great reasons to be innovative are others that may help mitigate investment risk.

Residential homes that combine energy efficient attributes as well as allergy friendly (low emission) attributes, can offer owner occupants, investors and tenants a range of benefits that intertwine to achieve positive health, environmental and financial outcomes.

The following diagram illustrates an overview of heath and productivity gains of healthy sustainable properties.

Pathway to Health and Economic Gains

1. Allergy friendly (minimised pollutants) home
2. Energy efficient home

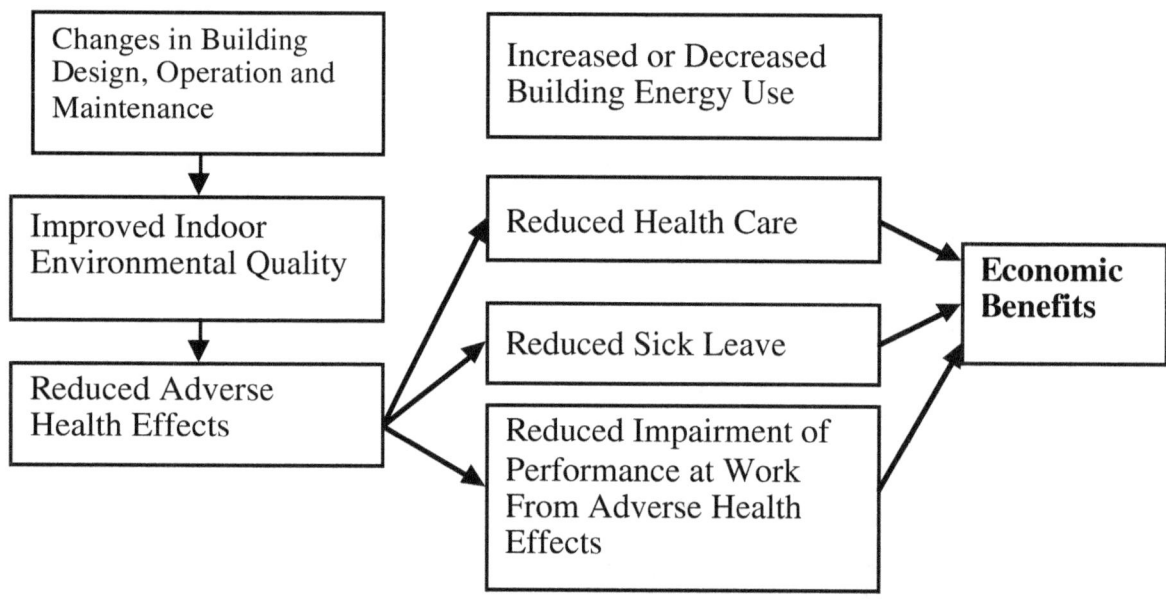

Supplied by William J Fisk, Health and Productivity Gains from Better Indoor Environments and Their Implications for the U.S Department of Energy

The building landscape is changing globally to embrace 'green' design initiatives. The World Green Building Council report in 2013 has highlighted that in markets where green is becoming more mainstream, indications of 'brown' discounts are occurring (where buildings that are not green may sell or rent for less).

For the savvy property investor, assessment of potential investment risks and staying ahead of the pack to hold investments that are sought after makes financial sense.

The following are some identified reasons as to why investing in healthy, sustainable properties reduces property investment risk:

Regulatory risk

The Business Case for Green Building report of 2013 indicates 'consensus that governments will implement regulations that target sustainability factors far more aggressively than has previously been the case, and investors will need to understand what the consequences will be.'

Investors need to consider their property sustainability profile, compared to other buildings and the perceived value as we move into the future.

Will legislators regulate at some stage for mandatory disclosure of energy efficiency performance information within the residential sector? This is already mandatory in the ACT where the energy efficiency rating must be available for any residential property sold or rented. This may expand to other states and territories in the future. Ensuring your property investment has a 'sustainable profile' is positive risk management. There is currently legislative mandatory reporting in the USA and the UK.

Even if legislated mandatory disclosure is not enforced, voluntary disclosure has the potential to affect property profile demand criteria.

Currently there is no mandatory 'indoor health' rating system or requirements for homes in Australia (other than those specified in Volume II of the National Construction Code of Australia), despite the increasing awareness of this potential health issue, (especially since Australian housing is changing to more air tight construction). Could this change in the future?

Market risk

The Business Case for Green Building report refers to a commercial property market risk of tenancy as 'likelihood that tenants might leave a building, or not lease it in the first place, because of its inadequate sustainability performance is recognised as a key risk by investors.'

This is relevant to the residential sector. If tenants have a choice between rental accommodation that offers a healthy indoor environment along with energy efficient attributes to keep costs of living down, it is common sense that this property will be preferred over another similar property without those attributes. It's worth noting that properties with higher star ratings in the ACT obtain a higher market price of between 3-5 percent per star rating above the traditional ratings (thought to be around two stars). For more information, refer to the Energy Efficiency Rating and House Prices in the ACT study 2006.

Commercial buildings with high NABERS (National Australian Building Energy Rating System) ratings or that are Green Star rated are achieving significantly better returns than traditional buildings.

Sustainability and health credentials of a property provide an additional feature, further to other desirable features such as location, age and quality of a property.

With the evolution of certification bodies in the green industry there are organisations that can provide ratings or certificates on sustainability elements of a home, including energy efficiency, building material and finishes, and product environmental impacts and attributes. These independent bodies can provide investors with certification certificates for various products used on a property, providing investors with third party validation of property attributes to use for marketing their investment in the rental or sales market. An example is Homestar in NZ and eTool in Australia.

Physical risk

The physical ability of buildings to withstand environmental challenges such as extreme weather events is a significant factor, particularly for those with investments in locations subject to damaging events and extreme heat.

Investors will increasingly need to factor in the ability of buildings to withstand predicted climate impacts into their decision-making. Chief amongst these impacts will be extreme weather events, flooding, subsidence and the ability of buildings thermal envelope and systems to cope with increased ambient temperatures and changing rainfall patterns.

Insurance limitations or inability to acquire insurance could reduce a property's value considerably, so consideration of potential future impacts of insurability of buildings given climate change potential is important. An example of this is the move by some Australian insurance companies to deny some properties flood cover relevant to property location.

Properties that can provide interior comfort through extreme weather events ensures that a property remains desirable to tenants into the future regardless of weather conditions, which minimises potential vacancies and cash flow issues.

Environmental risk

Investors need to consider how their property investment will compete with other property investments in the same tenancy pool, in relation to energy efficiency, water efficiency and indoor health attributes. Investing in 'green' properties is now a key consideration for commercial investment funds and superannuation organisations. The residential market is likely follow suit.

Technology risk

There are risks in utilising new innovative technologies, however there is also significant risk in avoiding new technology such as LED lighting and solar technologies. Resistance to implementing new technologies can increase the risk of missed opportunities for operational costs and create a less desirable choice for potential tenants.

Environmental and technology risk issues are already being experienced in the commercial area where inefficient properties are suffering a 'discounted' market value and higher vacancy rates, compared with efficient properties obtaining lower vacancy rates and higher sales prices.

In this interconnected world, technology is a key player: home automation systems, energy monitoring and management systems and products that provide multiple services (i.e. heaters that cool and solar PV that also provides hot water) are the new reality.

The healthy home quiz

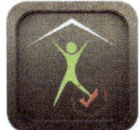 With the increase in asthma, allergies, chemical sensitivities and other illnesses related to indoor pollutants, a healthy home has never been more important. Families are being encouraged to seal homes for greater energy efficiency. Being an energy efficient consumer is advisable and beneficial, however when restricting passive ventilation we then need to follow through with minimising pollutants within the home.

The general public is largely unaware of reports such as the US National Institutes of Health report Reducing Environmental Cancer Risk - What we can do now? (2008 – 2009). The Healthy Home app captures information such as this and makes it available for families to take action. The following quotes are from the Reducing Environmental Cancer Risk report and an insight into some of the tips included in the app:

'It is vitally important to recognise that children are far more susceptible to damage from environmental carcinogens and endocrine-disrupting compounds than adults. To the extent possible, parents and child care providers should choose foods, house and garden products, play spaces, toys, medicines, and medical tests that will minimise children's exposures to toxics. Ideally, both mothers and fathers should avoid exposure to endocrine-disrupting chemicals and known or suspected carcinogens prior to a child's conception and throughout pregnancy and early life, when risk of damage is greatest.'

'Storing and carrying water in stainless steel, glass, or BPA and phthalate-free containers will reduce exposure to endocrine-disrupting and other chemicals that may leach into water from plastics.'

'Exposure to pesticides can be decreased by choosing, to the extent possible, food grown without pesticides or chemical fertilisers and washing conventionally grown produce to remove residues.'

'Exposure to antibiotics, growth hormones, and toxic run-off from livestock feed lots can be minimised by eating free-range meat raised without these medications if it is available.'

'Individuals can choose products made with non-toxic substances or environmentally safe chemicals'.

'Reducing or ceasing landscaping pesticide and fertiliser use will keep these chemicals from contaminating drinking water supplies.'

'Properly disposing of pharmaceuticals, household chemicals, paints, and other materials will minimise drinking water and soil contamination.'

'Driving a fuel-efficient car, biking or walking when possible, or using public transport also cuts the amount of toxic auto exhaust in the air.'

'...removing shoes before entering the home'

'...washing work clothes separately from other family laundry.'

'Filtering home tap ...water can decrease exposure to numerous known or suspected carcinogens and endocrine disrupting chemicals.'

'Individuals also can influence industry by selecting non –toxic products and, where these do not exist, communicating with manufacturers and trade organisations about their desire for safer products.'

The following pages include content from The Healthy Home app that was written by health-focused interior designer Melissa Wittig and released in 2012 to assist families to identify healthy home assets and challenges and create a home with minimised pollutants.

The app's content is collated from many reports and sources, bringing together a substantial healthy home reference resource. This section contains quiz questions from the app that allow you to walk through your home room by room and identify 'healthy home' assets or challenges. You can complete this quiz in this book or refer to the app available in the App Store. The app provides additional resources in the form of note-taking capability for reference when shopping, a score dial, favourite capability, camera for image references and functionality to assess multiple homes.

Giving your home a 'healthy home' overhaul has never been easier. Take the quiz and create your very own action plan to make healthier decisions in and around your home that suit your budget and living arrangements.

Quiz categories

Outdoors

Interior general

Entry

Bedrooms

Kitchen

Living zone

Bathrooms

Laundry

Lifestyle practices

Outdoors

Q1. Is your home located next to a busy road or business where cars idle?

Yes – challenge / No – asset

Traffic

If you live on a busy road or where cars idle you are likely to be subjected to higher levels of motor vehicle pollutants. Motor vehicles emit exhaust gases into the air such as carbon monoxide, oxides of nitrogen, hydrocarbons and particulates, along with evaporative emission otherwise known as fuel vapours. An Australian Environmental Protection Agency study (EPA Publication 789) found a link between high levels of fine particles, ozone, nitrogen dioxide and carbon monoxide and an increase in the number of hospital admissions for respiratory and cardiovascular disease. If opening your windows subjects you to these fumes, you may like to opt for an air purifier to assist you to keep your indoor air clean.

Q2. Do you use chemical pesticides around the exterior of the house or garden?

Yes – challenge / No – asset

Outdoor pesticides

Let's state the obvious – pesticides are designed to kill pests! Many pesticides can also pose a risk to human health. In some instances you will not find ingredients listed on the product label as the manufacturer may be protecting their secret formula. But this means you don't really know what chemicals you are using in your home. Just because a product is being sold does not mean it is safe. In many countries products such as these are not tested for human health. Children are more susceptible to pesticides given their size and there is much documented about the connection between pesticides and health issues. We like the work on this site: www.pesticides.org/docs/website-home-use.pdf

Q3. Do you have any asbestos around the home – exterior cladding, interior cladding, interior tiles, eaves, in heaters, on your shed/garage?

Yes – challenge / No – asset

Asbestos

If you don't know, we strongly suggest you contact a local licensed asbestos assessor to give you a report about where you may have this material. Asbestos can be found in many areas of a home such as cladding board, eave boards, interior lining board, behind tiles, floor tiles, insulation in ceilings or heating units, lagging around plumbing and more. Asbestos should not be disturbed. If removal is required it must be done according to local laws and must be done using the correct safety equipment to protect your health. Once it has been removed it requires safe disposal to avoid harming others. Asbestos exposure can be fatal in the years after exposure. Asbestos has been named a carcinogen in many countries. For more information relevant to your area contact your local building authority. Some general information can be found here www.asbestos.act.gov.au/about_asbestos

Q4. Is there evidence of mould around the outside of the house?

Yes – challenge / No – asset

Exterior mould

Mould around the exterior of the house can impact on the interior materials and quality of air inside the home. Check that land drainage is adequate, that spouting and downpipes are in good working order, that there are no cracks or holes in the roof or wall structures. Excess moisture around the home can lead to mould growth and material deterioration. Preventing problems early will save you money and prevent mould growth that may impact on your health.

Interiors general

Q1. Do you think the quality of the air you breathe is important?

Yes – asset / No-challenge

Indoor air

We often forget to consider the impacts that products we buy may have on the air that we breathe within our home. What we build our homes with, what we fill them with and our lifestyle practices all culminate to create the quality of the air we breathe indoors. As people around the world are sealing their homes to create energy efficient houses to reduce costs, it is vital to remember that the air we are sealing within our homes is what we are breathing. Studies confirm that indoor air within homes is being polluted by building materials, furnishings and lifestyle practices and can impact on occupant health. Learn more about the health concerns linked to indoor air quality here www.epa.gov/iaq/ia-intro.html#Sources

Q2. Do you think that all products sold in shops have been tested as being safe?

Yes – challenge / No – asset

Product safety

Not all products sold are tested first to ensure they are safe for human health. The global sale of cigarettes is a great example of this as they are still sold despite an understanding cigarettes cause cancer. Many products for the home are being sold that use chemicals that have not been tested and deemed safe for human health. Products are often recalled from sale after a health problem has been identified. Therefore consumers need to be informed and ask what products are made from and how they are made before buying them to ascertain if we really want to live with a product.

Q3. Do you know that household dust can contain chemicals from furnishings and lifestyle practices?

Yes – asset / No – challenge

Dust

Chemicals used to create products that we buy can in some instances migrate into household dust. Flame retardant chemicals and phthalate chemicals (plastic softeners), among others have been found in household dust studies. Flame retardants can be found in foams, textiles, lighting, building materials and electrical goods. Dust within a home is airborne as people move around the house and can be circulated by heating and cooling systems, resulting in inhalation or ingestion of pollutants. Dust can be a trigger for asthma, allergies and respiratory conditions. Read more about hazardous dust and health concerns at **www.ewg.org**

Q4. Do you know what a VOC is?

Yes – asset / No-challenge

VOC

Volatile Organic Compounds (VOCs) are chemicals that evaporate releasing fumes into the air. It is common for indoor air to contain a range of VOCs or fumes as a result of building materials, furnishings, consumer products and lifestyle practices within the home. Not all VOCs have an odour. VOCs contribute to indoor air pollution and have been linked to a range of health concerns, from eye and respiratory irritation, headaches, lethargy, to more serious health concerns. Read more **www.epa.gov/iaq/ia-intro.html#Pollution_and_Health**

Q5. Has your home been freshly painted within the last two years?

Yes – challenge / No – asset

Freshly painted

Freshly painted surfaces are higher in VOCs in the period of time directly after painting. The level of VOCs emitted from paintwork in the home will depend on the type of paint. When choosing paint, consider opting for products low in toxicity and low VOC. You can choose from naturally derived paints or petroleum based paints. If choosing a petroleum based paint, water based paints are healthier options rather than solvent based paints. If starting a painting project it's a good idea to keep children out of freshly painted areas for at least the first few weeks while the space is aired out and until the highest levels of VOCs have dissipated. Paints made from naturally derived ingredients are a good option as they generally allow the building surface to breathe.

Q6. Do you have any plasticised wall paper on your walls?

Yes – challenge / No – asset

Wallpaper

Plasticised wallpapers can contain PVC. PVC contains volatile organic compounds (VOCs) that off-gas. PVC also contains phthalate chemicals that are found in plastics. Some phthalate chemicals have been found to migrate into household dust and have been linked to asthma. Opt for paper based wallpaper or fabrics such as linen, silk, sisal, or jute with a water-based low VOC adhesive.

Q7. Are any of your walls made from asbestos sheeting?

Yes – challenge / No – asset

Asbestos walls

Decorating and renovating is an exciting time. Before drilling or hammering into walls make sure that the lining board is not asbestos. Asbestos is known to cause serious health problems. Asbestos was used to create various products used in housing prior to the mid-1980s and may still be used in some countries. Asbestos sheeting was used for many purposes, often for wet area surfaces hidden behind tiles, for walls, or eaves around a house. Asbestos contains small particles that if disturbed can cause potentially fatal health problems. Have an asbestos audit done on your home and ensure that you know where the asbestos is located or have it safely removed by a specialist. It should always be avoided, and treated with caution. www.asbestosadvisor.net/What_does_asbestos_look_like.aspx

Q8. Is there cracked and peeling paint on any of the walls?

Yes – challenge / No – asset

Peeling paintwork

Houses painted before 1970 in Australia may have been painted with paint containing lead. Up to the 1950s, Australian paint could contain as much as 50 percent lead. Modern household paints contain less than 1 percent lead, however renovating or repairing old paint surfaces can expose lead from old paint and can contaminate surfaces and cause lead poisoning. Small amounts of lead can cause serious health problems particularity for children. Lead has been associated with a wide range of health issues such as behavioural, growth and cognitive issues in children and nervous system, cardiovascular and kidney health issues among others for adults. Grab a lead test kit from the local hardware store and test if your old paintwork contains lead before your disturb it. Lead is only a danger once it is disturbed. Consider repainting the surface without disturbing the original surface or replace the substrate or hire a professional to remove the lead paint safely. Refer to the six-step guide to painting your home www.environment.gov.au/atmosphere/airquality/publications/leadpaint.html
www.lead.org.au
www.greenpainters.org.au/Consumer-Information/Lead-Paint.htm

Q9. Do you have vinyl floor coverings that are in poor condition ?

Yes – challenge / No – asset

Vinyl floor coverings

If yes, it's worth noting that a study of phthalates in indoor dust and their association with building characteristics by Gustaf Bornehag and others published by Environment Health Perspectives found a dose response relationship between concentrations of phthalates (plastic softeners) in bedroom dust and the likelihood of being diagnosed with asthma, rhinitis or eczema. Studies suggest that plastic softeners can find their way into household dust and be inadvertently inhaled. Opting for products free from plastics is a safer alternative for people and the environment. Learn more about asthma – www.asthma.org.au/Resources.aspx

Q10. Can you see any mold on any of the walls or ceiling in your home ?
Yes – challenge / No – asset

Mould on walls

Mould can cause a range of health issues such as fatigue, weakened immune system and contribute to allergy symptoms. Mould in the home indicates a problem with moisture and could be a result of a structural problem such as leaks, poor drainage, flooding, rising damp, condensation or humidity. Removing and preventing mould will assist with minimising maintenance expenses but importantly will prevent mould spores from growing and impacting on indoor air quality and your health. When moulds are disturbed they release spores into the air. When cleaning mould ensure you wear a suitable face mask. To remove mould use an 80 percent naturally fermented white vinegar to 20 percent water solution. www.mould.com.au/mythsaboutmould.htm

Q11. Do your windows open and close properly?
Yes – asset / No - challenge

Windows

Opening windows can assist with reducing indoor air pollution that has accumulated from building materials and finishes, furniture, household items and lifestyle practices. According to a 2012 report by leading global interdisciplinary design firm Perkins+Will, 374 substances that may be found in the home environment were highlighted as known or suspected asthmagens.

Q12. Are window and door screens in good repair?
Yes – asset / No – challenge

Screens

Opening doors and windows regularly helps with ventilation, pushing stale and often polluted indoor air out. Screens allow for air flow and minimises insects and pests from entering. Minimising access of pests also minimises the need for pest repellents.

Q13. Is there cracked or peeling paint around the windows?
Yes – challenge / No – asset

Paintwork dust

Old houses may have been painted with paint containing lead. If paintwork is deteriorated, chemicals from paintwork are more likely to find their way into household dust that may inadvertently be inhaled or ingested. Buy a lead test kit from the hardware store before undertaking any DIY repair work as lead paintwork needs to be repaired using protection. Use a HEPA filter vacuum regularly to minimise the spread of dust throughout the house.

Q14. When raining does water enter the windows when they are closed?
Yes – challenge / No – asset

Leaking windows

Mould needs moisture to start growing – prompt maintenance to repair the water leaks is needed now!

Q15. Do you have plasticised window coverings such as blinds or curtains?

Yes – challenge / No – asset

Plasticised window coverings

Plastics when heated release VOCs (volatile organic compounds), better known as gases or fumes. Plasticised window coverings receive direct sunlight and heat up in the window and contribute to poor indoor air quality. Some plasticised fabrics can contain phthalate chemicals (plastic softeners) that have been found to migrate into household dust and linked with health concerns. Opt for window furnishings free from plastics. Natural fibres or naturally treated timber are a great option.

Q16. Do you use a HEPA vacuum cleaner to remove dust from your house?

Yes – asset / No – challenge

HEPA vacuum

HEPA stands for high-efficiency particulate air. A HEPA filter is a type of mechanical air filter; it works by forcing air through a fine mesh filter that traps harmful particles. A HEPA filter vacuum used to clean the home minimises the spread of household dust that may be polluted with chemicals that have migrated from household products, as well as eliminating pollens, pet dander and dust mites.

Q17. Do you have fluorescent lighting in your home?

Yes – challenge / No – asset

Fluorescent lighting

Compact fluorescent lighting generally contains mercury. When fluorescent lighting is broken, mercury vapour is released into the air and has been linked to health concerns. The long life and low power consumption of these lamps tends to make them a popular choice for homeowners. Opt for maximising natural lighting within a home through the use of windows strategically placed to gain maximum sunlight or installation of skylights (roof windows). LED lighting is an energy efficient option for those seeking an alternative lighting solution. If you break a fluorescent lamp within the home, this should be disposed of with care. You can find more information here - **www2.epa.gov/cfl/cleaning-broken-cfl**

Q18. Have you investigated radon levels in your home?

Yes – asset / No – challenge

Radon

Radon is a colourless, odourless, radioactive gas. It forms naturally from the decay of radioactive elements, such as uranium, which can be found at different levels in soil and rock throughout the world. Radon gas in the soil and rock can move into the air and into homes and has been associated with lung cancer. Different locations around the world have differing levels of radon. You can check radon levels in your home to determine if you need to take action. Do-it-yourself radon detection kits can be ordered through the mail or purchased in some hardware stores. The kits are placed in the home for a period of time and then mailed to a lab for analysis. Read more about radon and health concerns - **www.who.int/ionizing_radiation/env/radon/en**

World Health Organisation's Handbook on Indoor Radon - **http://whqlibdoc.who.int/publications/2009/9789241547673_eng.pdf**

Entry

Q1. Do you have a door mat?

Yes – asset / No - challenge

Door mat

Door mats assist to trap unwanted potential pollutants such as heavy metals, bacteria and fine particles from entering the home and accumulating in household dust. The dust within our homes gets circulated by movement of occupants, heating and cooling systems. What is even better than a door mat? Take shoes off at the front door.

Q2. Do you take your shoes off when entering the house?

Yes – asset / No – challenge

Shoes

Taking shoes off at the front door prevents germs, bacteria, chemical residues and heavy metals from being walked into the home. Young children spend significant amounts of time on the floor surface and have lots of hand to mouth action which can result in pollutants being easily ingested from surfaces. Designing a space for shoes to be stored near the door most used is a healthy and practical solution, such as a shoe rack, shoe basket, bench seat with shoe storage or a shoe cupboard.

Q3. Upon entering the house do you smell fragrances e.g. air fresheners, incense, candles?

Yes – challenge / No – asset

Fragrances

Avoid air fresheners, petro chemically produced candles and incense – opt for natural essential oils, plants or flowers.

Q4. Do you smell a musty, damp mould smell?

Yes – challenge / No – asset

Musty odour

A damp, musty smell indicates that moisture is accumulating somewhere it should not be. Investigate where the odour is coming from and eliminate the source. Musty odours may be a result of something leaking or moisture build up within the home or may be the result of poor drainage or moisture outside the home structure. Quick action to resolve a musty odour could save you money and prevent any health issues from developing.

Q5. While walking around the house can you smell cleaning products?

Yes – challenge / No - asset

Clean smell

If you can smell cleaning products you are smelling VOCs. Many cleaning products do not list all their ingredients on the label and can contain chemicals that are considered toxic. Cleaning products leave residues on surfaces around the home creating opportunities for chemicals to be absorbed through the skin, inhaled or ingested. A clean odour can have 'no' odour. Select products that are transparent - understand the ingredients list of your cleaning products such as these www.healthyinteriors.com.au/featured-products

Q6. Do you smell cooking odours?

Yes – challenge / No - asset

Cooking odours

Check your exhaust fan over your cooktop in the kitchen is working properly. Try the tissue test – can your exhaust fan pull a ½ ply tissue sheet towards it? If not, the extraction force of the fan could be improved. Is your exhaust fan flued to the exterior to prevent combustion pollutions circulating inside the home or within the roof space?

Bedroom

Q1. Do you have plastic in or around your bed eg. plasticised fabric on the bed frame, plasticised mattress protector?

Yes – challenge / No - asset

Beds and plastic

Further to releasing VOCs, plastics can contain phthalates, otherwise known as plastic softeners. Some phthalates have been found to migrate into household dust and been linked to endocrine-altering health issues and allergies. A study by Bornehag CG et al, 'The association between asthma and allergic symptoms in children and phthalates in house dust' showed that 'phthalates, within the range of what is normally found in indoor environments, are associated with allergic symptoms in children'. Opt for natural fibre fabrics such as hemp, cotton, linen and wool. Mattress protectors made from organic cotton or wool are great options. Read more: www.ncbi.nlm.nih.gov/pubmed/15471731

Q2. Do you have a mattress that has been treated with a chemical flame retardant?

Yes – challenge / No - asset

Flame retardants

Some flame-retardant chemicals have been found to migrate into household dust and have been linked to a host of health concerns relating to nervous system health, hormonal and thyroid function health among others. Before buying bedding ask questions to understand the manufacturing process so that you understand what you are sleeping with such as flame-retardants, adhesives, stain resistant treatments etc. Read more: www.ewg.org/release/new-research-finds-highly-toxic-flame-retardants-widespread-homes-furniture

Q3. Do you have a mattress that has been treated with a chemical stain guard treatment?

Yes – challenge / No - asset

Stain treatments

Per fluorinated chemicals (PFCs) are widely used water, grease and stain repellents. PFCs have been associated with health concerns such as immune suppression, reproductive problems and hormonal disorders. PFCs can be found in carpets and furnishings as well as non-stick food packaging. Opt for products that have not been chemically treated.

Q4. Are you sleeping on a foam mattress?

Yes – challenge / No - asset

Matress

Foams are made from petrochemicals that can off-gas into the air that you breathe while sleeping, and many foams contain flame retardant chemicals.

Choose a mattress made from untreated, non-toxic natural materials ideally containing no synthetic chemicals or fire retardants. Opt for a mattress made from natural fibres with no chemical treatments. If a new mattress is not an option buy a wool or organic cotton mattress topper.

Q5. Do you have unsealed particle board or MDF furniture in your bedroom ? Eg particle board that is not sealed by a coating or finishing product.

Yes – challenge / No - asset

Fibre board products

The adhesives used to make particle board and medium density fibreboard (MDF) often contain urea formaldehyde. Formaldehyde can off-gas into indoor air. Formaldehyde has been documented to contribute to eye, nose, and throat irritation; wheezing and coughing; fatigue, skin rashes among other more serious health conditions. When purchasing pressed board products opt for LFE E0 board, meaning 'Low Formaldehyde Emission'. This product is manufactured using a modified glue to reduce formaldehyde emissions. Formaldehyde is classified as carcinogenic to humans by the International Agency for Research on Cancer (IARC). If MDF is used for products inside your home ensure that all the raw surfaces are sealed. Other furniture material options are solid timber, metal or glass furniture. Read more: **www.epa.gov/iaq/formaldehyde.html**

Q6. Do you have synthetic carpets in your bedroom?

Yes – challenge / No - asset

Carpet

Toxic chemicals can be found in fibre bonding materials, backing glues, fire retardants, dyes, fungicides and stain resistant treatments. Opt for carpets made from natural fibres such as wool, sisal, coir or seagrass to minimise VOCs. Avoid chemical treatments such as stain resistance, mothproofing and fungicides. Carpets with woven or jute backing is preferable to rubberised options. Read more: **www.epa.gov/iaq/voc.html**

Q7. Do you use organic bed sheets?

Yes – asset / No – challenge

Organic linen

Opt for organic bedding that is produced in accordance with global organic textile standards where possible. If this is not possible try to buy bed sheets that are Oeko-Tex certified. Avoid textiles that have been chemically treated such as stain resistant, crease free and antibacterial chemical treatments.

Q8. Do you dry clean your clothes, blankets or other items?

Yes – challenge / No - asset

Dry cleaning

Tetrachloroethene is a toxic chemical that is widely used in the dry-cleaning of fabrics. Other names for tetrachloroethene include perc, tetrachloroethylene, perchloroethylene or PCE. Perc can contribute to poor indoor air quality and for those with skin sensitivities can contribute to allergy symptoms. Opt for perc-free cleaning methods such as steam cleaning or hand washing of items. If you must dry-clean hang the item outdoors until the odour is gone. Read more: **www.atsdr.cdc.gov/tfacts18.pdf**

Q9. Is there air flow under your mattress / bed?

Yes – assett / No – challenge

Bed airflow

Unobstructed space under a mattress encourages air flow circulation and discourages moisture build up in the mattress. A bed design with slatted timber supports works well as long as the space under the mattress is free from clutter.

Q10. Do you sleep with a clock radio or any other electrical device turned on, eg. electric blanket?

Yes – challenge / No - asset

Electromagnetic fields

Could your bedroom design be preventing you from having a restful sleep due to electromagnetic fields (EMFs)? The issue of EMFs is receiving increasing attention globally in relation to health concerns and health sensitivities. Many hours are spent sleeping. Eliminating sources in the bedroom is a precautionary approach to ensure you get a healthy, good night's sleep. Remove electrical devices from the bedroom; avoid metal bed frames and mattresses with metal as metal tends to intensify electromagnetic fields. Are there appliances on walls adjoining the bedroom? Keep beds away from appliances on adjoining walls. Demand switches and other shielding options are available for those who wish to take further action. You may like to read more about this contentious issue here - **www.magdahavas.com/international-experts%E2%80%99-perspective-on-the-health-effects-of-electromagnetic-fields-emf-and-electromagnetic-radiation-emr**

Q11. Do you have sufficient concealed storage in your bedroom?

Yes – asset / No – challenge

Storage

Minimising dust in the bedroom helps to promote good indoor air quality for optimal health, as dust can circulate with movement, heating and cooling. Dust can contribute to allergies and asthma. Creating storage that is concealed prevents surface dust from collecting on items over time. Opt for shelving with doors, storage boxes with lids and minimise clutter.

Q12. Do you open the window in your bedroom weekly?

Yes – asset / No – challenge

Open windows

Research has shown that air inside the home is often many times more polluted than the air outside the home. Opening windows regularly will assist to flush out the build-up of VOCs that have accumulated in the indoor air. Even in cooler months a quick burst of outdoor air can help to maintain healthier indoor air for our lungs. Well maintained indoor plants have also been documented as assisting to clean indoor air. To learn more visit the Resource Library **www.healthyinteriors.com.au**

Q13. Do you let pets sleep in your room?

Yes – challenge / No - asset

People who suffer from pet allergies or asthma should ideally keep the cat or dog out of the bedroom. Bedding can trap allergens that are difficult to remove. Pets can also spread bacteria throughout the home. Wash pets regularly where possible and use a HEPA vacuum cleaner to remove pet dander and fur. Read more: **www.allergy.org.au/patients/product-allergy/pet-allergy**

Kitchen

Q1. Do you have a good exhaust fan over the cooking area?

Yes – challenge / No - asset

Tissue test

An easy and cheap test you can do to see if you have good air extraction from your exhaust fan is the tissue test. Use a ½ ply tissue; hold it a few centimetres away from the vent. When the fan is on does it draw the tissue up to the vent easily? If not, the extraction force of the fan could be improved. Effective extraction of cooking gases helps to minimise combustion pollutants that can build up in your indoor air. Combustion pollutants have been linked to health issues.

Q2. Are there any signs of mould or mildew in the kitchen, including under the sink?

Yes – challenge / No - asset

Removing mould

Tip - 'Occupants of damp or mouldy buildings are at increased risk of experiencing health problems such as respiratory symptoms, respiratory infections, allergic rhinitis and asthma.' Identify and eliminate the source of moisture. There are various ways to clean mould – we like the 80% naturally fermented white vinegar solution with 20% water. Read more: www.euro.who.int/__data/assets/pdf_file/0003/78636/Damp_Mould_Brochure.pdf

Q3. Do you use non-stick cooking items eg pots and pans?

Yes – challenge / No - asset

Non stick

Perfluorochemicals (PFCs) are commonly used to create non-stick cookware. There is information available that PFCs are highly toxic, which is of concern. Opt for stainless steel, cast iron or glass cookware. Read more: www.healthybuilding.net/healthcare/2009-04-20PFCs_fact_sheet.pdf

Q4. Do you use antibacterial hand or dish soap?

Yes – challenge / No - asset

Antibacterial

Tricolsan is a chemical found in many consumer products including many antibacterial soaps and liquids. According to the Environmental Working Group triclosan has been 'linked to liver and inhalation toxicity, and low levels of triclosan may disrupt thyroid function.' Opt for soaps that use natural ingredients and look for ingredients that you can understand on the label.

Q5. Are the garbage recycling and any compost bins covered?

Yes – asset / No – challenge

Rubbish bins

Pests like food, moisture and shelter and an open recycling bin is the perfect home. Keep bins covered to avoid attracting pests. Pests can create a mess, multiply and spread germs.

Q6. Are there any signs of pests eg droppings, moths etc in the kitchen?

Yes – challenge / No - asset

Pests

Clean up spills quickly and keep surfaces such as benchtops and inside cupboards clean. To minimise the temptations for pests, ensure bins are sealed, containers used to store food are kept closed and screens on windows and doors are in good working order. If you must use a product to help rid your home of pests opt for chemical free options such as physical traps or nontoxic applications.

Q7. Do you have a carbon monoxide detector in the kitchen?

Yes – asset / No – challenge

Carbon monoxide

If no, it's worth noting that these are inexpensive and may help you detect a gas leak. Carbon monoxide, known as CO, is found in combustion fumes such as those from stoves, gas cooking, gas heating and engine fumes. CO can build up in enclosed spaces without an odour and can cause poisoning. Common symptoms associated with CO poisoning is headaches, weakness, nausea, vomiting, confusion and chest pain. High levels of carbon monoxide can cause loss of consciousness and death. Detectors help keep your home safe and alert you to any CO leaks.

Q8. Do you use plastic containers to store your food in?

Yes – challenge / No - asset

Food storage

Plastics contain plastic softeners known as phthalates. Phthalates have been known to migrate into food sources while food is being stored. Some phthalates have been linked to hormone disruption health concerns. Opt for alternatives such as glass, stainless steel or ceramic storage containers.

Q9. Do you use plastic in the microwave?

Yes – challenge / No - asset

Microwave oven

Plastics should not be heated especially near food, as chemicals can migrate into the food. DEHP is a phthalate (plastic softener) found in some plastics and can migrate into food - particularly fatty food - when heated. Avoid using plastic in the microwave.

Q10. Do you drink or eat from pottery items?

Yes – challenge / No - asset

Pottery kitchenware

Use ceramic cookware from large reputable suppliers. Look at the label to see if the item guarantees it is lead free. Lead can be used in the glazing process of ceramics and if ingested is harmful. Don't use old glazed ware for cooking, keep these as decorative items. Lead test kits can be purchased from the hardware store. Wash ceramic cookware by hand and if you notice cracks or chipping replace the item.

Q11. Do you check the containers you buy your food in – do they have the plastic ID numbers 3,6,7 ?

Yes – challenge / No - asset

Plastic ID

Get to know your plastics by checking your food packaging for a small triangle indicating the type of plastic. Numbers 3, 6 and 7 have been associated with hormone disrupting chemicals. Hormone disrupting chemicals have been linked to early puberty, obesity, development disorders, diabetes and cancer. Read more at the plastics pocket guide – **www.ecocycle.org/files/pdfs/pocket_guide_singleprint.pdf**

Q12. Do you choose organic or pesticide free food options?

Yes – asset / No – challenge

Fresh produce

Organic food can be expensive. If you are not able to eat organic produce make sure you wash your fresh produce well to remove any pesticide, fungicide or herbicide residue. A solution of 10 percent vinegar with 90 percent water can be used to soak vegetables and fruit before rinsing to help remove contaminants.

Q13. Do you eat canned goods?

Yes – challenge / No - asset

Canned food

Many canning companies place a lining inside cans that contains Bisphenol A, otherwise known as BPA. BPA has been linked to hormonal disruption health concerns. Studies have found that BPA can migrate into the canned food which is then eaten. Given the concern over BPA some companies are using a BPA alternative known as Bisphenol S (BPS), however there is concern mounting that this alternative may not be safe either. Opt for fresh or frozen food instead.

Q14. Do you use plastic drinking bottles?

Yes – challenge / No - asset

Plastic drink bottles

To avoid potential plastic softeners from leaching into your beverage, opt for stainless steel water bottles free from any internal lining.

Q15. Do you filter your drinking water?

Yes – asset / No – challenge

Water

Water supplies around the world vary greatly as does the type of treatment given to public water supplies. Using a water filter can remove bacteria, pesticides, lead, copper, iron, chlorine, nitrates and fluoride (depending on the filter used). Clean water is essential for good health. In instances where family members have skin conditions removing harsh irritants such as chlorine can also be beneficial. Fluoride is added to some water supplies around the world yet has been linked to a range of health concerns.

Bathroom

Q1. Is there a musty mould smell in the bathroom?

Yes – challenge / No - asset

Bathroom mould

Safely remove the mould and fix the cause. Tips to avoiding mould in the bathroom including taking shorter, cooler showers to minimise the build-up of steam and using a ceiling exhaust fan during and shortly after showering to remove steam and help dehumidify the air. If the bathroom has a window keep it open when possible for air circulation. Wipe down wet surfaces after finishing in the bathroom. Clean the bathroom regularly to avoid mould growth. Hang towels where they will dry as wet towels in a bathroom all day create a damp environment.

Q2. Do you see any signs of water damage?

Yes – challenge / No - asset

Water damage

Mould thrives in damp areas. A common area for mould growth in the bathroom is under silicone sealant around tiles. Remove the sealant, clean the area well, ensure it is dry and then reseal with a wet area low VOC sealant. Tea tree oil is effective in cleaning mould. A three percent solution or two teaspoons in a spray bottle with two cups of water (shake well) can be used as an alternative to a vinegar solution.

Q3. Does water condense on the inside of the window?

Yes – challenge / No - asset

Water condensation

Condensation is a common cause of dampness in buildings, often occurring on walls, windows, and floors, but it can also occur in roof spaces and in sub-floor areas.

To minimise condensation, increase passive and mechanical ventilation throughout the home. This can be done by opening windows and using effective exhaust fans throughout the home where moisture vapour occurs. Exhaust fans should always be used above the cooktop and over showers. If using a clothes dryer appliance ensure it is vented to the outside of the home (not the roof cavity). In cooler months indoor temperature throughout the home should ideally be kept at a reasonably constant temperature. Remove additional moisture sources from within the home, such as drying wet clothes indoors. Use a dehumidifier if required.

Q4. Is there a working exhaust fan over the shower?

Yes – asset / No – challenge

Bathroom exhaust

To test if the exhaust fan is working properly do a tissue test.

Divide a tissue (so that it is ½ ply) and hold it approximately 10 cm under the fan and see if the fan draws the tissue to the vent. If you do not have an exhaust fan in the bathroom, put this on your to do list as it is essential in minimising indoor moisture and potential mould growth. Allow natural airflow from windows to flow into the bathroom space after use where possible to assist with drying surfaces, weather permitting.

Q5. Do you have a plastic or PVC shower curtain?

Yes – challenge / No - asset

Plastic shower curtain

A Study by the Center for Health, Environment & Justice (USA) found PVC shower curtains can release as many as 108 volatile organic compounds (VOCs) into the air.

Opt for PVC-free shower curtains made out of safer materials such as organic cotton, nylon, polyester. www.chej.org/showercurtainreport/documents/Volatile%20Vinyl%20Executive%20Summary.pdf

Q6. Do you use antibacterial hand soap?

Yes – challenge / No - asset

Soap

Triclosan is an anti-bacterial chemical used in many anti-bacterial soaps/products.

Tricolan has been linked to liver, thyroid and endocrine (hormone development) disorders in children. The overuse of antibacterial products may lead to germs becoming immune to them and develop into superbugs that are not easily treated with antibiotics. See how the World Health Organisation advises to clean hands. www.who.int/gpsc/clean_hands_protection/en

Q7. Do you use non toxic, natural ingredient hair products?

Yes – asset / No – challenge

Hair products

What we use to wash our hair with impacts on our skin and can be irritating.

Avoid sodium lauryl sulphate which is a widely used synthetic detergent found in many personal care items.

Check out David Suzuki's dirty dozen guide http://davidsuzuki.org/dirty12/#wrapper

Q8. Do you use non toxic, natural ingredient personal care products?
Yes – asset / No – challenge

Personal care products
Have you read the label? Do you really know what you are using?
Your skin is your body's largest organ and is capable of absorbing products used.
Did you know that formaldehyde is used in many personal care products?
Did you know that formaldehyde is classified a probable carcinogen? Opt for products made from natural organic ingredients where possible. Look for products that are independently certified. Look for companies that are transparent with their ingredients. For more tips about personal care products visit the Environmental Working Group Skin Deep database **www.ewg.org/skindeep**

Laundry

Q1. Do you use non toxic washing products?
Yes – asset / No – challenge

Washing
Many ingredients used to create washing powders are not mentioned on the product label and are untested for human health. Harsh washing powders can irritate the skin. Fabric softeners, and scented drying products made from toxic chemicals, subtly coat the washing. Synthetic fragrances are among the world's top allergens and are suspected of being endocrine disruptors. Opt for products with no synthetic surfactants, no artificial fragrance, no bulking agents or fillers.

Q2. Does water condense on the walls and ceilings when using appliances in the laundry?
Yes – challenge / No - asset

Laundry moisture
Efficient ventilation and an exhaust fan is needed in the laundry to prevent moisture damaging the laundry room or making its way into other rooms of the house and encouraging mould growth.

Q3. If you have a dryer is it vented outside the house?
Yes – asset / No – challenge

Drying appliances
Venting the air externally will prevent excess moisture indoors. If the unit is not vented it may cause condensation and encourage mould growth. Venting into the roof cavity can also cause moisture issues to insulation and building materials. Opt for external release of moisture sources where possible.

Q4. Do you store paints and garage related products in your laundry?
Yes – challenge / No - asset

Garage items inside
Products can off-gas while being stored.
Keep paints, coatings and chemicals safely stored outside the house to avoid off-gassing and polluting indoor air.

Lifestyle practices

Q1. Do you dry clean your clothes?

Yes – challenge / No - asset

Dry cleaning clothes

Tetrachloroethylene is often used in the dry-cleaning process and this chemical is classed as a category 3 carcinogen and has been documented as having the potential to cause skin irritation. If dry cleaning is necessary, hang dry cleaned clothes outside for a while after collecting to minimise the fumes before putting them away indoors.

Q2. Do you use microfibre cloths for dusting?

Yes – asset / No – challenge

Dusting

Microfibre clothes attract dust to the cloth surface and reduce dust from being airborne. Many household chemicals migrate into dust such as flame retardants, stain resistant and insecticide chemicals.

Q3. Do you use a HEPA filter vacuum?

Yes – assett / No – challenge

HEPA filter

HEPA stands for High Efficiency Particulate Air filter. Air and dust is forced through a fine mesh filter trapping small particles of dust, pollens, pet dander and other pollutants to improve indoor air quality.

Q4. Do you use environmentally friendly cleaning products?

Yes – assett / No – challenge

Eco cleaning

Look for manufacturers that list all their ingredients on the label.

Contact the consumer number on the label and ask for a copy of the material safety data sheet so you understand what you are using and the hazards.

Q5. Do you ask guests to take their shoes off at the door?

Yes – challenge / No - asset

Visitor shoes

Put a large door mat outside doors. People walk all sorts of pollutants such as pesticides, heavy metals and germs indoors via dust on their shoes.

Q6. Do you use fragrance products inside the home eg stand alone scents, plug ins?

Yes – challenge / No - asset

Natural frangrance

Synthetic fragrances are one of the world's top allergens and are also suspected of being endocrine disruptors. Opt for natural fragrances such as flowers.

Q7. Do you leave your car idling in the driveway?

Yes – challenge / No - asset

Car

Exhaust fumes can potentially contain carbon monoxide, nitrogen dioxide, benzenes, sulphur dioxide, lead, formaldehyde and particulate matter. Vehicle emissions are toxic and can make their way indoors if stationary for extended periods of time.

Q8. Do you have and use an open fire in your home?

Yes – challenge / No - asset

Wood fire

Wood smoke is a mixture of gases and particles that are airborne. Wood smoke has been documented by many organisations as impacting on human health particularly on susceptible people such as those with heart and lung disease, asthma and small children.

Q9. Do you have indoor plants?

Yes – assett / No – challenge

Indoor plants

A study by NASA has shown that Indoor house plants have been shown to remove various toxins from indoor air such as formaldehyde, benzene, xylene among others.

To learn more about the type of plants studied read How to Grow Fresh Air available here - **www.healthyinteriors.com.au/shop/products/great-books**

Q10. Does anyone smoke indoors?

Yes – challenge / No - asset

Smoking

Tobacco smoke will pollute indoor air and has been shown to cause cancer. A healthy family is a great reason to quit or ask visitors to smoke outdoors away from windows and doors to prevent smoke entering the house.

Q11. Do you spray pesticides in the house or use the pest free plug ins?

Yes – challenge / No - asset

Pesticides

Airborne pesticide products pollute indoor air and can potentially be inhaled. Opt for natural pest remedies where possible or physical type baits or traps that do not spread chemicals throughout the home.

Healthy home action plan

From the identified challenges, these are issues of priority for me:

....

....

....

....

....

....

My top three priorities to action in the next three months:

....

....

....

....

....

You can download 'The Healthy Home' app from iTunes where you can store your answers to these quiz questions along with your notes, photos and favourite tips to use when shopping. Visit **www.healthyinteriors.com.au** for a direct link through to the app.

Checklists

Healthy home checklist

Ten tips to a healthy home	Can do	Done it
1. Beware of volatile organic compounds – VOCs VOCs are chemicals that escape or 'off-gas' into surrounding air. VOCs can be emitted from materials, finishes and products within the home and can trigger or contribute to illness.		
2. Understand the connection between environmental pollutants and health Did you know that the Australian Government and the CSIRO among many other organisations have documented that our indoor environment can cause and contribute to a range of illnesses?		
3. Look for nontoxic environmentally friendly products Opt for products that have minimised chemical intervention. Products that are nontoxic are better for your health, the health of your home and a better cleaner option for the environment.		
4. Look for independent certification on products Independent certification labels on products help you find items that have legitimate health or environmental credentials and help you avoid 'green washing'.		
5. Good ventilation and air flow Ventilation is essential to exhaust unwanted odours, water vapour and pollution, and replace them with fresh air. Use exhaust fans in wet areas and when cooking. Open windows and doors where possible to help remove indoor pollutants.		
6. Moisture Control – Avoid dampness and mould Avoid mould growth by lessening moisture levels in your home. This can be achieved by providing adequate ventilation. Mould can contribute to a range of health issues.		
7. Opt for natural materials and fibres Many natural materials and fibres have their own beneficial characteristics e.g. wool naturally has flame resistant and antibacterial properties.		
8. Avoid soft furnishings chemical treatments Question if soft furnishings have been chemically treated before you buy. Avoid stain resistant, UV resistant, antibacterial and flame retardant chemicals as these can break down into household dust and be ingested or inhaled. Contaminated dust has been documented as contributing to asthma, allergies and endocrine altering illnesses among others.		
9. Avoid plastics Plastics can contribute to indoor air pollution through off-gassing. Plastics can also release chemical pollutants into household dust.		
10. HEPA cleaning Use a vacuum appliance with HEPA (high efficiency particulate air) filtration when cleaning to trap fine dust particles and prevent them from being released back into indoor air when cleaning.		

Copyright © Healthy Interiors 2014.

Asthma & allergy home checklist

Bedding	Can do	Done it
Wash bedding such as sheets and pillow cases once a week in water at a minimum of 55-60°C if possible to kill mites.		
Tumble drying bedding on a hot setting for in excess of 10 minutes will also kill mites, if you are unable to wash in hot water or leave items in hot sun (indoors to avoid pollens).		
Place pillows and blankets in the hot sun (for minimum of three hours) or air them on a regular basis to kill mites. Dry the items to prevent mould that may occur from perspiration moisture (especially in summer months).		
Keep soft toys in the bedroom environment to a minimum (ideally none in the bed).		
Wash soft toys regularly at 55-60°C or place soft toys in the freezer overnight to kill dust mites.		
Opt for organic cotton bed sheeting and natural fibre blankets such as organic cotton or wool.		
Avoid PVC mattress protectors.		

Floors	Can do	Done it
Vacuum weekly using a HEPA filter vacuum cleaner.		
Take shoes off at the front door to prevent walking allergens through the house.		
If buying new carpet, opt for a low pile carpet to minimise the area for dust and particles to be hidden.		
Use nontoxic natural cleaner to reduce the residue, VOCs and spread of chemicals throughout the home.		

Windows	Can do	Done it
Open windows regularly to flush the build-up of indoor pollutants (gases from furnishings etc.) out.		
If suffering from hay fever, opening windows in high pollen seasons is not helpful, in this instance opt for an air purifier to clean indoor air as well as removing pollen pollutants.		
Heavy curtains are not recommended as these are difficult to clean and can harbour dust. Blinds that are easily cleaned are a good alternative to drapes/curtains.		
Opt for blinds made of natural materials free from plasticisers and chemical treatments.		

Furniture	Can do	Done it
Avoid vinyl furniture as it contains phthalates (plastic softeners) that may migrate into household dust and will off-gas when new.		
Dust mites are attracted to fabric so vacuum fabric furniture regularly using a HEPA filter vacuum.		
Opt for furniture that has not had stain resistant and flame retardant treatments, as these treatments can break down over time and be released into the home environment.		
Remove any raw MDF (medium density fibreboard) or particle boards as these often contain formaldehyde, a known respiratory irritant.		

Décor	Can do	Done it
Clutter provides an environment for dust to accumulate – reduce clutter and store items away.		
Children's toys and games can be stored in baskets or boxes made from natural fibres such as sea grass to minimise plastics indoors and keep toys free from dust.		
Avoid plastics where possible.		
Avoid soft furnishings that accumulate dust; opt for easy to clean products		

Bathroom	Can do	Done it
Mould can contribute to allergies and in some cases other illnesses – an effective air extraction fan is needed to remove steam and moisture from the air when water is being used.		
Opt for fabric shower curtains rather than plasticised options – PVC shower curtains can release toxic gases when they are heated by hot water.		
Regularly clean bathroom surfaces with nontoxic cleaners to avoid chemical exposure.		
Attach a filter to shower and/or bath outlets to remove chlorine (fluoride removal is more expensive) from the water. Chlorine is harsh on the skin and hot water containing chlorine can result in VOC emissions while showering.		

Kitchen	Can do	Done it
Clean using nontoxic cleaners as surfaces wiped can inadvertently be ingested after food preparation.		
Drink filtered water.		
Ensure that an effective exhaust fan/rangehood is being used over the cooktop when cooking to remove combustion pollutants, cooking fumes and moisture.		
Excess moisture in the kitchen can cause mould growth - wipe kitchen surfaces after use to prevent food contamination, germs and remove the temptation of crumbs to pests.		
Use a bin that has a lid to minimise the attraction to household pests and pets.		

Cleaning	Can do	Done it
Wiping dusty surfaces with a damp cloth will minimise dust being airborne when cleaning.		
Use a HEPA vacuum to reduce dust & pollutants being airborne when vacuuming.		
Use nontoxic cleaners preferably non-fragranced for all surfaces to minimise pollutant triggers.		
Avoid using fragranced air freshener products, including essential oils.		
Use sensitive washing powder free from artificial fragrances, optical brighteners, phosphates, petrochemical surfactants and enzymes. Opt for plain soap powder and rinse well.		
Avoid hanging clothing or bedding outside to dry for those with pollen or severe dust allergies.		
Wash pillow cases regularly to remove pollutants and place pillow in hot sun on still, no breeze days to air (this is not suitable for hay fever sufferers – place pillow in a sunny spot inside to avoid pollens)		
Wash work clothes separate to family washing.		
Do not wear dry cleaned clothing straight away, ideally avoid this cleaning method unless dry cleaned without toxic chemicals e.g. steamed.		
Wash all new clothing and linen before using.		
Remove mould as soon as visible, identify cause and rectify (follow removal instructions in the maintenance section).		
HEPA vacuum soft furnishings & window furnishings regularly (with clean attachment).		

Household practices	Can do	Done it
Take shoes off at the front door to prevent walking pollutants through the house.		
Opt for natural personal care products such as hair products, soaps & deodorant to avoid absorbing, inhaling or ingesting product chemicals.		
Avoid synthetic fragranced air products, opt for natural fragrances such as fresh cut flowers.		
Avoid scented products such as cosmetics, stationery, potpourri, incense sticks and burnt oils.		
Avoid burning petro chemically derived candles - opt for bees wax candles with lead free wicks if needed (although best to avoid where possible).		
Avoid tobacco smoke – no smoking in or around the home.		
Avoid combustion pollutants from open fires or un-flued gas heaters – opt for clean air heating such as hydronic heating, electric heating or flued gas heating (ducted heating can increase dust distribution).		
If direct neighbours' cigarette smoke or open fire combustion pollutants are in the air keep windows closed.		
On days where bushfire or building smoke is in the air, close up doors and windows and use an air purifier if available.		
To minimise the spread of pollen (for hay fever sufferers) indoors, place worn clothes in the laundry straight after wearing them outside (not in the bedroom).		
Keep shoes out of the bedroom, create a space (box, cupboard, basket, stand) for them near the door.		

General	Can do	Done it
Remove shoes at the front door to avoid walking pollutants through the home.		
Keeping the indoor environment at a fairly constant temperature will help minimise condensation or humidity which can result in excess moisture and mould growth.		
Wipe surfaces with condensation quickly to remove moisture and eliminate any interior moisture sources such as drying wet clothes inside or ineffective cooking or drying exhaust systems.		
A dehumidifier can be used in the home where humidity is constantly high.		
Keep internal doors open throughout the house to assist with even temperature distribution which will assist to reduce condensation.		
Regularly clean exhaust fans to ensure they remain efficient.		
Repair any indoor water damage immediately.		

Home maintenance	Can do	Done it
Repair any leaks or moisture damaged surfaces quickly to prevent moisture and mould growth.		
Regularly clean filters on heating and cooling units to prevent air pushing past trapped dust and mould that can be recirculated in the home.		
Regularly clean exhaust extraction fans to allow them to work efficiently.		
Regularly air and vacuum mattresses.		
Regularly vacuum floors and window coverings to remove dust.		
Opt for natural physical pest management products where needed such as traps and baits; avoid sprays that can be inhaled and pollute indoor air while leaving a chemical residue around the home.		
If renovating or buying new materials or products for the home opt for low emission, natural materials where possible.		

Pets	Can do	Done it
Pet allergens are often reactions to the pet's saliva or skin cells that are regularly shed. If you are allergic to an animal that resides in the home, the most effective strategy is for the animal to live outside of the house or be re-homed depending on severity.		
If rehoming is not an option, keep contact with the pet to a minimum and keep pets out of the bedroom.		
Don't keep unwashed clothing in the bedroom.		
Shower before bed and change into clean bedding to minimise pet skin cells being carried into the bed.		
Change pillow cases frequently to minimise the inhalation of collected dust.		
Vacuum carpets, mattresses and upholstery regularly with a HEPA filter vacuum.		
Using a saline nose spray before bed may help remove any inhaled allergens to assist with a good night's sleep.		

Garden	Can do	Done it
If suffering from allergies associated with pollens, keep windows and doors closed during peak pollen times.		
Wear glasses or sunglasses when outdoors to minimise airborne pollens entering the eyes.		
Keep windows and doors closed when nearby lawns are being mowed.		
Avoid gardening – ask someone else to attend to the garden during pollen seasons.		
When landscaping opt for allergy friendly plant species to reduce pollens directly around the home.		
Shower and change clothing after spending time in the garden during pollen seasons to minimise the spread of pollens indoors.		
When working in the garden be sure to wear protective clothing to prevent any bites or stings.		

Copyright © Healthy Interiors 2014.

Healthy home renovating checklist

Ten tips to renovating safely	Can do	Done it
1. **Asbestos inspection** – have a pre-renovation asbestos inspection to identify any asbestos and have it removed in accordance with safety guidelines by an approved removalist before starting a renovation.		
2. **Avoid hazardous chemicals** – specify low emission and low toxicity product options to be used where possible.		
3. **Research non toxic** – Identify environmentally friendly products before commencing the project to avoid using whatever is convenient at the time.		
4. **Look for independently "Certified" products** – certifications assist with product claim verification.		
5. **Designated waste area** – separate recyclable product to other waste. Recyclable products can at times be sold or when separated can cost less to have removed.		
6. **Remove hazardous materials** – remove from site quickly in accordance with industry standards to prevent site contamination, such as soil.		
7. **Have disposable N-95 masks on hand** – mask up when inspecting the site during dusty phases, especially for children, available from the hardware store.		
8. **Designated cutting area** – designate an area close to works where cutting is to occur to prevent trades from using multiple sites on different days. This will minimise the spread of dust from various materials.		
9. **Ventilation** – where possible have windows and doors open during work for maximum air flow to reduce indoor VOCs.		
10. **Clean trades** – request that all trades clean up after themselves as they go to minimise the spread of pollutants and minimise the need for harsh cleaners to be used on surfaces at the completion of works.		

Copyright © Healthy Interiors 2014.

Extreme heat healthy home checklist

With extreme weather events occurring more frequently and the forecast for hotter summers, the following tips can help prepare the home and family for times of extreme heat.

Tips for resilience and staying healthy in extreme heat	Can do	Done it
Establish an emergency action plan with family in the event that telecommunication services are not available and family are not able to get home for any reason e.g. fire or cancelled transport services.		
If you live in an area subject to fire risk ensure you have a fire plan, to learn about how to create a fire plan, visit **www.cfa.vic.gov.au/plan-prepare/fire-ready-kit**		
Have a supply of drinking water stored in the event that tap water is not drinkable, e.g. due to fire contamination.		
Have water filled bottles in the freezer ready for use in an esky/cooler should the power be disconnected and food needs to be kept cold. When the water has melted it can also be used as drinking water if necessary.		
Have an electrolyte product (dehydration prevention) and first aid supplies at home. If power is turned off in the area, pharmacies may close and access to these types of products may be limited.		
Arrange to work from home if possible to avoid delayed or cancelled public transport.		
Investigate if there is a fire app for your area and use this along with local radio or television to keep informed in case situations arise that you may need to respond to.		
If there is smoke outdoors as a result of fires, keep doors and windows closed. Using the air conditioner will assist to filter the indoor air. If you have an air purifier using these will also assist to purify combustion pollutants from the indoor air.		
If outdoor temperatures fall at night (assuming there is no smoke from fires), open doors and windows to the house where possible to help cool the interior of the home. Leave these open for as long as possible (exhaust fans can help draw out hot air) and close doors and windows just before the outdoor temperature starts to rise above the temperature in the house.		
People who suffer from respiratory or cardiac complaints should remain indoors when smoke is in the air to avoid inhaling irritants.		

Table continued next page.

Tips for resilience and staying healthy in extreme heat	Can do	Done it
Keep internal window coverings closed during the day to assist with keeping heat out.		
Also keep external awnings down over windows during the day to prevent the sun reaching the window and heat being absorbed into the house. If you have windows without window coverings use temporary coverings to shield the interior from the sun's heat. For those without external awnings in single level buildings, temporary awnings may also be an option.		
Keep a set of P2 masks (available from the hardware store) in your car and in the house. These should be used in any situation where you may be exposed to concentrated pollutants such as encountering a fire in your travels.		
Keep a torch near the bed as extreme weather events can result in electricity being disconnected at any time.		
Stay out of regional bush areas with limited access at times of extreme heat as fire risk is high.		
Pack away any outdoor furniture as extreme heat can cause damage.		
Move portable potted plants into a shaded area together to protect them. Water plants in the evening or morning avoiding the hottest part of the day.		
Avoid being outdoors during the day. Stay indoors where possible to avoid the heat. If you don't have air conditioning in your home, visiting venues that are cooled is an option to stay cool such as a shopping centre, movie theatre, restaurant, gallery, entertainment centre or visit with friends and family.		
Keep family cool and hydrated by drinking small amounts of fluids often, especially children and the elderly. Cool baths or showers can help cool body temperature and frozen fruit pieces can be fun, hydrating and cooling for children. Keep pets cool with a constant supply of water.		

Copyright © Healthy Interiors 2014.

Healthy home maintenance checklist

Ongoing home maintenance can prevent costly repairs and assist to keep the interior of a home operating efficiently while maximising health attributes.

Tips for home maintenance	Can do	Done it
1. Dust – dust using a damp cloth to prevent dust containing pollutants from being airborne		
2. Air – Air pillows and mattresses regularly		
3. Heating & cooling – clean filters regularly to prevent trapped pollutants from being recirculated and keep the unit operating efficiently		
4. Repairs – action home repairs quickly to prevent deterioration and potential structural damage e.g. moisture damage and mould. Repair upholstered items without delay to avoid exposed foams		
5. Replenish – replenish surface coatings as needed to prevent deterioration which may lead to pollutants contaminating household dust		
6. Check – check batteries in alarm devices – smoke alarm, carbon monoxide alarm		
7. Remove – remove dust from soft furnishing regularly with a HEPA filter vacuum – lounge suites, window coverings, rugs and mattresses		
8. Extraction – check all exhaust fans (laundry, kitchen, bathroom) to ensure they are working properly and clean the covers to maximise air extraction		
9. Clean – clean seals and filters in appliances to remove trapped pollutants or bacterial growth – washing machine, clothes dryer, dishwasher		
10. Water – replace water filters in accordance with manufacturer's instructions to prevent compromised water quality		
11. Guttering – clean guttering regularly to prevent the build-up of debris that may force water into the building structure that can result in water damage, moisture and mould growth		
12. Utilities – turn off water and gas meter and note the reading before going on a short holiday. Check meters on return to check there are no leaks in the system. Only turn off water if no automated watering systems		
13. Gas heating – have internal gas heating units serviced in accordance with manufacturer's guidelines to ensure combustion pollutants are not leaking into the indoor air		

Copyright © Healthy Interiors 2014.

Draught-proofing checklist

How to use this checklist

This checklist has been created to help you find and fix the draughts in your home. The list is zoned into the various areas of a home to make it as easy as possible to identify where to look.

The first step is to work through the list and seal the obvious gaps. You'll need this checklist and a pen. Work through this list, checking off what you find needs draught-proofing, then check it off when fixed. When you have fixed all the obvious gaps, you can progress to the next step.

The second step is to depressurise the home by closing all doors and windows, and turn off any heating and cooling systems. You'll need a notepad, pen and incense stick. Turn on all externally vented exhaust fans and the kitchen rangehood. Choose a windy day if you can. Then light the incense stick and use it to find air movement where smoke is blown back into the home as this signifies an air leak. Note the location and seal it after checking all areas of the home.

Indoor checklist

General – It might be difficult to check this but if you can...	Found	Fixed
Ducting – check for gaps in insulation and joins in any ducting		

Kitchen	Found	Fixed
Doors and windows between architrave frame and wall		
Doors and window between door/window and architrave		
Gaps between floorboards, walls and skirting		
Cracks in walls or ceiling		
Gaps around power points and where services go through walls		
Gaps/leaks around skylights		
Exhaust fans (should be closed when not in use)		
Heating/cooling vents (particularly evaporative cooling vents)		
Fixed open vents (wall or ceiling)		
Downlights		

Family / Living / Lounge Rooms	Found	Fixed
Doors and windows between architrave frame and wall		
Doors and window between door/window and architrave		
Gaps between floorboards, walls and skirting		
Cracks in walls or ceiling		
Gaps around power points and where services go through walls		
Gaps/leaks around skylights		
Exhaust fans (should be closed when not in use)		
Heating/cooling vents (particularly evaporative cooling vents)		
Fixed open vents (wall or ceiling)		
Down lights		
Pet doors		
Chimneys		

Table continued next page.

Laundry	Found	Fixed
Doors and windows between architrave frame and wall		
Doors and window between door/window and architrave		
Gaps between floorboards, walls and skirting		
Cracks in walls or ceiling		
Gaps around power points and where services go through walls		
Gaps/leaks around skylights		
Exhaust fans (should be closed when not in use)		
Fixed open vents (wall or ceiling)		
Downlights		
Pet doors		
Loft / roof space entrance		

Bathrooms and Toilets	Found	Fixed
Doors and windows between architrave frame and wall		
Doors and window between door/window and architrave		
Gaps between floorboards, walls and skirting		
Cracks in walls or ceiling		
Gaps around power points and where services go through walls		
Gaps/leaks around any skylights		
Exhaust fans (should be closed/self-sealing when not in use)		
Fixed open vents (wall or ceiling)		
Downlights		

Bedrooms	Found	Fixed
Doors and windows between architrave frame and wall		
Doors and window between door/window and architrave		
Gaps between floorboards, walls and skirting		
Cracks in walls or ceiling		
Gaps around power points and where services go through walls		
Gaps/leaks around skylights		
Exhaust fans (should be closed when not in use)		
Heating/cooling vents (particularly evaporative cooling vents)		
Fixed open vents (wall or ceiling)		
Downlights		
Chimneys		

Outside checklist

Garage / carport	Found	Fixed
Gaps around the door between garage and house		
Gaps under garage door		
Gaps around other doors/windows in the garage area		

Outside services	Found	Fixed
Gaps and cracks where plumbing and services come through walls		

Build and renovate checklist

To make a new home a more cost efficient and comfortable, consider including the following sustainable features when you next build or renovate. If you can, you'll reap the benefits for years to come. This is a guide only, for specific advice speak with a sustainability advisor.

What	Do during building	Cheaper during building but can do later	Anytime
Orientate main living areas to north side	✓		
Plan north facing roof line for future solar appliances	✓		
Ensure appropriate eaves all-round the home	✓		
Insulation in ceiling, walls and under floor	✓		
Keep all wet areas together	✓		
Lag all hot water pipes	✓	✓	
Use recycled/renewable materials if you can	✓	✓	
Include rainwater tanks, plumb into toilets and laundry (what stage is the best depends on the home)	✓	✓	✓
Include sealed skylights for natural light to internal areas		✓	
Install appropriate window types and glazing for the local climate		✓	
Low energy lighting (LED is best, then CFL). Avoid downlights		✓	
Ensure all exhaust fans are self-closing and externally vented		✓	✓
Get a light (white/light cream) coloured roof		✓	
Light colours outside of the house on walls		✓	
Install an efficient hot water system		✓	
Install 5+ star energy rated appliances (e.g. fridge)		✓	✓

Table continued next page.

What	Do during building	Cheaper during building but can do later	Anytime
Set up grey water system to plants (not food)		✓	✓
Install ceiling fans (some have lights)		✓	✓
Install dual flush toilets		✓	
Install water efficient shower heads and tapware		✓	✓
Heating/cooling, best to have zoned system or separate unit in each room (6+ star rating)		✓	✓
Use heavy backed close fitting curtains or roman blinds with pelmets on windows			✓
Use solar garden lighting and security lights			✓

For later consideration	Do during building	Cheaper during building but can do later	Anytime
Select renewable energy from your energy provider			✓
Install renewable energy (solar power, wind turbine)		✓	✓
Use shade sails, blinds or deciduous trees to protect in summer			✓
Plant fruit trees and herbs			✓
Set up a vegetable patch			✓
Set up a compost heap and/or worm farm			✓
Plant drought tolerant plants elsewhere			✓

What to look for in a home checklist

How to use this Checklist

This short checklist has been created to help you identify some of the key resource efficiency items in a home (think energy and water use items), so that you know what to look for and what to ask about when you are looking for a new home. Further information on key items can be on the page following and are highlighted in **bold** below.

Take this with you when you look at homes and check off the relevant items as you go. Use the 'Cost' column to note if any retrofit item would be high or low cost to do. The more of these features, the more resource efficient a home should be.

The general building	Got it? Yes/No	Option to retrofit? Yes/No	Cost? High or Low
Is there......			
A Star Rating for this house? If so what is it?		n/a	
External shading on north and west facing windows and walls?			
Solar PV electricity generation? If so, what size?			
Any unshaded north facing roof space (potential for future solar)			
Are window types appropriate for the climate?			
Windows that can be opened for natural ventilation?			
Draught seals on all external doors and windows?			
Good insulation in the ceiling? (you'll need to ask)			
What is the...			
Hot water system? (refer notes over page)			
Heating system? (refer notes over page)			
Cooling system? Shading and fans are better than air conditioners			

Kitchen & family living areas	Got it? Yes/No	Option to retrofit? Yes/No	Cost? High or Low
Is there.....			
North facing living areas (that could be shaded in summer)?		n/a	
Good natural lighting?			
Low energy lighting in the area?			
Water efficient taps?			
Water and energy efficient appliances? (check star ratings)			

Outdoor area	Got it? Yes/No	Option to retrofit? Yes/No	Cost? High or Low
Is there.....			
An external clothes line?		n/a	
Room for herb pots or a veggie garden?			
Any productive fruit trees?			
Any rain water tanks and/or grey water recycling units?			

What's close	Walk? Yes/No	Bike? Yes/No	Need to drive? High or Low
Can you walk or bike ride to...			
Local public transport?		n/a	
Local shops and cafes?			
Amenities that you use often? (schools, community centres etc.)			

Items noted in **bold** can significantly affect the running cost of a home.

Star ratings

These provide information on the expected thermal performance of a home and relate to the building envelope (floor, walls, windows and roof) only. It does not take into account any other features of the home (e.g.: any solar power, heating systems, hot water, lighting etc.).

Any home built since 2003 should have a star rating of at least 5 stars. Homes built since May 2012 should be 6 star or higher. Older homes are unlikely to be rated and generally perform at around one star which is very inefficient. The difference is in the amount of energy required to heat and cool the home to keep it comfortable (referred to as 'active' heating or cooling). For example:

0-1 star rated home – estimated annual cost to heat/cool is around $ 4,080 pa

5 star rated home – estimated annual cost to heat/cool is around $ 1,344 pa

6 star rated home – estimated annual cost to heat/cool is around $ 1,056 pa

If you're building, consider:

Eight star rated homes have an estimated annual cost to heat/cool of around $528 pa

A 10 star rated home is considered to be thermally comfortable without the need for active heating or cooling. Estimated annual cost to heat/cool $ 0.

Good insulation in the ceiling

If the home is star rated as noted above, the ceiling (and external walls) should be well insulated. If the home is older ask the owner how old the insulation in the ceiling is (if any). Insulation that is older than 20 years is likely to need replacing. Insulation can reduce your heating and cooling costs by up to 55 percent and is a worthwhile investment.

Heating system

The type of heating system in the home can affect the running costs by up to 50 percent. Electric under floor heating is the most expensive to run. Highly efficient zoned heating is the most cost effective. In our view, gas boosted solar (or gas fired) zoned hydronic heating is the best, closely followed by a highly efficient zoned ducted gas system or reverse cycle (inverter type) electric units in each room. Pellet fires and some wood burners are also extremely effective and would be suitable in certain situations.

Hot water

Gas boosted solar is the cheapest to run, costing on average $115 pa, efficient gas is the next cheapest to run at $317 pa, off peak electric costs from $807 upwards while electric peak costs from $1,296 pa. These estimates are from Sustainability Victoria and based on usage of 260 litres/day. Note that energy prices change regularly and technology is rapidly improving so check the details each time you need to replace a hot water unit.

North facing living areas

If a home has north facing living areas, you generally have good natural lighting and access to passive solar heating which can help you to reduce heating costs during winter. For each square metre of glass the sun directly hits, it radiates in around 35 percent more which provides heat to your room. Think of your car parked out in the sun on a cool day – it's warm when you get in, isn't it! It's the same for a home.

Good natural lighting

Natural light is not only good for our health; it saves on electricity by not having to turn lights on. It can usually be easily accessed through windows, glazed doors, solar tubes and sky lights. If there are dark areas in the home, often hallways, bathrooms, toilets, kitchens and laundries, see if it's possible to incorporate some natural light. The right solution will depend on the home.

Energy smart checklist

This checklist has been created to help you reduce energy waste and save money. The list is zoned into the various rooms of a home to make it easy to go through the home.

With a few simple actions you can make a difference to your energy bills. Be smart, be efficient and spend the savings on something fun!

Indoor checklist

Whole of house items	Can do	Done it
Always buy energy and water efficient appliances		
Hot water (storage systems) check temp is set to 65°C		
Insulate hot water pipes where possible		
Insulate any ducting and check there are no leaks		
Draught-proof the home (see our DIY Draught-Proofing Checklist)		
Reduce the set temperature on the heating in winter (aim for 19°C)		
In winter, close window coverings to help maintain warmth in the home		
In summer, shade the windows to minimise heat gain in the home		
Increase the set temperature for cooling in summer (aim for 25°C)		
Use energy saving lighting (LED, CFL or fluoros) and turn off when not needed		

In the Kitchen	Can do	Done it
Only fill the kettle with enough water for the number of drinks you are making		
Cook with the lid on saucepans and turn the temp down on the cooker		
Use the microwave or bench to defrost food (not hot water or the oven)		
Minimise oven use where possible and keep door closed when in use		
Only run the dishwasher when full and use the 'short' or 'eco' cycle		
Turn chargers, computers and electronics off at the power when not charging		
Check the seals on the fridge and ensure it is well ventilated		
Check fridge temperature is 4°C, freezer is -18°C		

Family / Living / Lounge Rooms	Can do	Done it
Use standby power cut out switches to reduce standby power waste		
Make sure all gaming equipment is off when not in use		
Use a fan before turning on the air conditioner		
Use a fan in conjunction with an air conditioner and turn up the set temp		

Laundry	Can do	Done it
Only run washing machine when full and spin on high to assist fast drying		
Minimise use of the dryer; air dry on the line or a drying rack instead		
Wash in cold water when you can		

Bathrooms & Toilets	Can do	Done it
Use water saving shower heads and basin taps, it reduces hot water energy		

Bedrooms	Can do	Done it
Turn off any chargers at the power point when not charging the device		
Use low energy lamps for reading		

Outside checklist

Garage / carport / shed	Can do	Done it
Beer fridge (empty into kitchen fridge and turn off when not needed)		
Turn off any electrical tools etc. at the power point when not in use		

Pools and spas	Can do	Done it
Use the cover when it's not in use		
Minimise pool pump running times when you can		
If heated, opt for solar heating and turn it off for winter and when away		

Irrigation systems	Can do	Done it
Check timer settings appropriate for expected weather		

Other	Can do	Done it
Install solar garden lighting, it's easy and costs nothing to run		
Consider green roofs or vertical gardens to shelter the building from sun		

© Green Moves Aust.Energy Smart Checklist 2014.

Water smart checklist

This checklist has been created to help you find and fix any water leaks in your home. The list is zoned into the various wet areas of a home for checking. The second page gives you tips on how to reduce water use around the home.

First, work through the checklist and fix any drips/leaks you find. Look for tell-tale signs of water marks or dampness.

Second, apply the tips on the next page to save even more!

If you think you have a leak you can't see, use the water meter to find out. Read the meter before and after a 6 hour (or longer) period when no water is being used in the home (make sure everything is off and the toilet is not flushed). If the meter has a different reading there is probably a leak somewhere.

Stop leaks checklist

Inside checklist

Kitchen	Leak FOUND	Leak FIXED
Kitchen tap ware		
Kitchen plumbing under the sink (include garbage disposal units)		
Dishwasher connections and plumbing		
Refrigerator connections (if plumbed into mains water)		

Laundry	Leak FOUND	Leak FIXED
Laundry tapware		
Plumbing under the laundry sink		
Connections and taps feeding washing machine		

Bathrooms & Toilets	Leak FOUND	Leak FIXED
Toilet leaks (use a few drops of food dye to see if dripping into bowl)		
Toilet – check around base		
Basin tap ware		
Basin under sink plumbing		
Bath tapware		
Check bath plug does not leak		
Shower tapware and shower head		

Outside checklist

Around the house	Leak FOUND	Leak FIXED
Garden taps		
Rain water tank connections and feeder pipes		
Grey water connections and feeder pipes		
Irrigation system lines and drippers		

Pools and spas	Leak FOUND	Leak FIXED
Check filter and pump connections		

Water smart checklist

General things	Could do	Doing it
Always buy water efficient appliances and tapware		

In the kitchen	Could do	Doing it
Only use dishwasher when full		
Rinse dishes in a sink of water, not under running water		
Wash veggies in a large bowl then put the used water onto plants		
Install a flow restrictor on the kitchen tap		
Only use enough water to cover the veggies for cooking and use the lid		
Thaw frozen foods in the microwave or on the bench instead of running water		
Keep a container of cold water in the fridge (to contain the water that you otherwise waste while waiting for hot water to arrive)		
Minimise use of garbage disposal units, use a compost bin, green cone or worms		

In the laundry	Could do	Doing it
Only run the washing machine with a full load, adjust the water setting if not full		
Minimise washing by wearing clothes more than once (if not smelly or too dirty)		
Divert rinse water to the garden (not food plants) if you can		
Front loaders are more energy and water efficient		

Bathrooms and toilets	Could do	Doing it
In the toilet, use the ½ flush when appropriate		
Get the boys to wee on the citrus trees in the garden once a day (good for the garden and saves a flush)		
If you don't have a dual flush toilet, place a 1.5L bottle of water in the cistern to displace water, or replace with a dual flush model		
Turn the tap off when brushing teeth and shaving (rinse razor in the sink)		
If the basin tap isn't water efficient, install a flow restrictor		
Take shorter showers and turn the water off between soaping up and rinsing off		
Catch the water in a bucket while the shower's warming up and reuse on plants		
Use a shower timer, especially with kids!		
Share a bath with a friend or kids can share to save water		

Around the house	Could do	Doing it
Plant drought resistant plants		
Use mulch in garden beds and around trees to minimise evaporation		
Use irrigation systems and water plants sub surface		
Use a broom or blower to clean driveways and paving, not a hose		
Wash the car on the grass using a bucket, use the hose only to rinse off		
Install a rain water collection tank and use it on the garden, pool, toilet or laundry		
Reuse grey water where you can		

Pools and spas	Could do	Doing it
Use a cover when not in use to minimise evaporation		
Top up from rain water tanks if you can		
Discourage splashing and activities that spill water		

© Green Moves Aust. Water Smart Checklist 2014.

Conclusion

The saying 'buyer beware' rings loud when it comes to purchasing products for the home. Until labelling laws are overhauled to disclose all materials used within a product and highlight those that cause harm to human health, consumers need to think about and question the ingredients and materials in consumables to consciously create a healthy home and minimise environmental pollutants indoors.

The reality for Australian families is that sustainable living success (or not) largely emanates from personal lifestyle decisions, many concerning the home environment.

Many of the sustainability initiatives communicated to the community are actions promoted for 'future' benefits – a message of act today to ensure the health of the future.

There is largely a lack of understanding that making healthy sustainable decisions on a daily basis is essential and beneficial for all of us who are alive now (not just future generations). The exciting news for families as outlined in this book is that families are privileged to have choice, the ability to take preventative action each day to preserve or improve their quality of life. Creating a healthy, sustainable home today is beneficial for individuals now and the greater environment for the future – a message of act today for today and tomorrow.

Families want to know how to make wise product decisions for themselves, however as illustrated in these chapters there are fundamental issues that are making this extremely difficult – such as inadequate product labelling and product standard inadequacies in many sectors.

This book has touched on some industry insights, information families need to make informed, healthy, sustainable lifestyle choices. A life lesson mentioned early in the book was, 'money makes the world go around', and this very sentiment is likely the reason products that are potentially harmful continue to be produced for sale and many products hide behind fancy labels with no specific information.

It is disturbing to see our hospitals continue to bulge at the seams, many disease statistics continue to rise, many with environmental triggers. Meanwhile families wade through a minefield of pollutants every day in the form of prettily packaged products that largely hide the facts that many are made using ingredients that are potentially harmful – in the form of foods, personal care products, cleaning products, household products, furnishings and building products.

The following are some consistent messages we hear from authorities – all with an interesting common thread:

- Our health care system is not coping with increasingly sick people
- Look after your health – be fit and healthy
- Be mindful of the environment and be energy-resource efficient
- We need to reduce pollution

The common thread above is consumption (products)!

The concerning question is - How do people make informed, healthy, sustainable product choices when products are not required to be 100 percent transparent about how they are made and what pollutants they contain?

While further Government intervention into product standards and labelling could make improvements to the status quo, so too can industry, suppliers and retailers if they chose to do so. Some products and brands are voluntarily more transparent than others, although sadly for many companies, chasing the dollar is more important than the health of their customers.

As individuals understand that daily choices impact on family health outcomes, a significant personal incentive evolves. A value can be identified as to the 'now' benefits of investing personal time, energy and money into healthy sustainable social change – healthy, efficient sustainable homes. The uptake of sustainable lifestyle choices for the benefit of personal health is:

- a win for human health
- a win for families
- a win for the health system
- a win for the environment

The knowledge in this book highlights that living simply is a solid foundation for a healthy, efficient, sustainable home.

We cannot avoid all the pollutants that surround us each day and it's not practical to try to do so. However, through making informed decisions and asking more questions, we can significantly reduce the pollutants that make their way into our home and body. A healthy sustainable home benefits you and your family and has a flow-on effect to the community through waste reduction, industry demand, pollution, water and air consequences.

In doing something positive for yourself and your family you are making a positive difference for the future.

A smart way to live!

Glossary of terms

Term	Meaning
Active Cooling	Cooling systems that are mechanical and require energy to run. i.e. air conditioners and fans
Active Heating	Heating systems that are mechanical and require energy, i.e. gas central heating systems, reverse cycle heating systems
Ammonia	Ammonia (NH3) is one of the most commonly produced industrial chemicals. It is used in industry and commerce, and also exists naturally in humans and in the environment. Ammonia is essential for many biological processes and serves as a precursor for amino acid and nucleotide synthesis. In the environment, ammonia is part of the nitrogen cycle and is produced in soil from bacterial processes. Ammonia is also produced naturally from decomposition of organic matter, including plants, animals and animal wastes
Beam angle	The outer angle of the light emitted form a light source at 50 percent of its centre beam intensity.
Benzene	Benzene is a chemical used as a constituent in motor fuels; as a solvent for fats, waxes, resins, oils, inks, paints, plastics, and rubber; in the extraction of oils from seeds and nuts; and in photogravure printing. It is also used as a chemical intermediate. Benzene is also used in the manufacture of detergents, explosives, pharmaceuticals, and dyestuffs.
Building envelope	The primary barrier between internal conditioned spaces, and the outside (external walls, roof, floor, windows and external facing doors)
Bisphenol A	Bisphenol A (BPA) is a chemical produced in large quantities for use primarily in the production of polycarbonate plastics and epoxy resins. Polycarbonate plastics have any applications including use in some food and drink packaging and dental products.
CFL	Compact Fluorescent Lighting, usually in a coiled type lamp. Note these contain mercury and special care is required for disposal and clean up if broken.
Colour Rendering Index (CRI)	The Colour Rendering Index (CRI) is a measure of how well a light source can accurately display colours compared to natural light. It is expressed as percentage.
Colour temperature	Measured in 'degrees Kelvin'. Kelvin temperature is a numerical measurement that describes the colour and appearance of the light produced by the lamp and the colour appearance of the lamp itself, expressed on the Kelvin (K) scale. This indicates the hue or colour of a light source.
Cooling load	The amount of energy required to cool an enclosed space at a constant temperature (i.e. 22°C). Generally specified in watts per square metre of floor area (W/m2)
Condensation	Air contains invisible water vapour. The higher the air temperature, the more water vapour it can hold. The lower the air temperature the less water vapour it can hold. When the air cools below a temperature known as the 'dew point', invisible water vapour condenses to visible water droplets on the cold surface. The water that is formed is known as condensate and the process is called condensation.
Earth Coupling	Building with a high value thermal mass product into the ground to take advantage of the earth's constant temperature at relevant depths.
Efficacy	The ratio of light output to power input measured in lumens per watt.
Emissivity	Often called Thermal Emissivity. A surface condition that emits low levels of radiant thermal heat energy. The value given to materials based on the ratio of heat emitted compared to a black body (emissivity of 1) on a scale from 1 to 0, where 0 is a perfect reflector.

Term	Meaning
Endocrine Disruptors	Endocrine Disruptors are chemicals that may interfere with the body/s endocrine system and produce adverse developmental, reproductive, neurological and immune effects in both humans and wildlife. A wide range of substances both natural and man-made are thought to cause endocrine disruption.
Formaldehyde	A colourless water-soluble gas. Due to its wide use, it is frequently considered separately from other VOCs. Materials containing formaldehyde include building materials, furnishing, and some consumer products. Formaldehyde has a pungent odour and is detected by many people at levels of about 100 parts per billion (ppb). Besides the annoyance, it also causes acute eye burning and irritates mucous membranes and the respiratory tract. The USA Environmental Protection Agency has determined formaldehyde to be a probable human carcinogen.
GHG	Greenhouse Gas
Heating load	The amount of energy required to maintain a constant temperature (i.e. 20°C) in an enclosed space. Generally specified in watts per square metre of floor area (W/m2)
Kilowatt (kW)	The power rating of an appliance
Kilowatt hours (kWh)	The amount of power used per hour by an appliance
LED	Light Emitting Diode
Light efficiency	This is the percentage of power that is converted to light.
Lumens	The amount of light that is emitted from a bulb. A high number of lumens means it has a brighter light; lower lumens is a dimmer light.
Lux	The measurement of the amount of light over a given area. Generally measured in lux per m2
NABERS	National Australian Building Energy Rating System
NatHERS	National House Energy Rating System
Passive House	A home that is highly efficient, that works with the local environment and requires very little, if any, active heating and cooling.
Passive Design	A design approach that uses natural elements, such as sunlight and wind, to heat, cool, or light a building.
Passive Heating	Using the heat of the sun to heat a structure without relying on mechanical heating systems.
Passive Cooling	Using design features to cool a building without the need for mechanical cooling systems.
Perchloroethylene (Perc)	Tetrachloroethylene, also known as perchloroethylene, or perc, is the predominant chemical solvent used in dry cleaning. Perc is also used in the cleaning of metal machinery and to manufacture some consumer products and other chemicals. It is a clear, colourless liquid that has a sharp, sweet odour and evaporates quickly. It is an effective cleaning solvent and is used by most professional dry cleaners because it removes stains and dirt from all common types of fabrics. Perc is also a toxic chemical with both human health and environmental concerns

Term	Meaning
Polybrominated Diphenyl Ethers (PBDEs)	Polybrominated diphenyl ethers (PBDEs) include the commercial versions of pentabromodiphenyl ether (c-pentaBDE), octabromodiphenyl ether (c-octaBDE), and decabromodiphenyl ether (c-decaBDE). Each of these commercial products is a mixture composed of several PBDE congeners. PBDEs are used as flame retardants in a number of applications, including textiles, plastics, wire insulation, and automobiles.
Polychlorinated Biphenyl (PCB)	PCBs belong to a broad family of man-made organic chemicals known as chlorinated hydrocarbons. PCBs were domestically manufactured from 1929 until their manufacture was banned in 1979. They have a range of toxicity and vary in consistency from thin, light-coloured liquids to yellow or black waxy solids. Due to their non-flammability, chemical stability, high boiling point, and electrical insulating properties, PCBs were used in hundreds of industrial and commercial applications including electrical, heat transfer, and hydraulic equipment; as plasticisers in paints, plastics, and rubber products; in pigments, dyes, and carbonless copy paper; and many other industrial applications.
Phthalates (THAL-ates)	A family of man-made chemical compounds developed in the last century to be used in the manufacture of plastics, solvents and personal care products. Ingestion, inhalation, skin absorption and intravenous injection are all potential pathways of exposure
P2 mask	A particulate filter personal respiratory protection device is a close fitting mask worn for airborne precautions, which is capable of filtering 0.3mm particles. A P2/N95 respirator must comply with AS/NZS 1716:2009.1 The difference between N95 and P2 classification for respirator face masks is the N95 classification means the mask complies with USA testing requirements and the P2 classification indicates compliance with European testing requirements. www.health.qld.gov.au/chrisp/resources/fit_check_factsheet.pdf
Solar heat gain	The amount of heat gained through a window as a result of direct sunlight hitting the glass.
Sustainably sourced	A product that is created from renewable materials and where the embodied energy is minimal
Triclosan	Triclosan is an antimicrobial active ingredient contained in a variety of products where it acts to slow or stop the growth of bacteria, fungi, and mildew. Triclosan is an ingredient added to many consumer products to reduce or prevent bacterial contamination. It may be found in products such as clothing, kitchenware, furniture, and toys. It also may be added to antibacterial soaps and body washes, toothpastes, and some cosmetics.
Toluene	Toluene is a common ingredient in degreasers. It's a colourless liquid with a sweet smell and taste. It evaporates quickly. Toluene is found naturally in crude oil. It's used in oil refining and the manufacturing of paints, lacquers, explosives (TNT) and glues. In homes, toluene may be found in paint thinners, paint brush cleaners, nail polish, glues, inks and stain removers. Toluene is also found in car exhaust and the smoke from cigarettes
Volatile Organic Compounds (VOCs)	Volatile organic compounds are organic chemical compounds whose composition makes it possible for them to evaporate under normal atmospheric conditions of temperature and pressure.

References

Melissa's story
Endrocine Society of USA, 2009. Statement. www.ncbi.nlm.nih.gov/pmc/articles/PMC2726844

Missing ingredient in healthy lifestyle mantra
World Health Organisation, 2006. *The Development of WHO Guidelines for Indoor Air Quality Report on a working group meeting*, Bonn, Germany 23-24 October, Pg1
Available at www.euro.who.int/__data/assets/pdf_file/0007/78613/AIQIAQ_mtgrep_Bonn_Oct06.pdf

Toxic soup social experiment
Lantz, Dr S 2009. *Chemical Free Kids*, Joshua Books, Australia
Bader, W 2007. T*oxic Bedrooms – Your guide to a good night's sleep*, Freedom Press, CA, pg 42

International concerns
World Health Organisation, 2011 – International, Environmental & Occupational Cancers Fact Sheet No 350.
www.who.int/mediacentre/factsheets/fs350/en
Accessed online: 17/3/14

World Health Organisation Europe, 2006, Development of WHO Guidelines for Indoor Air Quality, Germany
www.somamedical.net/articles/pdf/Development_of_WHO_Guidelines_for_Indoor_Air_Quality.pdf
Accessed online: 17/3/14

World Health Organisation, 2014. News Release – 'Seven million premature deaths annually linked to air pollution' 25th March, 2014, Geneva, online pg 1
www.who.int/mediacentre/news/releases/2014/air-pollution/en
Accessed online: 28/3/14

Brown SK, 1997. *Indoor Air Quality, Australia: State of the Environment Technical Paper Series (Atmosphere)* CSIRO and Environment Australia, pg 12
http://secure.environment.gov.au/soe/1996/publications/technical/pubs/12indora.pdf

Meek, SL 1991. *'Health Issues' in Indoor Air Quality in Homes: Synthesising the Issues and Educating Consumers* J. Laquatra & S.A. Zaslow [eds.]
American Association of Housing Educators and Building Research Council, Small Homes Council, University of Illinois at Urbana - Champaign. pp. 12-16

CSIRO, 2001. Australia State of Knowledge Report 2001, Department of the Environment and Heritage
Accessed online 17/3/14

Mendell MJ, 2007. 'Indoor residential chemical emissions as risk factors for respiratory and allergic effects in children: a review.' International Journal of Indoor Environment and Health, Volume 17, issue 4. Abstract, p1
www.ncbi.nlm.nih.gov/pubmed/17661923
Accessed online: 17/3/14

Icahn School of Medicine at Mount Sinai, 2013. 'New York State's Children and the Environment: A Report from the Children's Environmental Health Centre' p2
www.mountsinai.org/static_files/MSMC/Files/Patient%20Care/Children/Childrens%20Environmental%20Health%20Center/NYS-Children-Environment.pdf
Accessed online: 17/3/14

Mount Sinai Hospital website, 2014. 'Importance of Children's Environmental Health'
www.mountsinai.org/patient-care/service-areas/children/areas-of-care/childrens-environmental-health-center/childrens-disease-and-the-environment
Accessed online: 17/3/14

Doll, S, *Children At Risk Report* 2004. Oregon Environmental Council
www.oeconline.org/resources/publications/reportsandstudies/childrenatrisk.pdf
Accessed online: 17/3/14

The American College of Obstetricians and Gynaecologists, 2013. 'Environmental Chemicals Harm Reproductive Health' published on The American Congress of Obstetricians and Gynaecologists' website.
www.acog.org/About_ACOG/News_Room/News_Releases/2013/Environmental_Chemicals_Harm_Reproductive_Health
Accessed online: 17/3/14

Department of Health and Aged Care, Commonwealth of Australia, 2000. 'Indoor Air Quality – A Report on Health Impacts and Management Options'
www.health.gov.au/internet/main/publishing.nsf/Content/ABEE2143025D6775CA257BF00021DE7E/$File/env_indoorair.pdf
Accessed online: 17/3/14

Australian Government Department of Environment website, 2014. 'Indoor Air Quality – Health effects as a result of exposure to pollutants'
www.environment.gov.au/topics/environment-protection/air-quality/indoor-air#fn4
Accessed online: 17/3/14

National Institutes of Health, US Department of Health & Human Services 2010. 'Reducing Environmental Cancer Risk: What we can do now' 2008 – 2009 Annual Report, President's Cancer Panel p111
http://deainfo.nci.nih.gov/advisory/pcp/annualReports/pcp08-09rpt/PCP_Report_08-09_508.pdf

International recognition - your home air matters

World Health Organisation, 2014. News Release 'Seven million premature deaths annually linked to air pollution' 25th March, 2014, Geneva
www.who.int/mediacentre/news/releases/2014/air-pollution/en
Accessed online: 28/3/14

Department of the Environment, Water, Heritage & Arts 2008. *Home: Design for lifestyle and the future - Technical Manual* – 4th edition

USA Environmental Protection Agency (USA EPA), 2009. An Introduction to Indoor Air Quality (Online)
www.epa.gov/iaq/voc.html
Accessed online: 25/8/09

Whittle Waxes, 2013. Understanding V.O.C and Toxicity
www.whittlewaxes.com.au/news/5053/understanding-voc-and-toxicity
Accessed online: 27/11/13

Brown S K, 1997. *Indoor Air Quality, Australia: State of the Environment Technical Paper Series (Atmosphere)* CSIRO and Environment Australia, pg 8
http://secure.environment.gov.au/soe/1996/publications/technical/pubs/12indora.pdf
Accessed online: 18/3/14

World Health Organisation, 2006. Development of WHO Guidelines for Indoor Air Quality
Report on a working group meeting, Bonn, Germany, 23-24 October, Pg 3, Pg 1
www.euro.who.int/__data/assets/pdf_file/0007/78613/AIQIAQ_mtgrep_Bonn_Oct06.pdf

CSIRO, 2000. Media Release – 'New home owners breathe toxic cocktail', Oct 11, 2000
www.csiro.au/files/mediarelease/mr2000/prtoxichrome.htm
Accessed online: 5/10/09

World Health Organisation – International, 2008. Children's Health and the Environment - WHO Training Package for the Health Sector
www.who.int/ceh/capacity/Indoor_Air_Pollution.pdf
Accessed online: 15/11/13

Sterling EM, Arundel A, Sterling TD, 1985. Criteria for Human Exposure to Humidity in Occupied Buildings, *ASHRAE Transactions*, Vol.91, Part 1, Page 621
www.sterlingiaq.com/photos/1044922973.pdf

Living by assumptions

The Cancer Council, 2013. 'Tobacco in Australia - The Costs of Smoking'
www.tobaccoinaustralia.org.au/chapter-17-economics/17-2-the-costs-of-smoking
Accessed online: 3/10/13

National Industrial Chemicals Notification and Assessment Scheme (Online)
www.nicnas.gov.au/about-nicnas/about-us/community
Accessed online: 20/11/13

National Toxicology Program
http://ntp.niehs.nih.gov/?objectid=7201637B-BDB7-CEBA-F57E39896A08F1BB
Accessed online: 20/11/13

Andrews D, 2013. 'New chemicals: Sell first, Test for safety later?' Environmental Working Group, USA.
www.ewg.org/enviroblog/2013/05/new-chemicals-sell-first-test-safety-later
Accessed online: 20/11/13

Mount Sinai Children's Environmental Health Center, 2014. Fact Sheet – Acetone, pg 2. New York, NY
www.mountsinai.org/static_files/MSMC/Files/Patient%20Care/Children/Childrens%20Environmental%20Health%20Center/Acetone.pdf
Accessed online: 23/3/14

Mount Sinai Children's Environmental Health Center Fact Sheet – Ammonia, pg 2. New York, NY
www.mountsinai.org/static_files/MSMC/Files/Patient%20Care/Children/Childrens%20Environmental%20Health%20Center/Ammonia.pdf
Accessed online: 23/3/14

Mount Sinai Children's Environmental Health Center Fact Sheet – Benzene, pg 2. New York, NY
www.mountsinai.org/static_files/MSMC/Files/Patient%20Care/Children/Childrens%20Environmental%20Health%20Center/Benzene.pdf
Accessed online: 23/3/14

USA Pediatric Environmental Health Specialty Units (PEHSU), 2008. BPA Patients Fact Sheet. Association of Occupational and Environmental Clinics, pg 2
www.mountsinai.org/static_files/MSMC/Files/Patient%20Care/Children/Childrens%20Environmental%20Health%20Center/BPA_Patient_Factsheet.pdf
Accessed online: 23/3/14

Mount Sinai Children's Environmental Health Center Fact Sheet – Carbon Monoxide, pg 2. New York, NY
www.mountsinai.org/static_files/MSMC/Files/Patient%20Care/Children/Childrens%20Environmental%20Health%20Center/Carbon%20Monoxide.pdf
Accessed online: 23/3/14

USA National Library of Medicine, 2014. Tox Town – Chlorine
http://toxtown.nlm.nih.gov/text_version/chemicals.php?id=8
Accessed online: 23/3/14

American College of Allergy, Asthma and Immunology, 2014. 'Chlorine Allergy – Reality or Myth?'
www.acaai.org/allergist/allergies/Types/other-allergies/Pages/chlorine-allergy.aspx
Accessed online: 23/3/14

Mount Sinai Children's Environmental Health Center Fact Sheet – Endocrine Disruptors, pg 2. New York, NY
www.mountsinai.org/static_files/MSMC/Files/Patient%20Care/Children/Childrens%20Environmental%20Health%20Center/Endocrine%20Disrupters.pdf
Accessed online: 23/3/14

Mount Sinai Children's Environmental Health Center Fact Sheet – Formaldehyde, pg 2. New York, NY
www.mountsinai.org/static_files/MSMC/Files/Patient%20Care/Children/Childrens%20Environmental%20Health%20Center/Formaldehyde.pdf
Accessed online: 23/3/14

Mount Sinai Children's Environmental Health Center Fact Sheet – Lead, pg 1. New York, NY
www.mountsinai.org/static_files/MSMC/Files/Patient%20Care/Children/Childrens%20Environmental%20Health%20Center/Lead.pdf
Accessed online: 23/3/14

Mount Sinai Children's Environmental Health Center Fact Sheet - Mold, pg 1. New York, NY
www.mountsinai.org/static_files/MSMC/Files/Patient%20Care/Children/Childrens%20Environmental%20Health%20Center/Mold.pdf
Accessed online: 23/3/14

Mount Sinai Children's Environmental Health Center Fact Sheet – Particulate Matter, pg 1. New York, NY
www.mountsinai.org/static_files/MSMC/Files/Patient%20Care/Children/Childrens%20Environmental%20Health%20Center/Particulate%20Matter.pdf
Accessed online: 23/3/14

USA National Library of Medicine, 2014. Tox Town – Perchloroethylene (PCE, PERC)
http://toxtown.nlm.nih.gov/text_version/chemicals.php?id=22
Accessed online: 23/3/14

USA Environmental Working Group, 2003. 'PFCs Global Contaminants: PFOA and other PFCs come from common products in every home' pg 1
www.ewg.org/research/pfcs-global-contaminants/pfoa-and-other-pfcs-come-common-products-every-home
Accessed online: 23/3/14

USA EPA, 2013. Basic Information: Polychlorinated Biphenyls (PCBs)
www.epa.gov/epawaste/hazard/tsd/pcbs/pubs/about.htm
Accessed online: 24/3/14

Australian Government Department of Environment. Polybrominated diphenyl ether flame retardants (PBDEs), pg 1, pg 3
www.environment.gov.au/system/files/resources/8e81d7e1-a379-4590-b29619e14a72d909/files/factsheet.pdf
Accessed online: 24/3/14

USA EPA, 2014. 'Existing Chemicals: Polybrominated Diphenyl Ethers (PBDEs) Action Plan Summary', pg 1
www.epa.gov/oppt/existingchemicals/pubs/actionplans/pbde.html
Accessed online: 24/3/14

USA Pediatric Environmental Health Specialty Unit. PBDEs: Information for Pediatric Health Professionals, pg 2
http://icahn.mssm.edu/static_files/MSSM/Files/Research/Programs/Pediatric%20Environmental%20Health%20Specialty%20Unit/PBDE_National_%20factsheet.pdf
Accessed online: 24/3/14

USA Natural Resources Defense Council (NRDC), 2011. 'Chemical Culprits: PFCs', pg 1
www.nrdc.org/living/healthreports/chemical-culprits-pfcs.asp
Accessed online: 23/3/14

USA EPA, 2012. Perfluorooctanoic Acid and Fluorinated Telomers (PFOA) Risk Assessment, pg 1
www.epa.gov/oppt/pfoa/pubs/pfoarisk.html
Accessed online: 23/3/14

Mount Sinai Children's Environmental Health Center Fact Sheet – Pesticides, pg 2 New York, NY
www.mountsinai.org/static_files/MSMC/Files/Patient%20Care/Children/Childrens%20Environmental%20Health%20Center/Pesticides.pdf
Accessed online: 23/3/14

Mount Sinai Children's Environmental Health Center Fact Sheet - Phthalates, pg 1
www.mountsinai.org/static_files/MSMC/Files/Patient%20Care/Children/Childrens%20Environmental%20Health%20Center/Phthalates.pdf
Accessed online: 23/3/14

USA Centers for Disease Control and Prevention (CDC), 2013. Factsheet - Phthalates, pg 1
www.cdc.gov/biomonitoring/phthalates_factsheet.html
Accessed online: 23/3/14

Healthy Child Healthy World, 2013. 'Avoid Phthalates: Find Phthalate Free Products Instead', in Chemical
http://healthychild.org/easy-steps/avoid-phthalates-find-phthalate-free-products-instead%E2%80%A8%E2%80%A8
Accessed online: 23/3/14

National Pollutant Inventory, 2013. Polychlorinated Biphenyls (PCBs). Australian Government Department of the Environment pg 1
www.npi.gov.au/resource/polychlorinated-biphenyls-pcbs
Accessed online: 23/3/14

Mount Sinai Children's Environmental Health Center Fact Sheet – PCBs, pg 1-2. New York, NY
www.mountsinai.org/static_files/MSMC/Files/Patient%20Care/Children/Childrens%20Environmental%20Health%20Center/PCBs.pdf
Accessed online: 23/3/14

USA National Library of Medicine, 2014. Tox Town – Solvents, pg 1
http://toxtown.nlm.nih.gov/text_version/chemicals.php?id=28
Accessed online: 23/3/14

USA Agency for Toxic Substances & Disease Registry (ATSDR), 2000. Toxic Substances Portal – Public Health Statement for Toluene, pg 1 online
www.atsdr.cdc.gov/phs/phs.asp?id=159&tid=29
Accessed online: 23/3/14

Mount Sinai Children's Environmental Health Center Fact Sheet –VOCs, pg 1-2
www.mountsinai.org/static_files/MSMC/Files/Patient%20Care/Children/Childrens%20Environmental%20Health%20Center/VOC%20Fact%20Sheet.pdf
Accessed online: 23/3/14

USA EPA, 2012. An Introduction to Indoor Air Quality: Volatile Organic Compounds (VOCs), pg 1
www.epa.gov/iaq/voc.html
Accessed online: 23/3/14

USA Centers for Disease Control and Prevention, 2013. Biomonitoring Summary: Triclosan, pg 1
www.cdc.gov/biomonitoring/Triclosan_BiomonitoringSummary.html
Accessed online: 23/3/14

Beyond Pesticides, 2014. Triclosan: Health Effects pg 1 online
www.beyondpesticides.org/antibacterial/health
Accessed online: 23/3/14

Healthy Child, Healthy World, 2013. 'Skip the Triclosan and other antibacterial products', pg 1
http://healthychild.org/easy-steps/skip-the-triclosan-and-other-antibacterial-products
Accessed online: 23/3/13

Step 1 - Build It / renovate

Alternative Technology Association, 'Sanctuary' and 'ReNew' magazines
www.ata.org.au
Accessed online: 20/3/2014

Australian Building Codes Board, 2011, Australian Climate Zone Map
www.abcb.gov.au/~/media/Files/Download%20Documents/Major%20Initiatives/Energy%20Efficiency/Climate%20Zone%20Maps/2012%20Logo%20Updates/AUST_ABCB_Map_2012_v41.pdf
Accessed online: 10/3/2014

Readon, C 2013. 'Passive Design and Orientation' *Your Home: Australia's guide to environmentally sustainable homes*. Australian Government Department of Industry, 5th edition, March 2014.
www.yourhome.gov.au
Accessed online: 12/3/2014

McGee, C 2013. 'Shading' *Your Home: Australia's guide to environmentally sustainable homes*.
Australian Government Department of Industry, 5th edition, March 2014
www.yourhome.gov.au
Accessed online: 16/3/2014

Australian Government Department of Industry, 2014. 'Passive Cooling' Your Home: Australia's guide to environmentally sustainable homes. 5th edition, March 2014.
www.yourhome.gov.au

Australian Institute of Refrigeration, Air-conditioning and Heating 2011. *Evaporative Cooling Report 2011*
www.airah.org.au/imis15_prod/Content_Files/HVACRNation/2011/May2011/HVACRNation_2011_05_F02.pdf
Accessed online: 15/3/14

Clean Energy Council, 2014.
www.cleanenergycouncil.org.au
Accessed online: 20/3/2014

Fire Protection Association of Australia
www.fpaa.com.au

Commonwealth of Australia, Bureau of Meteorology, 2014. 'Wind Roses for Australian Sites'
www.bom.gov.au/climate/averages/wind/index.shtml
Accessed online: 15/3/2014

United Nations Centre for Human Settlements (Habitat), 1990. National Design Handbook Prototype on Passive Solar Heating and Natural Cooling of Buildings. Nairobi
www.unhabitat.org/pmss/getElectronicVersion.aspx?nr=1230&alt=1
Accessed online: 10/3/2014

Passive House Institute Germany, 2012.
http://passiv.de/en
Accessed online: 10/3/2014

Australian Passive House Association
http://passivehouseaustralia.org
Accessed online: 10/3/2014

CSIRO, 2014. The Evaluation of the 5-Star Energy Efficiency Standard for Residential Buildings
www.industry.gov.au/Energy/Pages/Evaluation5StarEEfficiencyStandardResidentialBuildings.aspx
Accessed online: 28/2/2014

Department of Environment and Heritage, NSW, 2014. Insulation FAQs
www.environment.nsw.gov.au/energy/insulatefaq.htm
Accessed online: 12/4/14

Brandjes Environmental Building Consultancy, Melbourne

Hollo, N. 2012. *Warm house: Cool house. Inspirational Designs for Low-energy Housing*, 2nd edition, Choice Books, Sydney

New4old, 2008. Technical Guidelines for Building Designers
European Renewable Energy Council
www.new4old.eu//guidelines/3_Introduction%20Technical%20Guidelines.pdf
Accessed online: 10/3/2014

Phase Change Energy Solutions
www.phasechange.com/index.php/en
Accessed online: 10/3/2014

NAHB Research Center, Southface Energy Institute and US Department of Energy, 2000. Passive Solar Design Fact Sheet.
http://apps1.eere.energy.gov/buildings/publications/pdfs/building_america/29236.pdf
Accessed online: 10/3/2014

US Department of Energy website, 2014. Passive Solar Home Design and Energy Saver sections
http://energy.gov/energysaver/energy-saver
Accessed online: 13/3/2014

Autodesk Sustainability Workshop, 2011. 'Total R-Values and Thermal Bridging'
http://sustainabilityworkshop.autodesk.com/buildings/total-r-values-and-thermal-bridging
Accessed online: 18/3/2014

Brindle, B, 28 March 2011. '10 Benefits of a Passive House' HowStuffWorks.com
http://home.howstuffworks.com/home-improvement/construction/green/10-benefits-of-a-passive-house.htm
Accessed online: 7/3/2014

Windows Energy Rating System, 2014
www.wers.net
Accessed online: 20/3/2014

Australian Window Association, 2014
www.awa.org.au
Accessed online: 20/3/2014

Glass and Glazing Association of Australia, 2014
www.agga.org.au
Accessed online: 20/3/2014

Choice Online, 2012.
www.choice.com.au
Accessed online: 24/3/2014

NatHERS, 2010. Nationwide House Energy Rating Scheme, 2010
www.nathers.gov.au
Accessed online: 17/3/2014

Wrigley, D. 2012. *Making your home sustainable: a guide to retrofitting*, revised edition. Scribe Publications, Brunswick, Victoria

Savewater website
www.savewater.com.au
Accessed online: 25/3/2014

Commonwealth of Australia 2013. Water Efficiency Labelling and Standards (WELS) Scheme.
www.waterrating.gov.au
Accessed online: 25/3/2014

Environmental Protection Authority (Vic), 2013.
www.epa.vic.gov.au/~/media/Publications/977.pdf
Accessed online: 25/3/2014

Australian Water Association, 2010.
www.awa.asn.au
Accessed online: 26/3/2014

Futerra Sustainability Communications, 2008. *The Greenwash Guide*
www.futerra.co.uk
Accessed online: 15/12/13

Gipe, P, 2011-2014. Wind Works Online Archive
www.wind-works.org
Accessed online: 28/3/2014

Australian Geothermal Energy Association, 2014.
www.agea.org.au
Accessed online: 26/3/2014

Homepower, 2014.
www.homepower.com
Accessed online: 26/3/2014

Australian Medical Association, 2014. Wind Farms and Health (statement).
https://ama.com.au/position-statement/wind-farms-and-health-2014
Accessed online: 30/3/2014

Australian Government, Department of Environment, Water, Heritage and the Arts, 2008.
http://ee.ret.gov.au/energy-efficiency/strategies-and-initiatives/national-construction-code/energy-use-australian-residential-sector-1986-2020
Accessed online: 14/3/2014

State Government of Victoria, 2013. Switch On website
www.switchon.vic.gov.au
Accessed online: 28/3/2014

Commonwealth of Australia, 2012. Energy Rating website
www.energyrating.gov.au
Accessed online: 26/3/2014

National Electrical Contractors Association of Australia, 2014.
www.neca.asn.au
Accessed online: 29/3/2014

Planet Ark, 2014. Recycling Near You website.
www.recyclingnearyou.com.au
Accessed online: 26/3/2014

Department of Environment, Water, Heritage and the Arts, 2008. *Energy Use in the Australian Residential Sector 1986-2020*.

Energy Consult Pty Ltd, 2012 (Amendment 2). *Video Game Consoles: Energy Efficiency Options* prepared for the Department of Climate Change and Energy Efficiency
www.energyrating.gov.au/wp-content/uploads/Energy_Rating_Documents/Library/Home_Entertainment/Video_Games_Consoles/FINAL-VGC-Efficiency-Options-with-Industry-mods-V2-2.pdf
Accessed online: 14/3/14

Site health tips

Asbestos

American Cancer Society, 2013. Asbestos – What is Asbestos? (online)
www.cancer.org/cancer/cancercauses/othercarcinogens/intheworkplace/asbestos
Accessed online: 6/4/14

Australian Government Asbestos Safety and Eradication Agency, 2013. Fact Sheet on Asbestos Safety
http://asbestossafety.gov.au/sites/asbestossafety.gov.au/files/Factsheet-on-asbestos-safety-August-2013.pdf
Accessed online: 6/4/14

Australian Government Asbestos Safety and Eradication Agency, 2014. Frequently Asked Questions (online)
http://asbestossafety.gov.au/publications
Accessed online: 6/4/14

Radon

American Cancer Society, 2013. What is Radon
www.cancer.org/cancer/cancercauses/othercarcinogens/pollution/radon
Accessed online: 6/4/14

ARPANSA (Australian Radiation Protection and Nuclear Safety Agency), 2012. Fact Sheet: Radon in Homes
www.arpansa.gov.au/radiationprotection/Factsheets/is_radon.cfm#
Accessed online: 6/4/14

Lead

Australian Government Department of Sustainability, Environment, Water, Population and Communities, 2009. *The Six Step Guide to Painting Your Home*, 4th edition, Commonwealth of Australia.
Accessed online: 28/4/14

Australian Government Department of the Environment, 2014. Lead alert facts: Lead in House Paint
www.environment.gov.au/resource/lead-alert-facts-lead-house-paint
Accessed online: 28/4/14

The LEAD Group, 2014.
www.lead.org.au/fs/fst38.html
Accessed online: 28/4/14

Step 2 – Products & furnishings – interior materials

Bornehag CG, Lundgren B, Weschler CJ, Sigsgaard T, Hagerhed-Engman L, and Sundell, J, 2005. 'Phthalates in Indoor Dust and Their Association with Building Characteristics' Environmental Health Perspectives. October; 113(10), 1399-1404.
www.ncbi.nlm.nih.gov/pmc/articles/PMC1281287

Timber vs steel

Sustainable Timber Action in Europe, 2012. Buying Sustainable Timber – A Guide for Public Purchases in Europe
www.sustainable-timber-action.org/fileadmin/files/STA_Toolkit/STA-guide-for-procurers-ENGLISH-www.pdf

Engineered Wood Products Association of Australasia, 2012 (revised). Facts about Formaldehyde Emissions from EWPAA Certified Products.
www.ewp.asn.au/library/downloads/ewpaa_formaldehyde_facts.pdf

Australian Timber
www.atfa.com.au/wp-content/uploads/2012/10/33_Hardwood-flooring-grades.pdf
Accessed online: 7/3/14

Australian Bureau of Statistics, 2010. 8731.0 Building Approvals, Australia, Feb 2010
Accessed online: 28/4/14

American Iron and Steel Institute, 2014. Steelworks - Recycling Construction Materials (online source)
www.steel.org/en/sitecore/content/Recycle-steel_org/Web%20Root/Steel%20Markets/Construction.aspx
Accessed online: 28/4/14

Timber coatings

Australian Timber Flooring Association, 2008. 'Coating Choices' Information Sheet #7
www.atfa.com.au/wp-content/uploads/2012/10/is-coating-choices.pdf
Accessed online: 7/3/14

Plastics and your health

Allsopp M, Santillo D & Johnston P, 2001. 'Poison Underfoot – Hazardous Chemicals in PVC Flooring and Hazardous Chemicals in Carpets'. Greenpeace Research Laboratories, University of Exeter pg 6
www.greenpeace.org.uk/MultimediaFiles/Live/FullReport/3218.pdf
Accessed online: 17/3/14

USA Centers for Disease Control and Prevention, 2013. Phthalates Fact Sheet (updated July 2013)
www.cdc.gov/biomonitoring/phthalates_factsheet.html
Accessed online: 28/2/14

American Cancer Society, 2013. Known and Probable Human Carcinogens. (revised July 2013)
www.cancer.org/cancer/cancercauses/othercarcinogens/generalinformationaboutcarcinogens/known-and-probable-human-carcinogens
Accessed online: 28/2/14

Bornehag CG, Sundrell J, Weschler CJ, Sigsgaard T, Lundgren B, Hasselgren M, Hägerhed-Engman L. 2004. 'The association between asthma and allergic symptoms in children and phthalates in house dust: A nested case-control study.' Environmental Health Perspectives 112:1393-1397.
http://ehp.niehs.nih.gov

Colborn T, Dumanoski D, Peterson Myers J, 1996. Our Stolen Future. Dutton, USA
www.ourstolenfuture.org/newscience/oncompounds/phthalates/2004/2004-0720bornehagetal.htm
Accessed online: 2/5/14

Bornehag, CG, Lundgren B, Weschler, CT, Sigsgaard, Hagerhed-Engman L and Sundell J, 2005.
Phthalates in Indoor Dust and Their Association with Building Characteristics. Environmental Health Perspectives 1399-1404.
http://ehp.niehs.nih.gov

Flooring

USA EPA, 2014. Vinyl Flooring
www.epa.gov/climatechange/wycd/waste/downloads/vinyl-flooring-chapter10-28-10.pdf
Accessed online: 5/3/14

Choice, 2010. Sustainable flooring: Environmental impacts to consider
www.choice.com.au
Accessed online: 7/3/14

USA Healthy Building Network, 2014. PVC Facts
www.healthybuilding.net/pvc/facts.html/HBN_FS_PVC_in_Buildings.pdf
Accessed online: 7/3/14

Natural Stone Council, 2014. Stone & Sustainability - Material Fact Sheets
www.naturalstonecouncil.org/education-training/stone-sustainability
Accessed online: 7/3/14

Australian Timber Flooring Association, 2014.
www.atfa.com.au/consumer-services/consumer-information
Accessed online: 7/3/14

Armstrong Commercial Flooring, 2014. 'What is in linoleum and how it is made?' USA & Canada
www.armstrong.com/commflooringna/what-is-linoleum.html?intcid=link_AFPUSCOM_flash_AllAboutLino
Accessed online: 12/3/14

Lowell Centre for Sustainable Production, University of Massachusetts Lowell, 2011. Technical Briefing - Phthalates and their alternatives: Health and Environmental Concerns.
www.sustainableproduction.org/downloads/PhthalateAlternatives-January2011.pdf

Lithner D, 2011. Environmental and Health Hazards of Chemicals in Plastic Polymers and Products. PhD Thesis, University of Gothenburg, Sweden.
https://gupea.ub.gu.se/bitstream/2077/24978/1/gupea_2077_24978_1.pdf

Carpet

USA Natural Resources Defense Council, 2014. Smarter Living: Chemical Index – Pyrethrins
www.nrdc.org/living/chemicalindex/pyrethrins.asp
Accessed online: 5/3/14

Allsopp M et al, 2001.'Poison Underfoot – Hazardous Chemicals in PVC Flooring and Hazardous Chemicals in Carpets.' Greenpeace Research Laboratories, University of Exeter pg 6
www.greenpeace.org.uk/MultimediaFiles/Live/FullReport/3218.pdf
Accessed online: 17/3/14

USA Centers for Disease Control and Prevention. Phthalates Fact Sheet (updated July 2013)
www.cdc.gov/biomonitoring/phthalates_factsheet.html
Accessed online: 28/2/14

American Cancer Society, 2013. Known and Probable Human Carcinogens (updated October 2013)
www.cancer.org/cancer/cancercauses/othercarcinogens/generalinformationaboutcarcinogens/known-and-probable-human-carcinogens
Accessed online: 28/2/14

Carpet Institute of Australia Limited, undated. Consumer Health Information: Allergens in the Home.
http://members.carpetinstitute.com.au/pubs/documents/allergens.pdf

USA EPA, 2006. (updated 2012). Permethrin Facts (Reregistration Eligibility Decision Factsheet) pg 1
www.epa.gov/oppsrrd1/REDs/factsheets/permethrin_fs.htm
Accessed online: 7/4/14

Cabinetry

Australian Competition and Consumer Commission, Product Safety Australia 2014. Formaldehyde in Consumer Products
www.productsafety.gov.au/content/index.phtml/itemId/973697
Accessed online: 12/3/14

Benchtops

USA Environmental Protection Agency, 2014. Radon and Radioactivity in Granite Countertops
http://radiation.supportportal.com/link/portal/23002/23013/Article/20952/What-about-radon-and-radioactivity-in-granite-countertops
Accessed online: 03/01/14

Rimex Metal Group, 2009. Stainless Steel, Architecture & the Environment.
www.rimexmetals.com.au/PDF_data_sheets/StainlessSteelArchitectureandtheEnvironment.pdf
Accessed online: 03/01/14

The Stainless Steel Information Center, 2014.
www.ssina.com/sustainability
Accessed online: 27/2/14

Paint

Environment Protection & Heritage Council & Environ Australia Pty Ltd, 2009. VOCs from Surface Coatings – Assessment of the Categorisation, VOC Content and Sales Volumes of Coating Products Sold in Australia.

Australian Paint Approval Scheme, 2006. APAS Document B181
www.apas.gov.au/PDFs/D181.pdf
Accessed online: 17/3/14

Good Environmental Choice Australia, 2013. Environmental Performance Standard – Paints & Coatings
www.geca.org.au/media/medialibrary/2013/03/GECA_23-2012_v2_2_final.pdf
Accessed online: 17/3/14

Australian Government Department of Sustainability, Environment, Water, Population and Communities, 2009. *The Six Step Guide to Painting Your Home, fourth edition*. Commonwealth of Australia, Canberra.
Accessed online: 28/4/14

Australian Government Department of the Environment, 2014. 'Lead alert facts: Lead in house paint'
www.environment.gov.au/resource/lead-alert-facts-lead-house-paint
Accessed online: 28/4/14

O'Brien E, 2014. Lead paint and ceiling dust management – how to do it lead-safely. The Lead Group Inc.
www.lead.org.au/fs/fst38.html
Accessed online: 28/4/14

World Health Organisation/United Nations Environment Programme, 2012. State of the science of endocrine disrupting chemicals – 2012. An assessment of the state of the science of endocrine disruptors. p viii; 195
www.who.int/ceh/publications/endocrine/en

European Union, Directorates General, Health and Consumer Protection, Public Health, 2014. 'Nanotechnologies: What are the uses of nanoparticles in consumer products?'
http://ec.europa.eu/health/scientific_committees/opinions_layman/en/nanotechnologies/l-3/5-nanoparticles-consumer-products.htm Source document: http://ec.europa.eu/health/ph_risk/committees/04_scenihr/docs/scenihr_o_003b.pdf
Accessed online: 28/4/14

National Industrial Chemicals Notification and Assessment Scheme (NICNAS), July 2013. Nano Titanium Dioxide Fact Sheet. NICNAS Nanomaterial health hazard review: health effects of titanium dioxide nanoparticles
www.nicnas.gov.au/communications/issues/nanomaterials-nanotechnology/nicnas-technical-activities-in-nanomaterials/nano-titanium-dioxide-human-health-hazard-review/titanium-dioxide-nanomaterial-factsheet
Accessed online: 28/4/14

Window coverings

Oeko-Tex
www.oeko-tex.com

Water ware and plumbing

Government of Western Australia, Department of Health 2009. Trihalomethanes (THMs) in Drinking Water.
www.public.health.wa.gov.au/cproot/2410/2/Trihalomethanes.pdf
Accessed online: 19/2/14

The American College of Allergy, Asthma and Immunology, 2010. Chlorine Allergy, Reality or Myth?
www.acaai.org/allergist/allergies/Types/other-allergies/Pages/chlorine-allergy.aspx
Accessed online: 19/2/14

Choi A, Sun G, Zhang Y, Grandjean P, 2012. 'Developmental Fluoride Neurotoxicity: A Systematic Review and Meta-Analysis' *Environmental Health Perspectives*, National Institute of Environmental Health Science Oct 2012; 120(10): 1362–1368.
www.ncbi.nlm.nih.gov/pmc/articles/PMC3491930

USA Centres for Disease Control and Prevention, 2013. Chemical Irritants (Chloramines) & Indoor Pool Air Quality
www.cdc.gov/healthywater/swimming/pools/irritants-indoor-pool-air-quality.html
Accessed online: 19/2/14

Lighting

EcoDecisions, 2014. Lighting plan information (supplied)
www.ecodecisions.com.au
Accessed: 28/3/2014

Australian Geothermal Energy Association, 2014.
www.ee.ret.gov.au/energy-efficiency/lighting
Accessed online: 26/3/2014

Beacon Lighting Australia, 2014
www.beaconlighting.com.au
Accessed online: 28/3/2014

Appliances

Alternative Technology Association. 'Sanctuary' and 'ReNew' publications
www.ata.org.au
Accessed online: 20/3/2014

Commonwealth of Australia, 2012. Energy Rating
www.energyrating.gov.au
Accessed: 26/3/2014

Commonwealth of Australia 2013. Water Efficiency Labelling and Standards (WELS) Scheme.
www.waterrating.gov.au
Accessed: 25/3/2014

Public Health Association of Australia, 2011. Hot tap water temperature and scalds policy
www.phaa.net.au/documents/130201_Hot%20Tap%20Water%20Temperature%20and%20Scalds%20Policy%20FINAL.pdf
Accessed online: 10/3/2014

Commonwealth of Australia, Department of Industry 2013. Your Home: Australia's guide to environmentally sustainable homes. 5th edition. March 2014.
www.yourhome.gov.au
Accessed online: 30/3/2014

US Department of Energy, Passive Solar Home Design and Energy Saver sections
http://energy.gov/energysaver/energy-saver
Accessed: 13/3/2014

Commonwealth of Australia, Department of Health, 2011. Regulatory approaches by Australian States and Territories to the Prevention of Legionellosis.
www.health.gov.au/internet/main/publishing.nsf/Content/7FDDB6DADD503805CA257BF0001F985F/$File/legapp1.pdf
Accessed online: 13/3/2014

Australian Consumer Association, 2014. Choice
www.choice.com.au
Accessed online: 13/3/2014

Osman P, Ashworth P, CSIRO, 2009. *The CSIRO Home Energy Saving Handbook*, Sydney, Pan McMillan Australia Pty Ltd.

Asthma Australia, 2014
www.asthmaaustralia.org.au
Accessed online: 30/3/2014

Solar Air Heating Association, 2014
www.solarairheating.org.au
Accessed online: 28/3/2014

Australian Consumer Association, 2014. Choice
www.choice.com.au
Accessed online: 13/3/2014

Australian Institute of Refrigeration, Airconditioning and Heating (AIRAH), 2014. Water efficiency for evaporative air coolers
www.airah.org.au
Accessed online: 20/3/2014

Estimated Hot Water Running Costs in Victoria – report August 2010, Energy Consult (for Sustainability Victoria).

Technology

International Agency for Research on Cancer, World Health Organisation, 2011. 'IARC Classifies Radiofrequency Electromagnetic Fields as possibly carcinogenic to humans' Press Release No 208, WHO, pg 1
www.iarc.fr/en/media-centre/pr/2011/pdfs/pr208_E.pdf

Australian Radiation Protection and Nuclear Safety Agency (ARPANSA) 2013. Radiofrequency Radiation.
www.arpansa.gov.au/radiationprotection/basics/rf.cfm
Accessed online: 27/3/14

World Health Organisation, 2014. Electromagnetic fields (EMF) – What are Electromagnetic fields?
www.who.int/peh-emf/about/WhatisEMF/en/
Accessed online: 27/3/14

Create Healthy Homes, 2014. Safer Use of Computers. California
www.createhealthyhomes.com/safercomputers.php
Accessed online: 27/3/14

Miller, O undated. 'Tips for a Healthy Home: Reduce Your Exposure to Electric Fields, Magnetic Fields and Radio Frequencies (EMFs)'. Environmental Design and Inspection Services, California pp 1 -16 online
www.createhealthyhomes.com/tips_for_a_healthy_home.php
Accessed online: 27/3/14

Heating and cooling systems

Alternative Technology Association, 'Sanctuary' and 'ReNew' publications
www.ata.org.au
Accessed online: 20/3/2014

Commonwealth of Australia, Energy Rating website, 2012
www.energyrating.gov.au
Accessed online: 26/3/2014

Public Health Association of Australia, 2011. Hot tap water temperature and scalds policy
www.phaa.net.au/documents/130201_Hot%20Tap%20Water%20Temperature%20and%20Scalds%20Policy%20FINAL.pdf
Accessed online: 10/3/2014

Commonwealth of Australia, 2013. Website of the Department of Industry. *Your Home: Australia's guide to environmentally sustainable homes*. 5th edition. March 2014.
www.yourhome.gov.au
Accessed online: 30/3/2014

US Department of Energy, 2014
http://energy.gov/energysaver/energy-saver
Accessed: 20/3/2014

Commonwealth of Australia, Department of Health, 2011. Regulatory approaches by Australian States and Territories to the Prevention of Legionellosis.
www.health.gov.au/internet/main/publishing.nsf/Content/7FDDB6DADD503805CA257BF0001F985F/$File/legapp1.pdf
Accessed online: 13/3/2014

Australian Consumer Association, 2014. Choice
www.choice.com.au
Accessed online: 13/3/2014

Commonwealth Scientific and Industrial Research Organisation (CSIRO) 2003- 2014
www.csiro.au
Accessed online: 25/3/2014

Asthma Australia, 2014
www.asthmaaustralia.org.au
Accessed online: 30/3/2014

Solar Air Heating Association, 2014
www.solarairheating.org.au
Accessed online: 28/3/2014

Australian Consumer Association, Choice, 2014
www.choice.com.au
Accessed online: 13/3/2014

AIRAH, Fairair, 2006
www.fairair.com.au
Accessed online: 13/3/2014

Australian Institute of Refrigeration, Airconditioning and Heating (AIRAH), 2014. Water efficiency for evaporative air coolers
www.airah.org.au
Accessed online: 20/3/2014

Commonwealth of Australia, Department of Industry, 2013. *Your Home: Australia's guide to environmentally sustainable homes*. 5th edition. March 2014.
www.yourhome.gov.au

Australian Government Energy Efficiency Rating of appliances
http://reg.energyrating.gov.au

Osman P, Ashworth P, CSIRO, 2009. *The CSIRO Home Energy Saving Handbook*, Sydney, Pan McMillan Australia Pty Ltd.

Asthma Australia
www.asthmaaustralia.org.au

Solar Air Heating Association
http://solarairheating.org.au

Australian Government, Department of Industry. Energy Efficiency, 2014, online
http://ee.ret.gov.au/energy-efficiency/water-heaters

Public Health Association of Australia, 2011. Hot tap water temperature and scalds policy
www.phaa.net.au/documents/130201_Hot%20Tap%20Water%20Temperature%20and%20Scalds%20Policy%20FINAL.pdf

Commonwealth of Australia, Department of Health, 2011. Regulatory approaches by Australian States and Territories to the Prevention of Legionellosis.
www.health.gov.au/internet/main/publishing.nsf/Content/7FDDB6DADD503805CA257BF0001F985F/$File/legapp1.pdf

USA Government energy website
www.energy.gov

Indoor plants

Wolverton Dr BC, *How to Grow Fresh Air*, Penguin Books, New York, 1996

Brethour C, Watson G, Sparling B, Bucknell D & Moor T, 2007. Literature Review of Documented Health and Environmental Benefits Derived from Ornamental Horticulture Products. George Morris Centre, Canada, pg 24
www.intogreen.nl/shared/files/28-q-federation_interdisciplinaire_horticulture_ornementale_qc_annexe3.pdf

Step 3 - Our behaviour - consumer choice

Environmental Defense Fund, 2014.
www.edf.org/health/where-are-toxic-chemicals-your-home
Accessed online: 15/11/13

Australian Competition and Consumer Commission, Product Safety Recall, 2014. Candles with Lead Wicks
www.productsafety.gov.au/content/index.phtml/itemId/974269

Shop wise

Australian Competition & Consumer Commission
www.productsafety.gov.au

The Chemical Maze
www.chemicalmaze.com

Food Standards Australia New Zealand
www.foodstandards.gov.au

Step 4 - Lifestyle practices
Family, Allergy & Asthma, 2014. Skin Allergy: Eczema
www.familyallergy.com/allergy/eczema
Accessed online: 7/4/14

Step 5 - Maintaining a home for efficiency & health
Government of Western Australia Department of Health, undated. Mould and Condensation in Your Home
www.public.health.wa.gov.au/cproot/2887/2/Mould%20Fact%20Sheet.pdf
Accessed online: 6/4/14

Low allergen and sustainable gardening
Asthma Australia
www.asthmaaustralia.org.au

Asthma Foundation of Victoria
www.asthma.org.au

Asthma Foundation NSW
www.asthmansw.org.au

Asthma Foundation WA
www.asthmawa.org.au

Weatherzone Australia - for air borne pollen index
www.weatherzone.com.au

Westmead Children's Hospital – for a list of poisonous plants
www.chw.edu.au

Mark Ragg, 1996. *The Low Allergy Garden* Hodder & Stoughton, Sydney

Australian Organic
www.austorganic.com.au

NSW Environment and Heritage – for composting information
www.environment.nsw.gov.au

Sustainable Gardening Australia – for sustainable gardening information
www.sgaonline.org.au

NSW Environment Protection Authority
www.epa.nsw.gov.au

Eden Gardens
www.edengardens.com.au

Plant This - for plant selector tool
www.plantthis.com.au

Metro regional government in Portland, Ore., Local Hazardous Waste Management Program in King County, Wash., 2009. *Grow Smart, Grow Safe: A Consumer Guide to Lawn and Garden Products*, sixth edition
http://library.oregonmetro.gov/files/gsgs_11-5_web.pdf
Accessed online: 2/5/14

University of California Agriculture and Natural Resources 2014. Integrated Pest Management Program website
www.ipm.ucdavis.edu/PMG/menu.homegarden.html

Investment sense
World Green Building Council, 2013. The Business Case for Green Building – A review of the costs and benefits for developers, investors and occupants.
www.worldgbc.org/files/2513/6277/6014/Business_Case_For_Green_Building_WEB_2013-03-08.pdf
Accessed online: 3/10/13

Fisk, WJ 1997. *Health and Productivity Gains from Better Indoor Environments and Their Implications for the U.S Department of Energy.* Lawrence Berkeley National Laboratory. Pg. 167
www.rand.org/content/dam/rand/pubs/conf_proceedings/CF170z1-1/CF170.1.fisk.pdf
Accessed online: 21/2/14

Department of the Environment, Water, Heritage and the Arts, 2006. Energy Efficiency Rating and House Price in the ACT.

Glossary

National Institute of Environment Health Sciences
www.niehs.nih.gov/health/topics/agents/sya-bpa
www.niehs.nih.gov/research/supported/assets/docs/j_q/phthalates_the_everywhere_chemical_handout_.pdf#search=phthalates
www.niehs.nih.gov/health/topics/agents/endocrine/index.cfm

United States Environmental Protection Agency
www.epa.gov/iaq/voc2.html
Accessed online: 14/4/14

Queensland Government Fact Sheet P2/N95 Mask Fit Checking
www.health.qld.gov.au/chrisp/resources/fit_check_factsheet.pdf
Accessed online: 14/4/14

United States Environmental Protection Agency
www.epa.gov/ttn/atw/hlthef/benzene.html
http://ofmpub.epa.gov/sor_internet/registry/termreg/searchandretrieve/glossariesandkeywordlists/search.do?details=&glossaryName=IAQ%20Glossary
www.epa.gov/oppt/existingchemicals/pubs/perchloroethylene_fact_sheet.html
www.epa.gov/waste//hazard/tsd/pcbs/about.htm
www.epa.gov/oppt/existingchemicals/pubs/actionplans/pbde.html
www.epa.gov/oppsrrd1/REDs/factsheets/triclosan_fs.htm
Accessed online: 14/4/14

Wisconsin Department of Health Services – Toluene Fact Sheet
www.dhs.wisconsin.gov/eh/chemfs/fs/toluene.htm
Accessed online: 14/4/14

US Food and Drug Administration
Triclosan - What Consumers Should Know
www.fda.gov/forconsumers/consumerupdates/ucm205999.htm
Accessed online: 14/4/14

ABCB and Australian Institute of Architects, 2011. Condensation in Buildings, ABCB, page 3
www.abcb.gov.au
Accessed online: 28/4/14

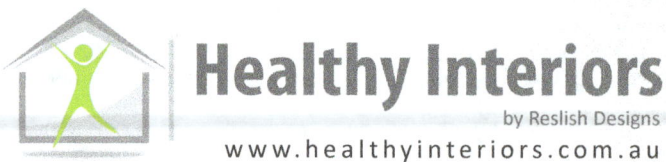

Healthy Interiors
by Reslish Designs
www.healthyinteriors.com.au

INTERIOR DESIGN - "HEALTH FOCUSED"

Relish Designs is www.healthyinteriors.com.au design service offering a range of interior design related services incorporating the importance of minimising pollutants in the home and using sustainable materials and finishes where possible subject to budget requirements.

Range of services available:

- Interior design - creative concepts consultation
- Décor concept scheme development
- Architectural or Individual project interior product & material specifications
- Product selection consultations
- Decorating consultations
- Materials and finishes digital concept boards
- Healthy Home design consultations

Benefits:

- Documentation of interior details allows for accurate project tender comparisons
- Reduce potential for project variation costs due to mid project changes
- Allows client to estimate budget
- Documentation for all parties to reference to minimise project communication issues
- Documentation for clients to reference into the future for maintenance purposes

Visit the website to view Featured Products - solutions to creating a healthy home

Healthy Interiors by Relish designs
Website : www.healthyinteriors.com.au
Email : info@healthyinteriors.com.au
Phone : 0417 122 399

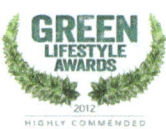

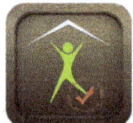

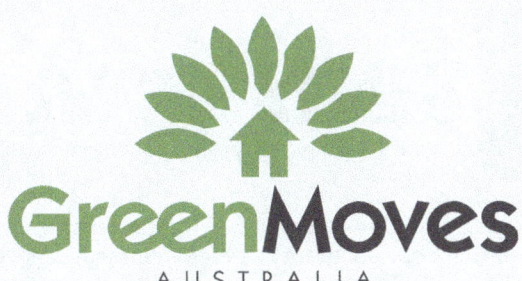

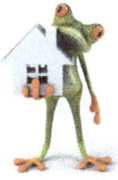

Residential services include:
- Expert consultations
- Energy Audits and Assessments
- Sustainability Assessments
- Building Plan reviews and advice
- Pre-purchase Home Reports
- Green Homes to Build listing

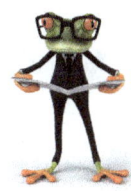

Resources available:
- Checklists
- Tips
- Training
- Speaking

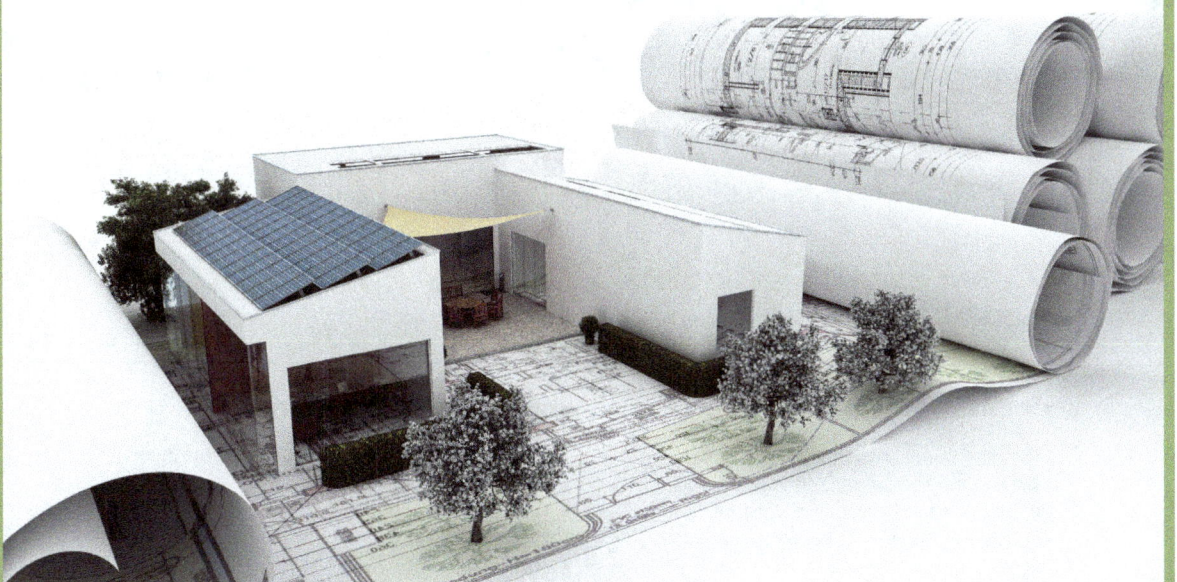

Helping you to create an efficient, healthy home

Green Moves Australia
P (03) 9024 5515 – 1300 898 742

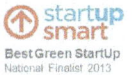
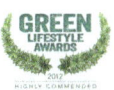

www.greenmoves.com.au

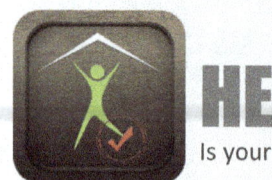

HEALTHY HOME APP

Is your home healthy? Would you know if it wasn't?

With the increase in asthma, allergies, chemical sensitivities and other illnesses related to indoor pollutants a healthy home has never been more important. Take a walk through your home and complete the quiz to identify health assets and challenges. Discover tips and resources to help you create a healthy home for your family.

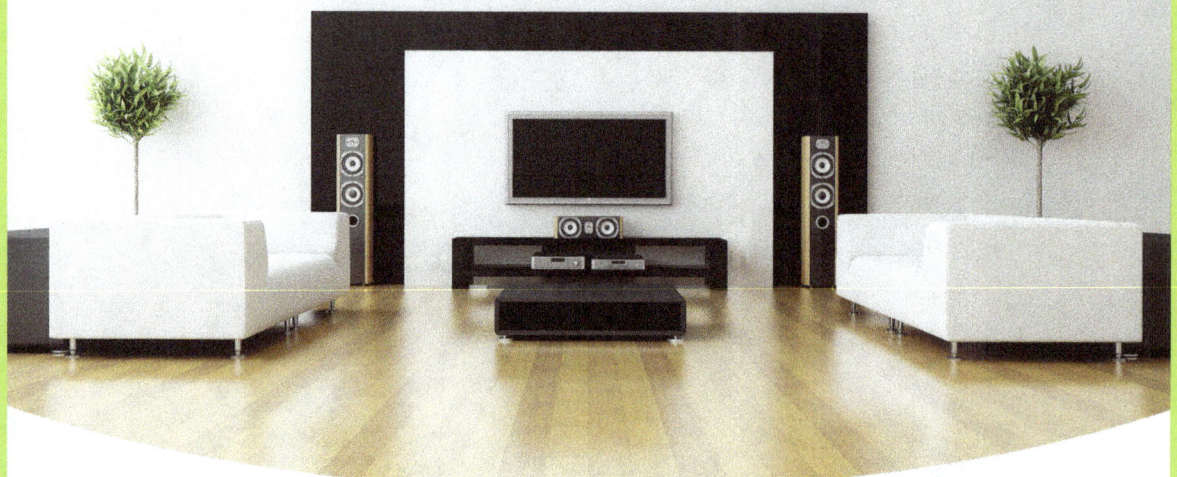

Take action and create a home that promotes wellbeing for your family.

Key Features of the Healthy Home App :

- Create multiple checklists as needed
- Take the interactive quiz that will highlight health issues to consider in your home
- Identify healthy home assets and challenges in your rooms
- Create notes
- Take photos
- Create asset and challenge reports

Would you benefit from the APP ?

- Expecting a baby and wanting to create a healthy home
- Families with children wanting to minimise indoor pollutants
- Renovating and want to create a healthy home
- Experiencing illness and want to reduce pollutants in your home
- You value good health and want to prevent illness and related lifestyle decisions that can make a positive impact on long term family health

Be empowered take the mobile quiz today!

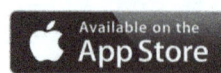
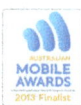

www.ingramcontent.com/pod-product-compliance
Lightning Source LLC
Chambersburg PA
CBHW080835230426
43665CB00021B/2845